The 10 Years
PREPPER'S SURVIVAL BIBLE

19 in 1

The Ultimate Encyclopedia of Food Canning & Preserving, Stockpiling, Water Harvesting, Survival Medicine, Worst Scenarios Surviving, and Home Defense

Tyler Gordon

TABLE OF CONTENTS

DEHYDRATOR
GUIDEBOOK FOR PREPPERS

1000 Days of Delicious Homemade Recipes for Fruit, Vegetables, Jerky, Mushrooms and More

Tyler Gordon

INTRODUCTION

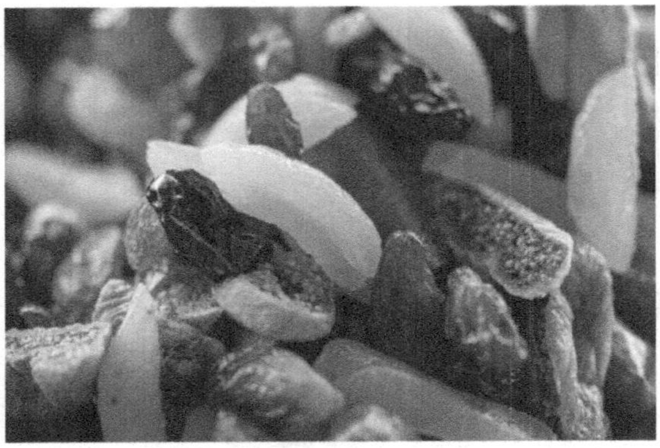

Dehydrated food retains many of the nutrients of fresh food far better than other methods of food preservation. Fresh food can lose up to 50 percent of its nutritional value sitting in the refrigerator. But dried food retains all the antioxidants and minerals of fresh food, and most of the vitamins. Dehydrated food weighs less and takes up less space in the pantry, making it ideal for road trips, hiking, emergency preparedness, and weekday meal prep. Let's dive in!

Dried food is typically brittle and can be snapped in half when bent. If food is still moist and pliable after drying, it should be returned to the dryer.

The easiest way to preserve food is by dehydrating or drying it. This method has been used for several years to help food last without being refrigerated. It is one of the least expensive and fastest ways to store your harvest for later use. Drying will also lighten the weight of foods prepared for backpacking and camping.

Dehydrating spectacularly lessens your food's moisture contents, making it last longer and still maintain its delicious taste. This is because it lessens the moisture contents of your food to between five to twenty percent, and the bacterium causing food decay cannot survive within that range. When you remove moisture from the foods you love to eat, you have also automatically extended their shelf-life.

As moisture leaves food, it often shrivels up and takes on a leathery, tough texture. The skin will wrinkle as the food inside shrinks. Compare a raisin to a grape taken straight off the vine and you get the picture. Grapes lose a lot of volume as the moisture inside them evaporates and they become raisins.

The health benefits of dehydrating are undeniable; this method retains up to 90 percent of the vitamins, minerals, and antioxidants in food. Preserving food by freezing retains about the same nutrition as dehydrating, but frozen food has a shorter shelf life. Dehydrated food is nutritionally superior to canned food; the high temperatures of the canning process deplete vitamin C, vitamin A, and many of the B vitamins.

Dehydrating allows you to control the ingredients in your food. You can choose how much sugar to put in the fruit leather or how much salt to put in your beef jerky. I especially like that you can also control cross-contamination with such common allergens as wheat, peanuts, or soy.

Drying food allows me to be creative both when preserving and using the ingredients in meals and snacks. It also bolsters my confidence, knowing my family is prepared for emergencies with safely stored healthy food, even if the power goes out.

This book is divided into three parts. In the first section, you'll find the basics to help you get started, even if you've never used a dehydrator. You'll learn about the equipment you need, some important techniques to ensure that your food is safe and free of bad bacteria, and how to pretreat food to ensure that the nutrients, texture, flavor, and color are preserved both in drying and in storage.

CHAPTER 1: UNDERSTANDING DEHYDRATING

Dehydration which is popularly known as 'drying' is a long-practiced method for preserving foods. It can also be referred as the process of removing water through evaporation from a solid or liquid food. The aim of this is to arrive at a solid material that has been sufficiently water-reduced. This process consists of reducing the level of food moisture into smaller levels in order to extend the lifespan of the food. It requires adding different forms of energy to the food.

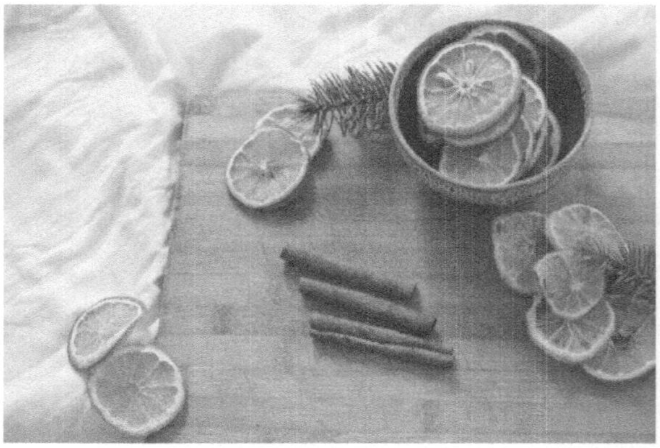

Note that dehydration does not include mechanical pressing of liquid foods. In most cases, Hot-air is used to add heat to the food and to reduce its moisture.

It is very easy for pathogenic bacteria to survive comfortably in the unfavorable environment of dried foods. This means that once your dried food is rehydrated and eaten, it could cause you food poisoning. Of course, you would not want to suffer food poisoning, all in the name of preserving your foods for later use.

What should you do then to prevent this when drying your food? Make use of high-quality materials with low contaminants when drying your foods. High-quality materials with low contaminants are materials and tools specifically made for dehydrating foods. Also, ensure proper sanitation of all tools and surfaces and ensure that the storage condition of the dried food is one that prevents contact with dust, rodents, insects and other house insects.

When you decide to dehydrate your food to make it last longer, then you have numerous options available for you. You could dry your food by air, vacuum, inert gas, steaming, or by directly applying heat to the food. Usually, the most popular and acceptable means of drying is by air. This is okay for obvious reasons. Using this method allows your food to dry gradually, plus it is very convenient. And, yes, air is very plentiful, and free! Allowing your food to dry gradually by using air prevents scorching and discoloration of your food, which is popular with other drying systems.

Dehydrating foods started as far back as times when early men spread their harvests or hunts out in the sun for sun drying. It is one of the oldest methods of preservation, as the prehistoric men were fond of drying some seeds before planting.

Fish, meats and food plants have been preserved over the years by drying them in the sun or naturally spreading them in the desert heat, across different desert areas.

In more recent times, American Indians stored their meats by laying them under the sun. The people of China also dried their eggs from the sunshine and the Japanese dried rice and fish under the sun's rays as well. During the Second World War, there was a great need to move food in bulk from place to place and this challenge ignited the developments of modern strategies on preserving foods, hence dehydration. In the year 1975 however, the French made a major breakthrough in the development of hot-air dehydration, which is the drying of foods through the method of blowing hot air over them.

Browning reactions are one of the most common chemical reactions that occur in dried foods. They occur when chemical compounds in the food being dried react with compounds in the air. Browning is usually considered undesirable because it can change the taste of the food as it changes its appearance. A little known fact about browning is it can sometimes damage the nutritional value of the food as the color changes.

Many fruits and vegetables undergo enzymatic browning when they're cut open and their flesh is exposed to the air. This sort of browning also occurs when produce is dropped, hit with something or otherwise damaged. It's a stress response brought on by the rapid conversion of chemical compounds in the flesh into brown melanin. The enzymes that cause browning can be deactivated through careful use of heat, acids or chemicals like sulphites. Blanching foods and/or exposing them to citric acids before setting them out to dry can inhibit browning enough to where it isn't much of a problem.

The Wonder of Dehydrating

A centuries-old technology, dehydrating removes moisture from fresh food so bacteria cannot grow. Dehydrating preserves your food for a year or more, without refrigeration. With 90 percent of the moisture removed, the food intensifies in flavor, concentrates its nutritional value, and takes up less room in your pantry.

In areas where the relative humidity is 30 percent or less, fruit naturally dries on the tree or vine, right in the garden. Airflow and heat are both essential to the dehydrating process. When left to nature, grapes turn into raisins slowly, dependent on local weather conditions. But in many areas the humidity is too high for this natural process to be successful. A food dehydrator controls the variables of temperature and humidity, speeding up the drying process and ensuring an end product that is safely preserved.

The first food-drying machine was invented in France in 1795 to aid Napoleon's war efforts. It used circulating airflow and temperature control to speed up the dehydration process. Dried food was useful for traveling armies because it was lightweight, retained its nutritional value, and took up less space than its fresh counterpart.

During the two world wars, dehydrated food was essential to provisioning the troops, leading to an increased demand and further innovation on an industrial scale. In fact, instant mashed potatoes were born from the war effort with the technology gained from dehydrating food for the troops.

Interest in home dehydrating was slower to take hold until the mid 1970s, when the back-to-the-land movement increased interest in home-scale food preservation. In response to this increased demand, several electric dehydrators for home use were patented that offered both airflow and heat.

When a recipe calls for blanching fruit or vegetables, it's usually done to stop or slow enzymatic action on the produce. Foods that need blanching should be processed quickly after cutting into them. The enzymatic action will initiate as soon as the flesh of the fruit or vegetable is exposed to oxygen. If you're planning on drying large amounts of produce, it's best to do so in smaller batches. Trying to do it all in one batch might result in the produce you cut in the beginning degrading to the point it can't be used by the time you get around to blanching it.

Color loss can also come about as a result of drying. This effect is especially pronounced when high heat or sunlight is used to dry leafy greens and brightly-colored vegetables that get their color from carotenoids, which are fat-soluble pigments. Pigments will often fade during drying and can further fade during storage.

Dried foods change texture when the moisture is removed. This is due to a number of factors, including the loss of moisture, changes to the cellulose material and degradation of some of the compounds found in the food. When foods are dried at too high a temperature, the outside of the food can dry before all the moisture leaves the inside, creating what's known as case-hardened foods. They appear dry on the outside, but there's still too much moisture inside the hard outer shell.

While it may sound like food drying is an invasive process that drastically changes food, it actually isn't that bad once you get past the physical changes. It's the least damaging food preservation technique and foods that are dried retain most of their nutritional value. Other preservation techniques involve the use of extreme heat or extreme cold, which is even more damaging to the structure and chemical composition of foods subjected to them.

From a technical standpoint, most food starts degrading as soon as it is harvested. Once a plant or animal is no longer alive, it starts to lose nutritional value. This loss is slow at first, but quickly accelerates into rapid degeneration once the food begins to spoil. Anything done to prepare the food like heating it, washing it, slicing it or otherwise processing it further damages the food.

Dehydrators for home use offer continuous circulating airflow, temperature control, food-safe tray materials, and special aftermarket add-ons like silicone sheets to make it easier to make leathers and snacks. The latest digital models allow for temperature control between sections of the dehydrator, as well as programmable temperature and time variations for different foods. With electronic precision, you can put the food in, set the cycle, and go about your day.

What Should (and Shouldn't) Be Dehydrated

Fruits and vegetables are the easiest and most forgiving foods to process. Dried fruit can be eaten without rehydrating. It's a nutrient-dense food that makes an ideal snack. It can be added to oatmeal, muffins, and hot cereal to improve the nutritional quality of simple meals.

Dried vegetables are convenient for soups, stews, sauces, and dips where they can be rehydrated in the cooking process. Aromatic vegetables such as onions, garlic, carrots, celery, and peppers can be used as ingredients in meals on their own or combined into spice blends to add flavor to other dishes.

Lean meat, poultry, and fish can also be dehydrated, provided a few precautions are taken with these high-protein foods. When dehydrating, temperatures should reach 165°F (74°C) to kill any spoilage organisms. If your dehydrator doesn't go this high, place the food in the dehydrator at 145°F for at least 4 hours, until it is done. Then put it in a preheated oven at 275°F for 10 minutes so that it reaches an internal temperature of 165°F (74°C).

Cured ham can be successfully dehydrated, but pork should never be dehydrated at home or used for jerky. The temperatures used in a home dehydrator cannot destroy the trichinella parasite nor other harmful bacteria that are commonly found in pork.

Raw eggs and milk products do not dehydrate well. They are prone to bacterial contamination at dehydrating temperatures.

Fatty and oily foods cannot be dried adequately in a home dehydrator. The fat won't dry properly and as a result, the food spoils quickly. This includes high-fat foods such as avocados and olives.

When dehydrating meat, you should remove all visible fat. Only lean meat, poultry, or fish should be used for dehydrating. Ground meat should be no more than 10 percent fat. Fish like salmon and mackerel have too high a fat content to make them good candidates for dehydrating; they can be dried for short-term storage, but they should not be used for long-term storage due to the increased risk of spoilage.

Foods high in sugar or alcohol won't dry properly. Foods like alcohol-soaked fruit, honey, or candy tend to absorb moisture from the air and resist dehydration.

Benefits of Dehydrating

Everyone comes to dehydrating for different reasons. Some like the convenience and portability of dried food. Others use their dehydrator to preserve their garden veggies. Still others use their dehydrator to make food for hiking or camping trips. I use my dehydrator to preserve produce in season, when it is at the peak of freshness and nutrition. But regardless of your reason for dehydrating food, there are several benefits to dehydrating food that are universal.

Reduction of Spoilage

Dehydrating helps reduce unnecessary food waste. You can stop putting leftovers in the refrigerator and then tossing them in the garbage or compost pile a week or two later when they grow green fuzz. Both leftover vegetables and main dishes can be dehydrated, preserving your investment in healthy food, plus you'll have future meals for busy days. Dehydrating also allows you to stock up on produce discounts like overripe bananas or onions past their prime. Many grocery stores and produce stands have discount bins where "seconds," like citrus fruit, apples, sweet peppers, and tomatoes are offered at significant savings. Dehydrating these foods helps you stock your pantry while saving money.

A church in my community collects excess produce from local grocery stores, dehydrates it, and turns it into dried soup mixes and dried fruit for food banks in several nearby towns. Using a commercial dehydrator with 20 trays, they divert 9,000 pounds of produce from the local landfill each month and convert it into nourishing food for hundreds of families.

Extended Lifespan

When foods are dehydrated, they last longer because the moisture is reduced and the dry food does not encourage the survival of bacteria. The absence of bacteria keeps food in good shape and this can last for as long as three months. When food items are dehydrated, they are sometimes converted into substances that can last a lifetime. Examples are spices such as cinnamon and curry powder which is derived from the dehydration and grinding of curry leaves. In most cases, spices like this can last for several years without getting spoiled.

Waste Reduction

When foods spoil, they reduce the amount of food available for consumption. Some food preservative methods usually give a very short extension before the spoilage of food. In many cases when we buy raw materials in the markets, the ability and knowledge to store them in good conditions help us keep the foods for a long time.

Improvement in Food Taste

The application of heat to reduce the water tastes in foods brings out the original taste of the other constituents of the food. The process of dehydration greatly improves the taste of food. When foods are water-filled, they are sometimes tasteless or acrid. When fruits are dried, the real taste is felt. In most cases, food tastes better when they are dehydrated.

Easy Storage

The fact that dehydrating foods make them easy to be stored is a great advantage of the process. When large bulks of foods are preserved in smaller packages, like the case of milk dehydrated into powder, it aids transportation and storekeeping. Through dehydration, storage is easier as it takes up lesser spaces.

Taste (and nutrition)

Dehydrated foods often taste better than when they're fresh, because their flavors are intensified. Moisture literally "waters down" flavor, so dried fruits taste much sweeter, even without added sugar. Dehydrated mushrooms are so flavorful that many chefs use them as a spice, not a vegetable, while a small handful of sun-dried tomato flavors an entire pasta dish. The icing on the cake is that dehydrated food also maintains their nutritional value. Removing the moisture doesn't destroy healthy vitamins, minerals, or calories.

Clean-eating

You can buy dried fruits, vegetables, and other snacks at the store, but more often than not, they're full of sugar and artificial ingredients. Even though dried foods last longer than fresh ones, packaged versions usually contain preservatives to make them last even longer. This is especially true for dried meats, which are not only highly-processed, they're usually extremely salty. Processed meat has also been classified as carcinogenic, which means it contains chemicals that might cause certain types of cancer! For all of this, you also pay a pretty penny. Making your own dehydrated snacks at home means you have total control over what goes in and what stays out.

Easy to carry around

There aren't a lot of truly portable snacks and the ones that are, like fruits and vegetables, got easily squished and bruised. When they're dry, they're hardened and much more durable. They also don't take up much space in a bag and they don't squirt juice everywhere when you're trying to eat them. Dehydrated food is the way to go if you're always on the run.

Dehydrating food at home saves money and space, makes clean and tasty snacks, and reduces food waste.

Preservation of Nutrients

Dehydrating food maintains the nutrients in the food before they are dehydrated. Nutrients such as minerals, vitamins and enzymes are absolutely preserved during dehydration. Dehydration is the only method that can ascertain the preservation of nutrients in food particles. Cooking and other preservative methods often lead to loss of nutrients. The entire essence of consuming food is to get benefits from the nutrients, if these nutrients are reduced; the essence of consuming the food has been lost.

Absence of Chemicals

The only substance needed to dehydrate food is the heat added to the food material. Unlike some other preservative methods, it does not involve the addition of chemicals. Dehydrating food therefore makes it safe from the fear of consuming poisonous substances because nothing but heat is added. The dehydrated food will only maintain its initial nutrients and that makes it perfect for consumption.

Economic and Financial Advantages

Dehydrating food makes food last longer. As such, people may buy food in bulk or harvest large quantity of produce and dehydrate it in batches, making it a very convenient method.

Reliability for Emergency Situations

Dehydrating keeps a person prepared for any emergency that requires immediate need for dehydrated food. Dehydrated food can be very useful for individuals traveling in extreme conditions, such as for mountain climbers and cross-country bike riders.

More Control over Food Contents

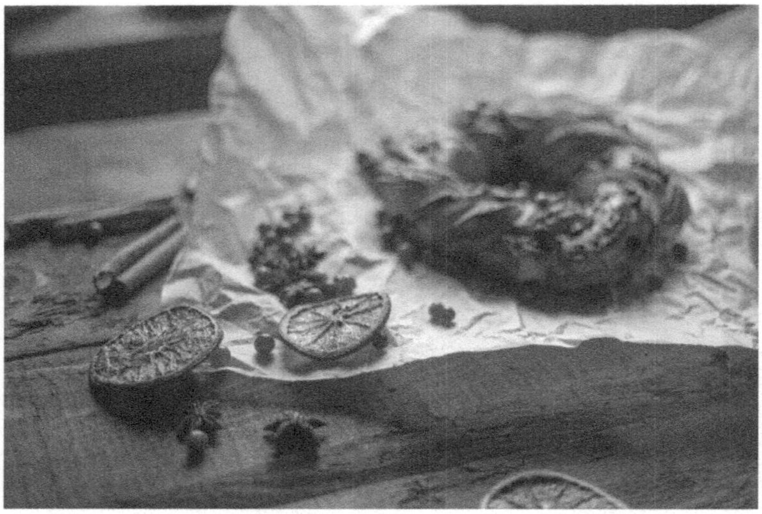

When you prepare your snacks and staple foods at home using your dehydrator, you control every step of the process—especially the ingredients. Healthy snack foods that are low in sugar and salt, or food without allergens, can be made easily in your dehydrator. You can adapt recipes to ensure there is no cross-contamination of food, making dehydrating ideal for families who deal with food allergies.

One member of my family has a serious wheat allergy. Almost all commercially dried or freeze-dried food has an ingredient warning "may contain wheat." But by drying our own produce and using our dehydrator for snacks and travel food, I have confidence that the food he eats is safe from cross-contamination, even when we are away from home.

Peanut, soy, milk, wheat, and other common allergens are easier to exclude when you provision your pantry with ingredients that you dehydrate yourself. When you make your own meals and snacks from scratch, you'll no longer need a magnifying glass to read ingredient labels!

You can also control the amount of sugar, starch, artificial colors and flavoring, and other chemical additives when you dry your own food at home. If you have dietary restrictions or preferences, using your dehydrator to make meals or pantry items can help you reach your personal goals.

Raw foodies can control the temperature at which the food is dried, ensuring high availability of enzymes, vitamins, and minerals for their special dietary needs.

Time, Space & Savings

Investing in a dehydrator ultimately saves you money. Buying produce in bulk—and in season—offers considerable savings over grocery-store prices. Fruit, vegetables, and nuts can be purchased in bulk directly from local farms, and then dehydrated while at their peak of flavor and nutrition, at significant savings over buying fresh or even frozen vegetables.

Last fall, I picked up a 20-pound bag of Walla Walla onions for $20 and a 25-pound bag of sweet peppers for $10 from the bargain bin at a farm stand. Walla Walla onions are $3 per pound at my grocery store, and sweet peppers are $4 to $5 per pound. That's a savings of almost $200! In just a few days, I dried all the onions in my dehydrator. I divided the peppers by color and dried the red ones first while waiting for the green ones to ripen.

The dried onions and peppers took up significantly less space in my pantry than the big bags of onions and peppers I brought home. Those two huge bags were reduced to four 1-quart jars and a pint jar that are much easier to store in my modest pantry.

Filling your dehydrator takes a little time, but it saves you time in the long run. Your dehydrated foods become convenience items once they are stored in jars in your pantry. It's so much faster to grab dried onions when you need them than to cut up a raw onion while making dinner. Think of the time it takes to prepare food for your dehydrator, and package it when it's done, as an investment in future convenience.

Emergency Preparedness

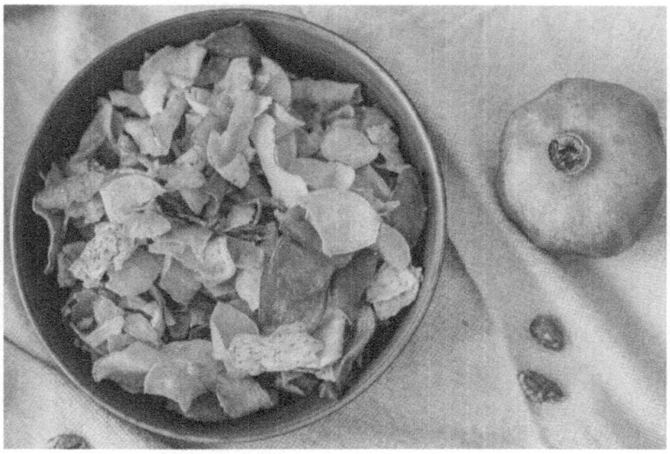

Dehydrated food is ideal for emergency food storage. Whether you are preparing for a weather event, a period of unemployment, or a natural disaster, having a 30-day supply of nutritious food on hand is wise.

Dehydrating food your family already eats ensures that you have as little disruption as possible in a real emergency. By stocking your pantry with dehydrated food that you've prepared from wholesome ingredients, you can be assured that your family's nutritional needs are met, even if you can't get to the grocery store.

Dehydrated food, when properly prepared and packaged for long-term storage, can form the foundation of a robust preparedness plan. Taking the extra step to package your dehydrated food in Mylar bags or glass jars with oxygen absorbers ensures that your dehydrated food will still be fresh and retain its nutrients in storage.

But even minor disruptions can be helped by having the convenience of dehydrated food in your pantry. An extra dinner guest, sickness in the house, or an unexpected bill doesn't have to shake your confidence. Having dehydrated ingredients to make your favorite comfort foods already in your pantry can help you move through even minor inconveniences with grace.

High Nutritional Value

When food is dehydrated, the water is removed, but the nutrition in the food remains stable. The flavor and nutrients become more concentrated, and the caloric value remains the same. Dehydrated food has the same calories, protein, fiber, and carbohydrates as fresh food. It also retains the same minerals, fatty acids, and antioxidants as fresh food, as well as most of the vitamins. Dehydrated food retains many of these nutrients in storage, even over several months and years.

There is some loss of vitamin C and some B vitamins during blanching, because some of these water-soluble vitamins are lost in the blanching water. Vegetables that are blanched before dehydrating have the same vitamins as frozen food, but dehydrated food has a longer shelf life. This vitamin loss can be minimized by blanching with steam before dehydrating, rather than immersing vegetables in boiling water prior to dehydrating.

Hikers and athletes benefit from the concentration of nutrients provided by dehydrated foods, allowing them to eat less while maintaining their energy levels.

To ensure that your dehydrated food retains the most nutrition, it should be dehydrated at its peak of ripeness, when the flavor, color, and texture are best. Vegetables that are past their prime and are fading in color, scent, or flavor will not make quality dried vegetables. Skip over the fading-green kale in the refrigerator vegetable bin. Choose the most vibrant-colored vegetables to get the most nutrition from your dehydrated food.

How to dehydrate

Preparing Fruits for Dehydration

Most dehydrating machines, no matter which brand or model you choose, are user-friendly. The first step in preparing fruits for the dehydration machine is selecting high-quality fruits.

Fruit should be fresh and at the peak of ripeness. Once you pick or purchase your produce, thoroughly wash it and discard any bruised or damaged pieces. Fruits may need to be peeled, cored or pitted, depending on the particular fruit you are handling.

After fruit has been peeled and sliced, it is advisable to apply a pre-treatment to maintain the color and freshness of the produce. Once certain fruits, such as apples, pears and peaches are sliced, their exposure to air initiates a chemical process called oxidation that results in discolored flesh. Using an antioxidant will temporarily halt the enzyme action and prevent further damage to the texture, flavor and appearance of the fruit. To make this solution, combine a small amount of ascorbic acid (1-2 tsp.) with one cup of water and coat the fruit evenly with the liquid.

Preparing Vegetables for Dehydration

When preparing your vegetables for dehydration, be sure to select high-quality, unblemished vegetables.

Particularly for certain vegetables such as root vegetables and potatoes, make sure they are thoroughly scrubbed and cleaned prior to dehydration. Similar to fruits, vegetables should be sliced thinly and uniformly for the best results.

Nearly all vegetables should be blanched first. Blanching vegetables halts enzyme action and thereby preserves the color and flavor of the food over time. Because some nutrients may be lost during the blanching process, place the vegetables in boiling water only for the required length of time.

After the vegetables are submerged in ice cold water, carefully dry the foods prior to placing them on trays. Note that a small number of vegetables, like mushrooms and onions, do not need to be blanched prior to dehydration.

Preparing Meat for Dehydration

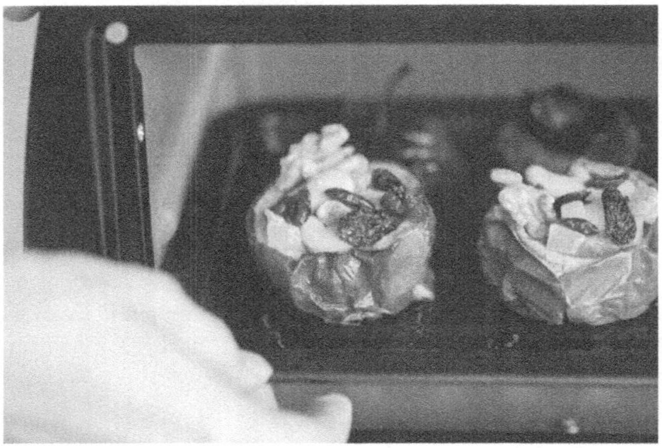

Dehydrated meats are delicious and simple to prepare, but do warrant special handling instructions. Only lean meats in excellent condition should be utilized for making jerky. When using ground meat for jerky, it should be at least 93% lean.

All other meat should have its fat thoroughly trimmed prior to slicing.

You might consider applying a marinade beforehand to flavor the meat. If so, keep marinated meats in the refrigerator or freezer before placing them in the dehydrator. After removing the meat from the refrigerator, blot its surface thoroughly to remove excess moisture and place on dehydrator trays. As always, raw meat should be kept away from other foods, and all surfaces and utensils that come into contact with raw meat should be thoroughly cleaned.

After using the dehydrator, experts recommend heating dried meat strips for ten minutes in a 275° F oven or for a longer time at a lower temperature. This additional step reduces any residual chance of contamination by eliminating pathogens, and also produces the most traditional style of jerky with respect to taste and texture.

Preparing Grains, Nuts, Beans and Seeds for Dehydration

Nuts, seeds, beans and grains can all be dehydrated using a similar two-step process. First, these foods must be soaked in a water solution. Soaking deactivates anti-nutrients, stimulates nutrients such as iron, potassium and magnesium, and is beneficial to your digestive system. Soak nuts or seeds in a salt brine solution for 12-18 hours. Add ½ tsp. high-quality sea salt for every cup of water. Since wet nuts and seeds are not appealing to most people, you can place the nuts in the dehydrator to create a delicious, crunchy, ready to eat snack. After soaking for the recommended time, drain the water and proceed with instructions for your dehydrating machine.

Using Your Dehydrator Machine

Once the fruits, vegetables, herbs, meat, nuts or grains have been prepped, spread them in thin layers without overlapping on the drying trays. Turn on the dehydrating machine and set the temperature. Drying times vary depending on the dehydrator model you own and the food you are dehydrating. Most dehydrators contain guides that provide recommended temperatures and times for dehydrating specific foods.

In general, it is recommended that fruits and vegetables be dried at 130°-140° F. Meats and fish should be dehydrated at the highest temperature setting on your machine, which is typically between 145°-155° F. When dehydrating meats, it is necessary to use dehydrator models with adjustable temperature controls to ensure a product that is safe for consumption. Dried herbs require a temperature not exceeding 90° F, as aromatic oils in herbs are sensitive to high heat. Nuts, seeds and grains, which also have a high oil content, dry optimally at 90°-100° F.

Determining Food Readiness

Foods should always be tested for adequate dehydration before removal. Many factors determine the length of time necessary to dehydrate foods, such as the temperature, humidity, type of food, amount of food on the tray, size of the food pieces, and total quantity of food in the machine.

In general, meats should be dehydrated to 20% moisture content, fruits to 10% and vegetables to about 5%. You can analyze the appearance and texture of foods for signs of readiness. It is important to test only a few pieces at a time and allow them to cool before determining whether they are ready.

Checking food for readiness is largely a matter of assessing its structure. Fruits should be pliable, but not totally brittle. Test fruits by cutting them in half; if you cannot squeeze out any moisture, then the fruit are fully dehydrated. Vegetables, however, should be brittle when they are done. Test vegetables by hitting them with a hammer to see if they shatter.

Most fully dehydrated vegetables should break into pieces. Certain vegetables, however, will retain a pliable and leathery texture upon complete dehydration. These include mushrooms, green peppers and squash. To test jerky, bend one piece and see how pliable it is.

The meat should bend, but not snap completely like a dry stick. The jerky should present as dark brown to black in color once it is fully dehydrated. Herbs are considered dried when they crumble easily. The stems of the herb should bend and break with little effort.

Recognizing Doneness

Food is done when it is dry enough to prevent bacteria from growing and spoiling the food. Different foods have different moisture requirements for safe food storage. The amount of moisture left in dehydrated food affects its flexibility. The more moisture, the more flexible your dehydrated food will be. You'll find specific guidelines in each produce entry and in each recipe to test for doneness so you won't be guessing. But here are some general guidelines for vegetables, fruit, herbs, and meat to get you started.

- Allow a sample to cool completely before testing for doneness. Most dehydrated food is flexible when warm but will firm up when cooled. If you are in doubt, dehydrate the food for a few more hours. It's better to dry longer than to stop drying too soon.
- Vegetables are usually done when they are leathery and brittle. When pressed between the thumb and forefinger, they should snap cleanly in half, without bending.
- Fruit is done when it is leathery but still flexible, and no soft pockets remain in the fruit. If you find soft, squishy sections, give the fruit more time. When the fruit is done, there will be no soft spots.
- Herbs are done when the leaves crumble when crushed. Stems should be hard and brittle. If the stems bend, they need more time.
- Meat should be dry and leathery with little flexibility when done, but specific meats vary in the test for doneness.

Storage

Once your food is properly dehydrated, your job isn't finished. It's important to package the food and store it to protect it from spoilage. Moisture, oxygen, and light can degrade your stored food, shortening the shelf life and allowing bacteria to ruin the food.

When stored properly and protected from moisture, heat, and light, dehydrated food can last for up to 10 years. The actual shelf life varies depending on the food, with fruit lasting longer than vegetables because the natural sugar in fruit helps extend its shelf life. (Consult the recipes for specifics on storage needs and the shelf life of individual foods.)

If you see any signs of spoilage, such as off-odors or mold, discard the contents of the package. It is not safe to eat.

Rehydrating

Rehydrating restores the moisture to dried food, returning it to its original size, form, and appearance. Rehydrated food retains its aroma, flavor, and texture as well as its nutritional content. There are several methods for rehydrating dried food, but in their simplest form, they all add moisture back into the food using either cold or hot liquids.

As a general rule, 1 cup of liquid reconstitutes 1 cup of dehydrated food. If the food hasn't softened enough after an hour, add more liquid. The liquid can be plain water, broth, juice, or milk. Fruit can also be reconstituted in liqueur or brandy.

Most fruit and vegetables reconstitute in one to two hours. However, larger pieces of food may take longer to reconstitute than powders or finely diced pieces. Generally, food that took longer to dehydrate also takes longer to rehydrate. Use only enough liquid as the food will absorb. Using too much liquid makes the food soggy and unappetizing.

Soaking does not take the place of cooking. Food still needs to be cooked after it is reconstituted by soaking.

Save the soaking liquid to add to soups, stews, or cereals. It contains the water-soluble vitamins and minerals leached from the dehydrated food.

Methods

There are two main methods of rehydrating: cold soaking and hot soaking.

Cold soaking should be used for foods that are commonly eaten raw, like fruit. It is a slower process that allows the tissues of the food to relax and absorb the liquid. Food that is reconstituted in room-temperature or cooler water retains its shape and texture better than food rehydrated using hot water.

The soaking liquid, like juice or yogurt, adds additional flavor as it rehydrates the food, but don't add additional salt or sugar to the soaking water, as they hinder the rehydration process. These can be added once the food is fully hydrated.

Use hot soaking when the food being rehydrated will be served cooked or added to a hot dish. Hot soaking breaks some of the plant cells as it rehydrates the food, causing the food to become softer. Hot soaking rehydrates food quicker than cold soaking.

Rehydrating the food while cooking it is fast and easy. Place dried vegetables in soups, stews, or sauces and rehydrate as the sauce cooks on the stovetop. Add dried fruit to sauces, puddings, and warm cereals during the cooking process and rehydrate it while the rest of the mixture cooks.

The Objectives of Food Dehydration

Impacting a peculiar feature, such as a different crispiness and flavor, to a food product: An example is the transformation of maize to cereal.

Shrinking the food material into smaller and more portable sizes to change their forms: Food materials, when the water has been reduced, become more portable and are easily packaged for transportation. Examples are the draining and grinding of curry leaves, thymes seeds etc. into spices.

Reducing the volume and the weight of the food: The volume of water poses a substantial addition to the volume and weight of the food, by reducing the water content, the weight and volume of the food particle is also reduced.

The conversion of food meals to a different form that is more convenient for storage, packaging and easy transportation: A great example is the conversion of milk or dairies to dry powder. When these products get to the places of consumption, they are reconverted to the previous forms through the addition of water.

The effect of water depression which leads to preservation and longevity of the nutrients.

Disadvantages of Dehydration

Time Consumption: Dehydrating food requires a lot of time in order to achieve perfect results. Some foods have a large amount of water content and to reduce the water will require a lot of time and meticulous observation. Taking so much time may be inconvenient for some individuals.

Unwanted Weight Gain: Dehydrated food might be rich in calories. Since it has shrunken in size, it may appear small; a little quantity consumed may seems insufficient while a large quantity consumed implies large nutrient consumption. The excess calories in the dehydrated food may lead to weight gain. People should be aware of it when consuming dried food.

Loss of Nutrients: Although when done correctly, dehydrating food can preserve nutrients, when done incorrectly it may lead to loss of nutrients in the food. Some nutrients can't stand high levels of heat. The degree of heat applied therefore determines the survival of the nutrients in food. If the dehydrated food is not stored properly too, nutrient can be lost due to excessive heat and poor storage condition.

Change in Taste and Look: With high heat, the appetizing appearances of common meals change. In most cases, people are easily turned off when foods don't wear the expected looks. When foods are dehydrated, the loss of water makes it shrink and the looks drastically change.

Technical Knowledge: Since not all foods are dehydrated in the same way or following the same pattern, dehydration requires technical knowledge in order to be carried out well. There is also the place of experience which gradually makes a person perfect in the art.

Why is Dehydration healthy?

Dehydration is healthy for consumption because of the following reasons:

Retains Nutrients: As mentioned earlier, when we dehydrate foods, the nutrients in the food is one of our primary concerns. Unlike other methods of preservation, dehydration saves the nutrients in the dehydrated food, when it is carried out effectively.

Bacteria Free: Dehydrated foods are germ-free. When we keep these foods for a long period of time, they still maintain their healthy state.

No Addition of External Chemicals: The heat used to dehydrate food is the only external requirement for the process. This heat contains no chemicals or acids that may be dangerous for the food. Unlike some preservative methods which engage the addition of preservative chemicals, dehydration is a healthy choice for storing food.

Safe Handling: Since dehydration has nothing to do with handling dangerous chemicals or intense equipment, it is safe for the user to easily dehydrate. Dehydration can be done with the simplest household mechanical devices like oven, microwave or a dehydrator. The smoke or steam that escapes from dehydrating food is not unhealthy to the environment, unlike regular burning of waste products. This makes the process healthy.

CHAPTER 2: DEHYDRATING METHODS

You can get started drying using items you probably already have in your kitchen.

The following items are essential to the drying process:

- Food.
- A source of heat.
- Trays or racks to dry the food on.

The trays should be slotted wood or mesh trays. Avoid using solid trays because they block air from circulating all the way around the food. In a pinch, you can cover a wood frame with cheesecloth and use it as a drying rack.

Containers to store the food in:

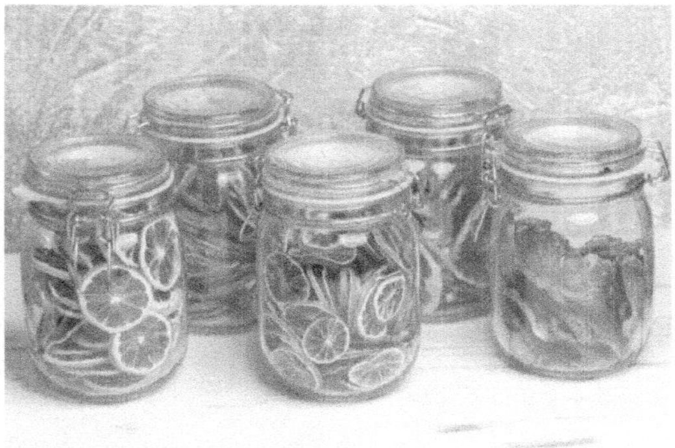

That's it. That's all you need to get started drying. There are other items you can use to make life easier on yourself, but the above items are the only absolute necessities.

You want to avoid trays made from the following materials because they can add harmful substances to your food during the drying process:

- Fiberglass.
- Vinyl.
- Aluminum.
- Copper.
- Plastic.
- Galvanized metal.
- The following items aren't required, but will make life easier on you:
- A commercial food dehydrator.
- A fan.
- A blancher.
- A sulfur box.
- A scale.
- A thermometer.

Now that we've established the items you need and the items you can buy to make life easier, let's take a look at the various methods used to dehydrate food.

Use a fan to circulate fresh air into the area where the food is drying.

Using Your Oven

If you have an oven (and who doesn't?), you have a tool you can use to dry foods.

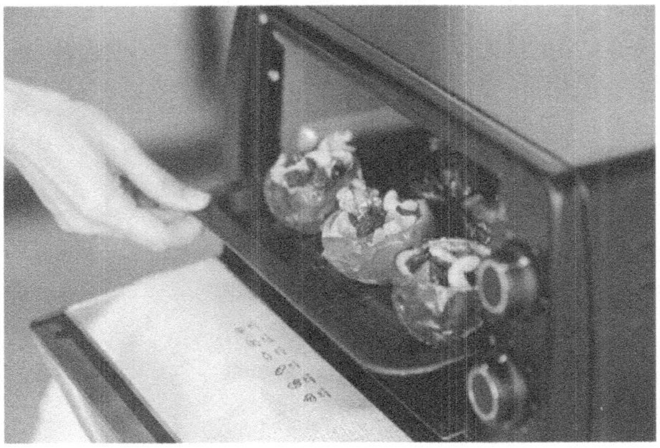

It isn't the best choice when it comes to drying, but it'll work in a pinch. The upside to using this method is it's one of the fastest methods of drying food. The downside is you can easily burn or scorch the food you're drying because it's difficult to keep the heat as low as you need it.

You can only dry small amounts of food in a normal kitchen oven. If you're planning on drying large amounts of food, buy a dehydrator and save yourself a lot of work.

You need to keep your oven temperature somewhere between 140 and 160 degrees F. To check oven temps, place an oven thermometer on the top rack and leave it there so you can monitor it. The temperature needs to be checked every 15 minutes to make sure it isn't getting too hot.

Place the food in a single layer on the drying trays. You can usually fit a couple pounds of food on each tray. Since most ovens have two racks, you're only going to be able to dry around 4 pounds of food at a time.

Here's a little trick you can use to fit more food in the oven: Place a couple 1 1/2-inch tall wood blocks on the bottom tray and set the next drying tray on the blocks. Then add a couple more blocks to the second tray and place another tray on it. You can fit up to four racks in your oven using this method, which will effectively double the amount of food you're able to dry at once. Since you're not heating the oven up too hot, you don't have to worry about scorching or burning the wood.

You need to prop the door open so there's a gap of 2 to 6 inches during the drying process. If you have a fan, set it up so it's blowing air into the oven through this gap. You need to keep the air inside moving so the oven doesn't fill full of humid air.

Set your oven at its lowest temperature

If you have a gas oven, you may be able to get away with just using the heat from the pilot light. Monitor the temperature to ensure it stays above 140 degrees F and below 160 degrees F.

The top rack is going to be a little cooler than the bottom rack. Additionally, the air isn't going to be the same temperature in the front of the oven as it is in the back, especially if you're using a fan to circulate air. For this reason, it's important to rotate the trays every 20 to 30 minutes. Rotate the top trays to the bottom and flip the trays around so the food that was in the front is now in the back. You're also going to want to periodically flip your food over or stir it on the tray because the side of the food that's facing down will dry at a slower rate than the side that's facing up.

The process used to dry foods in a toaster oven is same as with a conventional oven. Place the food on a tray and put it in your toaster oven. Set the oven on its lowest setting and prop open the door. If you have a fan, use it to circulate new air into the oven.

Since this sort of oven is smaller than a conventional oven, it's going to dehydrate the food you're drying faster than the larger oven. Make sure you watch it closely and soon you'll have a small batch of dried foods.

Here's a quick tip you won't see in too many other books about drying: Open the door of your oven every few hours to let out all the damp air trapped inside. Sure, it will cause the temperature to drop inside, but it will let all the moist air inside escape, replacing it with dry air. The hit you take in temperature is temporary and it's worth it to fill the oven with fresh air.

If you only dry occasionally, your oven will do the trick nicely.

Sun-Drying

A Sun-drying food is the oldest method used to dehydrate foods, predating ovens by thousands of years. This method is all-natural and doesn't require use of electricity or gas (to preserve the food or store it).

All you need is a nice, sunny day or two (or 5) in a row and you can use the power of the sun to dry your food.

In warmer climates, you can dry food using this method year-round. In cooler places or in areas where there's typically a lot of cloud cover, there may only be a handful of days a year this method can be used.

You need dry, clear weather with temperatures of at least 90 to 100 degrees F to sun-dry food.

If you live in an area where it's typically cloudy or there's a lot of moisture in the air, you're probably better off using one of the other methods of dehydrating. It's OK to move foods you've started sun-drying in and finishing the process in the oven or a dehydrator if it looks like inclement weather is on its way.

To sun-dry your foods, spread a layer out on a wood frame covered in cheesecloth. If you're worried about bugs or other animals getting to your food, you can place a layer of cheesecloth over the top of your food as well. Turn your foods regularly to assure even drying or the side left exposed to the sun will dry at a faster clip.

Alternatively, you can run a piece of string through your food items and hang them out to dry. Items like meat can be hung from hooks.

Spread food out in a single layer with at least a couple millimeters space between each piece so air can flow around it. Set the tray out in an area that gets sun for most of the day and has good circulation. Now, all you have to do is leave it there until the food is dry.

Leave the food out during the heat of the day, and then move it inside during the evening and night hours.

This accomplishes two things. It prevents the food from rehydrating due to condensation and it keeps the critters away. Animals enjoy dehydrated foods as much as you do and have been known to raid backyards at night. You don't want all of your hard work to be wasted at the hands of a marauding deer or raccoon.

Flip the food partway through each day. The bottom side gets less air and sun and will lose less moisture. Flip the food you're cooking over regularly so both side get equal amounts of sun.

There's no set time you need to leave food out to dry. All times shown in books and on the Internet are approximations of what it takes under "normal" conditions.

What exactly constitutes normal conditions is anyone's guess. What's normal in one place would be out of the ordinary somewhere else. That's probably why there's such variation in the dry times in different literature. I've tried to provide ranges in this book, but even the ranges can be off. The only way to make sure you dry your food correctly is to keep a close eye on it. When it gets close to the bottom end of the range, check it periodically.

The drying time varies based on the heat applied to the food, the humidity and the circulation of air in the area you're doing the drying. The hotter it is the faster food is going to lose moisture. The more humidity there is the slower moisture is going to be absorbed.

If you live in an area with a lot of vehicle traffic or high pollution levels, you shouldn't air-dry your food outside. Pollution particles can land on your food and contaminate it. Over time, the particulates you're eating can build up in your system and make you sick.

Dehydrating Equipment

Dehydration is mostly about prep work, so having the appropriate tools will make your job easier. Make sure you have the following tools on hand.

Baking sheet: If you don't already have one, a good-quality baking sheet that disperses heat properly and doesn't buckle under high heat is a great addition to your kitchen. Use it for roasting vegetables and fish.

Blender: Blenders are great for making purées for sauces, soups, and fruit leather. A food processor or immersion blender also works for this purpose.

Four-cup measuring pitcher: These pitchers are good for measuring liquids and for measuring the yield of dehydrated foods (if you don't have a kitchen scale).

Kitchen knife: Aside from the dehydrator itself, a kitchen knife is the most important tool for dehydrating. A good knife will make your prep work much easier. Perhaps you already have a favorite knife one that keeps a good edge, has a straight blade, and is comfortable to hold for extended periods. Good knives don't need to be expensive. In our kitchen we use the same knives many culinary schools offer; they are inexpensive but great tools for the job.

Kitchen scale: An inexpensive digital scale is very useful for measuring ingredients with precision and is also helpful for measuring and portioning the completed and dehydrated meals.

Parchment paper: Line baking sheets with parchment paper to prevent food from sticking to the pan. It also makes for easy cleanup.

How to dehydrate

Preparing Fruits for Dehydration

Most dehydrating machines, no matter which brand or model you choose, are user-friendly. The first step in preparing fruits for the dehydration machine is selecting high-quality fruits.

Fruit should be fresh and at the peak of ripeness. Once you pick or purchase your produce, thoroughly wash it and discard any bruised or damaged pieces. Fruits may need to be peeled, cored or pitted, depending on the particular fruit you are handling.

After fruit has been peeled and sliced, it is advisable to apply a pre-treatment to maintain the color and freshness of the produce. Once certain fruits, such as apples, pears and peaches are sliced, their exposure to air initiates a chemical process called oxidation that results in discolored flesh. Using an antioxidant will temporarily halt the enzyme action and prevent further damage to the texture, flavor and appearance of the fruit. To make this solution, combine a small amount of ascorbic acid (1-2 tsp.) with one cup of water and coat the fruit evenly with the liquid.

Preparing Vegetables for Dehydration

When preparing your vegetables for dehydration, be sure to select high-quality, unblemished vegetables.

Particularly for certain vegetables such as root vegetables and potatoes, make sure they are thoroughly scrubbed and cleaned prior to dehydration. Similar to fruits, vegetables should be sliced thinly and uniformly for the best results.

Nearly all vegetables should be blanched first. Blanching vegetables halts enzyme action and thereby preserves the color and flavor of the food over time some nutrients may be lost during the blanching process, place the vegetables in boiling water only for the required length of time.

After the vegetables are submerged in ice cold water, carefully dry the foods prior to placing them on trays. Note that a small number of vegetables, like mushrooms and onions, do not need to be blanched prior to dehydration.

Preparing Meat for Dehydration

Dehydrated meats are delicious and simple to prepare, but do warrant special handling instructions. Only lean meats in excellent condition should be utilized for making jerky. When using ground meat for jerky, it should be at least 93% lean.

All other meat should have its fat thoroughly trimmed prior to slicing.

You might consider applying a marinade beforehand to flavor the meat. If so, keep marinated meats in the refrigerator or freezer before placing them in the dehydrator. After removing the meat from the refrigerator, blot its surface thoroughly to remove excess moisture and place on dehydrator trays. As always, raw meat should be kept away from other foods, and all surfaces and utensils that come into contact with raw meat should be thoroughly cleaned.

After using the dehydrator, experts recommend heating dried meat strips for ten minutes in a 275° F oven or for a longer time at a lower temperature. This additional step reduces any residual chance of contamination by eliminating pathogens, and also produces the most traditional style of jerky with respect to taste and texture.

Preparing Grains, Nuts, Beans and Seeds for Dehydration

Nuts, seeds, beans and grains can all be dehydrated using a similar two-step process. First, these foods must be soaked in a water solution. Soaking deactivates anti-nutrients, stimulates nutrients such as iron, potassium and magnesium, and is beneficial to your digestive system. Soak nuts or seeds in a salt brine solution for 12-18 hours. Add ½ tsp. high-quality sea salt for every cup of water. Since wet nuts and seeds are not appealing to most people, you can place the nuts in the dehydrator to create a delicious, crunchy, ready to eat snack. After soaking for the recommended time, drain the water and proceed with instructions for your dehydrating machine.

Using Your Dehydrator Machine

Once the fruits, vegetables, herbs, meat, nuts or grains have been prepped, spread them in thin layers without overlapping on the drying trays. Turn on the dehydrating machine and set the temperature. Drying times vary depending on the dehydrator model you own and the food you are dehydrating. Most dehydrators contain guides that provide recommended temperatures and times for dehydrating specific foods.

In general, it is recommended that fruits and vegetables be dried at 130°-140° F. Meats and fish should be dehydrated at the highest temperature setting on your machine, which is typically between 145°-155° F. When dehydrating meats, it is necessary to use dehydrator models with adjustable temperature controls to ensure a product that is safe for consumption. Dried herbs require a temperature not exceeding 90° F, as aromatic oils in herbs are sensitive to high heat. Nuts, seeds and grains, which also have a high oil content, dry optimally at 90°-100° F.

Vegetables

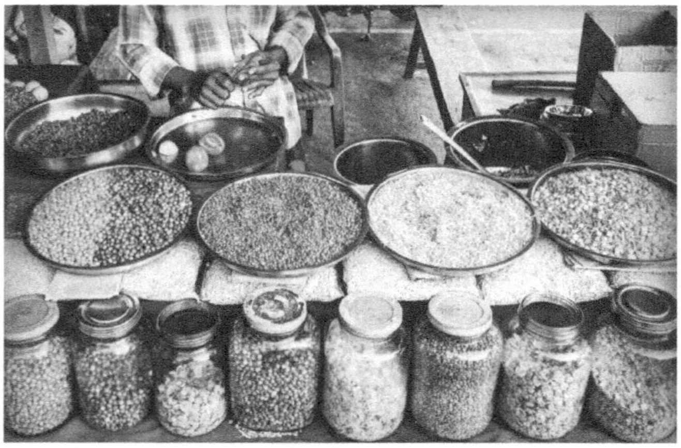

Dehydrating fresh produce entails a little more work. These need to be rinsed, peeled, and sliced into thin layers. Some may need blanching, boiling, coring and/or de-seeding.

Always dehydrate fresh produce in a conventional oven, with temperature set between 49° / 120° and 54° / 130° only. This allows gradual loss of moisture and prevents smaller pieces from burning.

When using the dehydrator, set the machine at lowest heat for delicate vegetables (e.g. leafy vegetables, onions, etc.); and at highest heat for hardier produce (e.g. legumes, root crops, etc.) or those that have thicker cuts.

Use approximately 1½ to 2 pounds per rotation.

Artichoke hearts, green peas, freshly shelled, etc.

Blanch with hot water and then dunk into an ice bath immediately to preserve color.

Drain well. Pat-dry using paper towels, if needed.

Follow recommended steps for oven drying or dehydrating. See: Oven drying: on page 28 and Dehydrating: on page 29. These may take between five to fourteen hours. These are done when these become brittle and wrinkled.

Beets, carrots, cassava, daikon (Asian radish,) potatoes, purple carrots, purple yam, sweet potatoes, yam, zucchini.

Scrub skins well.

Except for the zucchini, parboil (partially boil) veggies until slightly fork-tender (or when you can pierce outer layer with a fork.)

Remove from water and dunk into an ice bath immediately.

When veggies are cool enough to touch, peel, and slice into ⅛-inch thick disks. Drain well. Pat-dry using paper towels, if needed.

Follow recommended steps for oven drying or dehydrating. See: Oven drying: on page 28 and Dehydrating: on page 29. Beets may need three to ten hours of drying. These are done when individual disks feel dry and leathery to the touch. (Important: wear food-safe gloves to prevent beet juice from staining your hands.)

Carrots, potatoes, purple yam, sweet potatoes, and yam may need six to twelve hours. While the zucchini may need five to ten hours of drying. These are done when chips become crispy. Some pieces may have air pockets or browned edges, but these are normal.

Drying Herbs and Spices

Most herbs and spices are easy to grow at home, and many can be grown in small containers on your balcony, porch or any area of your house or yard that gets regular sunlight. In addition to being a considerable way to flavor foods, herbs and spices have a number of health benefits associated with them.

Drying is the convenient way to preserve herbs and spices because all you usually have to do is lay out the leaves, flowers or seeds and let them dry and then grind or crush them as you see fit. Herbs and spices should be dried in a dehydrator because drying them in the sun can bring them to lose some of their potency.

The following herbs and spices are good candidates for drying:

- Bay.
- Celery leaves.
- Chervil.
- Chicory.
- Chives.
- Cilantro.
- Cinnamon sticks.
- Cloves.
- Dill.
- Laurel.
- Marjoram.
- Mint.
- Oregano.
- Parsley.
- Peppercorns.
- Rosemary.
- Sage.
- Summer savory.
- Tarragon.
- Thyme.

Harvest herbs and spices by removing them from the plant in the early morning. Harvest them before the flowers open and be careful not to damage them during the harvest. Do not attempt to dry damaged pieces. The drying process isn't going to make damaged herbs and spices any better.

Lay the herbs or spices out in a single layer on the dehydrator tray and spread them out so there's a bit of space between them for air circulation. Most herbs and spices should be dried at temperatures between 115 and 125 degrees F, but be assured to check the documentation that came with your dehydrator to see what the recommended temperature for drying herbs and spices is.

The drying time for herbs and spices should be short. Most herbs and spices should be done drying in less than 4 hours. Herbs and spices are done when they feel crispy and are brittle to the touch. You should be able to crumble leaves, stems and flowers between your fingers.

Some herbs and spices can be hung out to air dry. Rosemary, thyme, sage and parsley can all be hung inside the house and left to dry. Basil, oregano and mint leaves need to be placed inside a paper bag before being hung out to dry. Air-drying can be done indoors or out, but be sure to hang the herbs and spices in a shaded area if drying them outside. Air-drying herbs by hanging them can take a week or two to properly dry the herbs.

Herbs and some spices can be dried in the microwave if you're in a hurry. Microwave them on high for 2 minutes and check them. If they're still wet, microwave them for 30 seconds and check them again. Continue microwaving the herbs in 30-second increments until they're done drying.

Storing Herbs and Spices

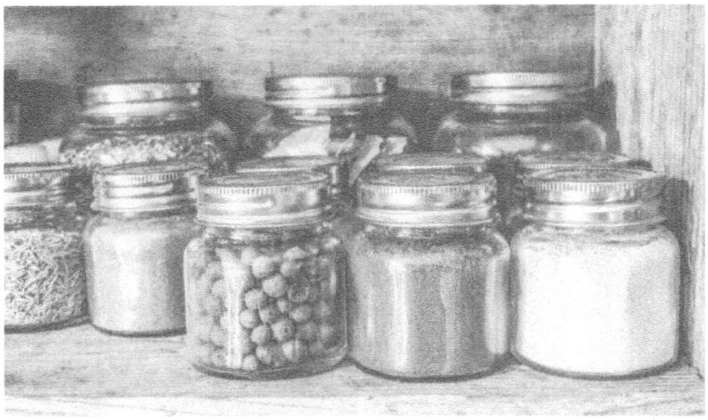

Here's the dilemma. Herbs and spices will last a lot longer when they're left whole, but they're usually ground or crushed when they're used in recipes. It's kind of a hassle to grind or crush your herbs every time you want to use them, especially when you're looking to make a quick meal.

What I do is dry a large batch of herbs and spices. I crush up half of it and store it that way, so I always have crushed or ground herbs and spices on hand. I then store the rest of it in the freezer whole. When I start to run low, I crush or grind the herbs I have in the freezer and I'm ready to go. I know when I pull a batch out of the freezer, I'm going to need to dry more soon or I'm going to run out.

Are nutrients lost during drying?

There are some nutrients lost during pretreatment and drying. Any time the food is exposed to heat, light or oxygen, there will be some degradation of nutritional value. The longer the exposure, the greater the damage. Most fruits start degrading as soon as they're harvested. This degradation is sped up by cutting into them or otherwise exposing the flesh to oxygen.

Many fruits contain enzymes that react to the air and cause browning and nutrient loss to begin as soon as they're cut into. If you've ever left an apple or a banana out for a while and seen it turn brown, you've seen these enzymes in action. This reaction to the oxygen in the air can be slowed to a crawl by pretreating or blanching the fruit after it's been cut.

The following vitamins can be damaged by too much heat, light or air exposure:

- Folate (heat).
- Riboflavin (heat).
- Thiamine (heat, light).
- Vitamin A (air, light).
- Vitamin B12 (heat, light).

Commercial foods that undergo intense treatment lose a lot more nutrients than fruit dried at home. While commercially dried foods can lose up to 80% of certain vitamins, foods dried at home usually don't come anywhere near that magnitude.

Take the following precautions to reduce the amount of vitamins lost while treating and drying produce:

Work on small batches of food at a time.

When you work on large batches and try to get a lot of fruit done at once, the pieces you cut into first are left to sit out while you process the rest of the produce. This can result in the earlier pieces degrading a lot faster than those cut later on.

Move food into pretreatment shortly after it's been cut.

Time is of essence when treating fruit that's prone to discoloration. It's important to slow down enzymatic reactions as early as possible to avoid nutrient loss.

Carefully regulate heat.

High heat can accelerate nutrient loss, so its important heat is monitored closely. Using a dehydrator allows you the most control over the amount of heat drying food is exposed to. Blanching also exposes food to heat and can damage nutrients, but may be critical to ensuring food can be properly stored. Blanching isn't as critical of a process with fruit as it is with vegetables.

Store dried food in an airtight container.

This will minimize the amount of air the food comes in contact with. If air is allowed into the container, the food can take up moisture from the air, drastically shortening how long the food will last.

Drying food in the sun exposes it to UV rays that can damage light-sensitive vitamins.

When vitamin retention is of concern, a dehydrator may be the better choice for drying.

Store food in small, single-serving containers.

Every time you open a container, more air is let in. Using single serving containers only exposes the food you plan on eating to new air.

No minerals are lost during the drying process, but pretreatment can cause some mineral loss. Boiling or otherwise exposing fruit to water may cause some of the minerals to leach out into the water. This can happen during blanching and again during rehydration. The drying process itself doesn't affect minerals.

Calories and sugar are largely unaffected by the drying process, but they will be concentrated into a smaller package. A raisin has the same caloric content and amount of sugar as it did when it was a grape, but it's now packed into the smaller raisin. Dried produce has more calories and more sugar than regular produce when compared by volume. For example, 100 grams of grapes have 15 grams of sugar and 70 calories. 100 grams of raisins have 60 grams of sugar and 300 calories. Raisins have 3 times the sugar and more than 4 times the calories than grapes when compared by volume.

For this reason, it's important not to overeat when it comes to dried fruit and vegetables. They can be a healthy part of most diets, but only if consumed in moderation.

The Best Techniques to Preserve Dried Foods

Over drying the dried food is just impossibility. So, when you are unsure if the food is completely dry or not, keeps drying it until you are entirely sure.

Never use granulated sugar in fruit leathers as the sugar will get crystallize over time. You can opt for honey or corn syrup if you need.

To be considered "dehydrated," foods must be at least 95% moisture-free. If they aren't and you try to store them, they'll quickly rot. How can you tell? If the food is soft, spongy, and sticky, it's back in the dehydrator they go. You can't really "over dry" food, so the harder and crunchier, the better. If you don't want certain foods to be that dry, you'll have to plan on eating them pretty much right away before bacteria has a chance to get at that moisture.

Store food properly

The last step you need to remember in the dehydration process is safe storage. All food should be stored in clean and dry containers, with airtight lids that can keep out moisture and bugs. If you're a prepper and don't plan on snacking frequently on your dehydrated foods just yet, vacuum-sealing is a great option.

Safe storage also means knowing how long a food is going to last, because even the most dehydrated food doesn't last forever. The only exception is freeze-dried foods, which can last decades, but most people don't have a special freeze-drier machine. Bear in mind that store-bought dehydrated foods last longer than homemade ones, because of the added preservatives. As an example, jerky you buy at the store lasts about a year, while home-dehydrated will only last 1-2 months when properly stored.

Health food stores usually stock bulk items such as rice, flour, pasta, millet, etc. Ask if you can buy them in bulk. Many stores will usually give a discount for whole case or whole bag purchases.

You will still have to store them in a bucket or some other container. You can use whatever food containers you have. Just make sure they were not used for toxic or hazardous materials. You don't want toxic residues to contaminate your food.

If you want, you can store your bulk items in plastic food storage bags available in any grocery store. The one-gallon and two-gallon sizes work well for this purpose. Squeeze the air out of the bag before sealing it. You can also add oxygen absorber packets before

After sealing the plastic bag, you can add an extra layer of protection by wrapping it with aluminum foil. This will act as a light bather. Then put this in another larger plastic bag, squeeze the air out and seal.

Mylar Bags (Metalized Liners)

To seal these bags, you can use foil tape. One brand is Refectix and should be available in hardware stores. If not, check with plumbing supply stores. A 30-foot roll costs around $4. If there is still air in the bag after you seal it, prick a little hole in it and push the air out. Then seal up the hole. Or you can use a portable heat sealer which can cost over 100 dollars.

If you don't want to use food buckets, you can store these packages in cardboard boxes – just make sure you have no mice. Or you can use the 18 gallon and 22 gallon storage tote containers sold just about anywhere (Wal-Mart, Kmart, Pamida, Gibson, hardware stores). Rubbermaid makes them as well as other companies. They cost around $5 to $7 each.

If there is a food service (restaurant) supplies store near you, go and see what is available that you can use.

The dryer the food is, the longer it can be stored for, so you'll want as much moisture in the food to be removed as possible. Airtight plastic bags and/or containers are great options for holding the food and resisting spoilage. Most of the nutritional value in dehydrated foods will be preserved, although it won't be as nutritious as it would be otherwise.

Remember that when storing any food for the long term, the food needs to be stored in a cool and dry location at room temperature. Any location that's humid or excessively hot should be automatically rejected for storing food because the food will be more likely to mold, even if it's been preserved.

How to Store Jerky

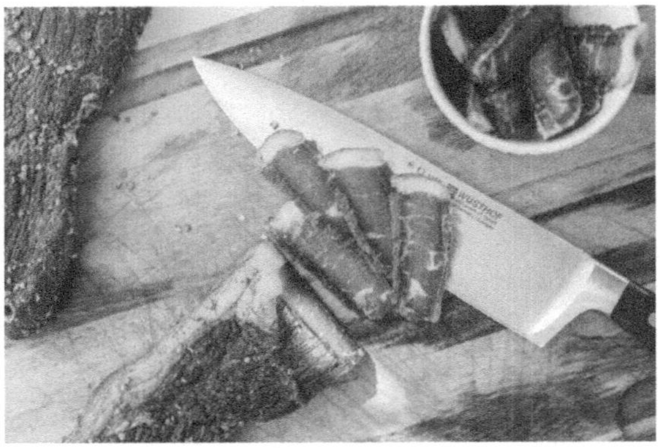

The best way to store jerky is to treat it like a fresh food item.

Limit the jerky's exposure to air.

Retain the quality of your jerky by placing it in an airtight container. Vacuum packing, sealable bags and plastic wrap can be used to wrap your jerky and are effective at keeping air out. The option that would allow the jerky to be most easily accessible is to place it in a storage container or jar that has a lid.

Label the container with the date at the beginning of the storage life so you know the age of the jerky and how long it has been stored.

Separate your jerky by type. Place different types of jerky in different containers to keep the flavors separate, ensuring top quality.

Eradicate any source of moisture.

Use a paper towel to dry your jerky. If you notice moisture or oil on your jerky, noted by wetness or a sheen on the surface, gently pat the surfaces of the meat with a paper towel.

Keep moisture at bay while the jerky is in storage by placing the jerky between layers of paper towel in the container. The towels will absorb any moisture from the jerky or container. Replace the towels when you notice any presence of moisture.

Know the shelf life of your jerky.

Time will take a toll on the quality of your jerky. With proper storage techniques, jerky can safely be stored for varying lengths of time depending on where you choose to store it.

Leave your jerky in a cool, dry place. When placed properly in an airtight container, you can leave your jerky on the counter top or another cool, dry place for no longer than 1 month.

Put your jerky in the refrigerator. Jerky can be stored in the refrigerator to be used within 6 months.

Store homemade jerky in the freezer. Jerky lasts up to 1-year when kept in your freezer

How to Store Herbs?

When completely dry, separate the leaves from the stems, and store the leaves (either whole or gently crumbled) in light-proof containers.

In terms of oven-drying, allow the dried herbs to cool, and gently crush the leaves. Store the dried herbs in light-proof containers.

Store all your dried herbs in a cool dark place, in airtight containers.

Never store your herb vinegars in the sun or on a lighted counter if you intend to use them, no matter how pretty they look. They should always be stored in the refrigerator.

FAQS

How long will dehydrated food last?

If prepared and stored properly, dehydrated food is can last 5 to 10 years. But it is advisable to use your own within four to six months.

Does dehydrating food remove (or preserve) nutrients?

Yes, some nutrients may be removed when food is dehydrated but no more than other methods of preservation. Heat and light are responsible for the breakdown of vitamins. By implication, the canning method of preservation tears down more nutrients than the low heat, low moisture dehydrating method. The amount of thiamin and vitamin A & C that diminishes from your vegetables can be reduced through blanching.

Does dehydrating food kill bacteria?

Provided that you dehydrate your vegetables and fruits until their moisture levels are anywhere between five and twenty percent, you have removed the bacteria that can cause food to decay. If you are concern about bacteria on meat, it is recommended by the USDA that you first heat your raw meat to 160°F temperature and then dehydrate at a steady temperature of 145°F.

Does Dehydrate Food Increase Sugar

In most cases, yes, because when you dehydrate food at a higher temperate, it will cause the death of enzymes. More dense foods may withstand higher temperatures without the enzymes being killed. But most enzymes will ultimately become dormant when the temperature rises between 140° to 160°F.

Can Cooked Food Be Dehydrated?

Yes. Meals can even be dehydrated, but some cooked food dehydrates better than others. If you are drying food for long-term storage, camping, or backpacking, you can prepare rice dishes, stews, and desserts and dry them by using nonstick sheets on the trays of dehydrator. And then remove the nonstick sheet when they have reached a moist, crumbly consistency.

How can I store dried food?

Dehydrated vegetables can last up to ten years and fruit up to five if properly stored. The best way to preserve your dried food for the long term is to vacuum seal using an oxygen absorber and keep it in a cool, dark place. If you are going to eat non-meat dried food within 12 months, store them in reusable storage bags or freezer bags with the air squeezed out.

If you will consume seafood and meat within a month, you can store in freezer bags and keep them in a cool, dark place; otherwise, the best thing is to vacuum seal and freeze them. Meat can last for up to a year if properly stored in the freezer.

The Best Ways, Temperature and Cooking Times to Dry Foods

Ways at Home

Pre-treating food

For best results, most of the food items need to be pre-treated before dehydration. Following are the commonly used pre-treatments:

Ascorbic acid or Vitamin C bath

By soaking fruits or soft vegetables in an ascorbic acid solution (one-part of ascorbic acid in 1 gallon of water) immediately after cutting will stop discoloring and browning. An exception is leafy greens, herbs, and broccoli as the acid will discolor them severely. For this, soak the cut fruits immediately in the solution for 8 to 10 minutes. Drain for dehydration.

Skin cracking

Fruits with tougher skins such as plums, cherries, grapes, figs, or berries may need their skins to be cracked before dehydration to pull moisture out from the fruit properly. For this, boil a pot of water and dip the fruit in it for 15 seconds. Remove and dip them in ice-cold water immediately. Drain water entirely before drying them.

Blanching

It is a process used for scalding vegetables in boiling water or steam, to stop the enzymatic action within the vegetables. Be cautious about the timing, as over blanching results in loss of nutrients and under blanching can cause food spoilage during or after the dehydration. For blanching, usually, two methods are used: boiling vegetables in water for some time, and scalding vegetables above the boiling water level, also known as steam blanching — steam from the boiling water scalds the vegetables.

Citric Acid bath

Citric Acid kills bacteria and stops food discolouration. For this, mix a teaspoon of citric acid in 2.5 cups of water, or you can mix equal parts of water and lemon juice. Soak the food for 8 to 10 minutes and drain entirely before dehydration.

Storage

Dehydrated foods can last for years if stored properly. To ensure maximum shelf life, you need to prevent dried food from moisture, heat, microorganism, light and oxygen. Essential steps of storage are:

Cooling

When the fruit is dry enough, remove it from the dehydrator and cool the fruit completely in a cool and dry place for half an hour; storing warm food will reintroduce moisture due to condensation. Make sure not to leave the dried food for too long as it will also result in moisture to come back into the food.

Conditioning

To ensure even distribution of moisture within the food, place the dried food in loose packaging and seal it for 2 to 4 days.

Packaging

As a final step of storage, you need to pack your dehydrated food in air-tight jars or cans. Store your jars or containers in a cool, dark, and dry place to maximise the shelf-life.

Types of Dehydrators

Although there are many methods to dehydrate food such as sun drying and oven drying, the most convenient method is by using an electric dehydrator. Why?

Because it is an easy and hassle-free way to dehydrate your food.

You can get commercial electrical dehydrators from the market that matches your needs, or you can go for DIY dehydrator at home.

DIY home dehydrator

You can construct your dehydrator, if you need to produce large batches of dried foods, from a wooden framed box. All you need is constant heat (gas burner) and airflow (a fan) and few shelves or trays to put food on. However, it becomes difficult to control the temperature levels if you are a beginner, and sometimes it results in a complete mess due to a complicated cleaning process. You need a lot of experimentation and testing to achieve the optimum temperature levels in DIY dehydrators.

Electric dehydrators

If you plan to dry your food regularly, then investing in a commercial electrical dehydrator is the best option. They can handle large quantities of food, and the best part is, you can control the temperature and air circulation without putting much effort. In a useful and well-made electric dehydrator, the temperature remains constant throughout the drying process with the help of a thermostatically-controlled heating system, and proper airflow is achieved through a built-in fan to ensure complete evaporation.

You can get a small unit with 4 or 5 trays under a hundred dollars if you want to dry small batches in one go. However, if you intend to dry a lot of food at once, you can get a commercial dehydrator with ten trays or more.

Dehydration Tool Kit

You have bought a good and suitable dehydrator, but there are still some other tools and products you may need to increase the productivity and the quality of your dried food. But remember to keep them simple and easy to use. You would need:

- Apple peeler and cherry pitter for quick and efficient work
- You will need a deep container with a tight lid for blanching
- A colander to fit into the container to hold food items for blanching
- Stainless steel knives for cutting food and meat
- Ascorbic acid or lemon juice to give Vitamin C bath to fruits
- Large pot or tub to hold Ascorbic Acid or lemon juice solution
- A blender to make fruit leathers, or to powder your dehydrated food
- Disposable latex or vinyl gloves to handle dried foods to prevent spoilage as handling dried foods with hands transform moisture and heat from your hands to the food.
- Nylon mesh to place on trays or shelves
- Air-tight containers for storing dehydrated foods such as mason jars or cans with air-tight lids, or zip lock bags that can be vacuum-sealed.
- A food processor for grating and slicing vegetables evenly
- A meat slicer to cut the meat evenly in desired thickness quickly and efficiently, and for slicing the fruits and vegetables evenly for making chips and crackers.
- .Sometimes you need to soak and spray the food with vitamin C or lemon juice before dehydrating to avoid browning. For this, a spray bottle is a mess-free option and do the work quickly.
- For making leathers, a squeeze bottle is quite useful. You can squeeze the puree out straight onto drying sheets, or you can even mix different colored purees to form a multi-colored design.

Using a dehydrator is the most effective way to remove moisture from food and extend its shelf-life.

DEHYDRATOR
COOKBOOK FOR PREPPERS

1000 Days of Delicious Homemade Recipes for Fruit, Vegetables, Jerky, Mushrooms and More

Tyler Gordon

CHAPTER 3: CRACKERS BREAD AND CHIPS

1. Carrot crackers

Preparation time: 20 minutes
Dehydration time: 6 hours
Servings: 10

Ingredients:

- 1 cup almonds, soaked overnight, rinsed, and drained
- 2 cups carrot pulp
- 1 tablespoon ground chia seeds
- 2 tablespoons ground flax seed
- 1 teaspoon italian seasoning
- 1 tablespoon coconut aminos
- ½ teaspoon smoked paprika
- 1 tablespoon dried onion
- ½ teaspoon red pepper flakes
- 2 cups water

Direction:

1. Add the almonds to a food processor or blender.
2. Pulse until crumbly.
3. Stir in the rest of the ingredients.
4. Pulse until fully combined.
5. Spread a thin layer of the dough in the cosori premium food dehydrator.
6. Dry at 125 degrees f for 2 hours.
7. Score the dough to form the crackers.
8. Dry at 115 degrees for 8 hours.
9. Storage suggestions: store in an airtight food container for up to 5 days.

Tip: soak the almonds overnight the day before processing.

Nutrition: calories: 122 fat: 7.4 g, carbs: 10.8 g protein: 3.9 g.

2. Sweet potato chips

Preparation time: 15 minutes
Dehydration time: 4 hours
Servings: 2

Ingredients:

- 2 sweet potatoes, scrubbed and sliced thinly
- Salt to taste
- 2 teaspoons onion powder

Direction:

1. Arrange the sweet potatoes in the cosori premium food dehydrator.
2. Process at 155 degrees f for 2 hours.
3. Flip and dry for another 2 hours.
4. Sprinkle with salt and onion powder.
5. Storage suggestions: store in a sealable plastic bag.

Tip: use homemade onion powder.

Nutrition: calories 195, fat 3, fiber 1, carbs 20, protein 4

3. Tomato & flaxseed crackers

Preparation time: 20 minutes
Dehydration time: 8 hours
Servings: 24

Ingredients:

- 1 cup flaxseed
- 8sun-dried tomatoes
- 1 bell pepper, chopped
- 1tablespoon olive oil
- Salt to taste
- 2 tomatoes, chopped
- 1 onion, chopped
- 1 clove garlic, crushed through garlic press
- ¼ cup dried oregano leaves, crushed
- Salt and pepper to taste

Direction:

1. Place the flaxseed in a bowl.
2. In another bowl, combine the remaining ingredients.
3. Stir in the flaxseeds.
4. Combine all the ingredients in the food processor.
5. Pulse until fully combined.
6. Spread the mixture in the cosori premium food dehydrator.
7. Process at 110 degrees f for 12 hours.
8. Storage suggestions: store in an airtight jar for up to 9 days.

Tip: soak the flaxseeds in water for 2 hours before processing.

Nutrition: Calories: 178, Fat: 13.3g, Carbs: 10.7g, Protein: 4.4g

4. Seed crackers

Preparation time: x hours
Dehydration time: x hours
Servings: 10

Ingredients:

- ¼ cup chia seeds
- ¾ cup flax seeds
- 1 cup water
- ¼ cup hemp seeds

- 1/3 cup sunflower seeds
- 2 tablespoons pumpkin seeds
- 1 tablespoon italian seasoning
- Salt and pepper to taste

Direction:

1. Soak the chia seeds and flax seeds in water for 1 hour.
2. Drain.
3. Transfer to a bowl.
4. Stir in the rest of the ingredients.
5. Process at 115 degrees f for 90 minutes.
6. Flip and break into smaller pieces.
7. Dry at 105 degrees f for 8 hours.
8. Storage suggestions: store in an airtight container for up to 7 days.

Tip: serve with hummus.

Nutrition: Calories: 178, Fat: 13.3g, Carbs: 10.7g, Protein: 4.4g

5. Apple chips with cinnamon

Preparation time: 15 minutes
Dehydration time: 8 hours
Servings: 4

Ingredients:

- 4 apples, sliced thinly
- ¼ cup sugar
- 1 tablespoon ground cinnamon

Direction:

1. Mix the cinnamon and sugar.
2. Coat the apple slices with this mixture.
3. Place the apple slices in the cosori premium food dehydrator.
4. Process at 135 degrees f for 12 hours.
5. Storage suggestions: store in an airtight food container.

Tip: use a mandoliner slicer to slice the apples thinly.

Nutrition: calories 195, fat 3, fiber 1, carbs 20, protein 4

6. Vegan bread

Preparation time: 30 minutes
Dehydration time: 6 hours
Servings: 4

Ingredients:

- 1 head cauliflower
- 1 teaspoon turmeric
- 2 tablespoons flax seed
- 1/2 cup psyllium hust
- 1/2 cup brewer's yeast
- 4 large zucchini
- Salt and black pepper

Directions:

1. Place cauliflower and zucchini in a food processor and pulse until they form a paste. Add the turmeric, flax seeds, psyllium, yeast, and a pinch of salt and black pepper. Pulse again until all ingredients are thoroughly combined.
2. Place paraflexx screens on the racks of your excalibur food dehydrator. Form the mixture into slices about 1/2-inch-thick, and place on the screens.
3. Set your excalibur to 150f and dehydrate for 6 hours. The bread should not be completely dry. One side should be slightly soft.

Nutrition: calories: 219 fat: 1.9 g, carbs: 61.6 g protein: 10.1 g.

7. Fluffy dinner rolls

Preparation time: 15 minutes
Dehydration time: 7 hours
Servings: 4

Ingredients:

- 2 cups almond flour
- 1 cup psyllium
- 3 tablespoons ground flax seeds
- 1 tablespoon onion powder
- 2 teaspoons garlic powder
- 1 tablespoon lemon juice
- 1 teaspoon salt
- 1/3 cup water

Directions:

1. In a large bowl, combine the flour, psyllium, flax seeds, onion powder, garlic powder, lemon juice, salt, and water. Mix well until combined.
2. Form the mixture into 6 round rolls.
3. Place paraflexx screens on the racks of your excalibur. Place the rolls on the screens so they are not touching. Dehydrate at 145f for one hour, and then lower the temperature to 110f for the remaining 6 hours. Remove from the screens and serve warm or allow cooling before storing.

Nutrition: calories: 319 fat: 7.1 g,carbs: 95.2 g protein: 3.5 g.

CHAPTER 4: VEGETABLES

8. Maple carrot straws

Preparation time: 15 minutes
Dehydration time: 6 hours
Servings: 4

Ingredients:

- 1 lb. Carrots, sliced into long strips
- 1 tablespoon maple syrup
- 1 tablespoon olive oil
- Salt to taste

Direction:

1. Combine all the ingredients in a bowl.
2. Arrange the strips in the cosori premium food dehydrator.
3. Process at 135 degrees f for 6 hours.
4. Storage suggestions: store in a food container.

Tip: use a peeler to slice the carrots.

Nutrition: Calories 214 Fat 3 g Carbs 41.4 g Protein 4.3 g

9. Dehydrated asparagus

Preparation time: 10 minutes
Dehydration time: 6 hours
Servings: 2

Ingredients:

- 4 cups asparagus, trimmed and sliced

Direction:

1. Arrange the asparagus in the cosori premium food dehydrator.
2. Process at 125 degrees f for 6 hours.
3. Storage suggestions: store in a sealable plastic bag.

Tip: you can also season the asparagus with salt or garlic powder.

Nutrition: Calories 434 Fat 39.4 g Carbs 20.9 g Protein 5.8 g

10. Fall carrot chips

Preparation time: 15 minutes
Dehydration time: 6 hours
Servings: 4

Ingredients:

- 1 pound of carrots, peeled
- 3 tbsp. Melted coconut oil
- ¾ tsp. Salt
- 2 tsp. Allspice (or combination of cinnamon, allspice or nutmeg)

Direction:

1. Wash, dry and slice carrots into uniform disks.
2. Mix together carrots, oil, salt and allspice.
3. Place carrots onto dehydrator trays and dry for 6-6 hours at 125 degrees or until crisp.

Nutrition: calories: 11, sodium: 337 mg, dietary fiber: 0.7 g, total fat: 0 g, total carbs: 2.7 g, protein: 0.2 g.

11. Herbed sweet potato chips

Preparation time: 15 minutes
Dehydration time: 6 hours
Servings: 4

Ingredients:

- 3 medium to large sweet potatoes
- 4 tbsp. Olive oil
- 2 tbsp. Fresh lemon juice
- 2 tsp. Dried thyme
- 1 ½ tsp. Salt
- ¼ tsp. Pepper

Direction:

1. Slice sweet potatoes into thin, uniform slices.
2. In a bowl combine sweet potato slices, oil, lemon juice, thyme, salt and pepper. Toss until well coated.
3. Place slices on dehydrator trays.
4. Set the temperature to 140 degrees. Dehydrate for 6-6 hours, or until crisp to touch.

Nutrition: calories: 35, sodium: 721 mg, dietary fiber: 1.9 g, total fat: 0.2 g, total carbs: 8.3 g, protein: 0.6 g.

12. Dried cauliflower popcorn

Preparation time: 15 minutes
Dehydration time: 8 hours
Serving: 1

Ingredients:

- 2 cups cauliflower florets
- 4 tablespoons hot sauce
- 3 tablespoons coconut oil
- 1 teaspoon smoked cayenne
- ½ teaspoon ground cumin
- 1 tablespoons paprika

Direction:

1. Toss the cauliflower florets in hot sauce and coconut oil.
2. Sprinkle with the smoked cayenne, cumin and paprika.
3. Add the seasoned cauliflower to the cosori premium food dehydrator.
4. Dry at 130 degrees f for 8 hours.
5. Storage suggestions: store in an airtight plastic bag.

Tip: add more cayenne pepper for spicier cauliflower popcorn.

Nutrition: calories: 9, sodium: 0 mg, dietary fiber: 0 g, total fat: 0 g, total carbs: 2.1 g, protein: 0.2 g.

13. Zucchini snacks

Preparation time: 45 minutes
Dehydration time: 12 hours
Servings: 4

Ingredients:

- 8 zucchinis, sliced into rounds and seeds removed
- 1 cup grape juice concentrate
- 1 cup water

Direction:

1. Add all the ingredients to a pot over medium heat.
2. Bring to a boil.
3. Reduce heat and simmer for 30 minutes.
4. Drain the zucchini and let cool.
5. Add the zucchinis to the cosori premium food dehydrator.
6. Process at 135 degrees f for 12 hours.
7. Storage suggestions: store in the refrigerator for up to 1 week.

Tip: do not overcook the zucchinis.

Nutrition: calories: 9, sodium: 0 mg, dietary fiber: 0 g, total fat: 0 g, total carbs: 2.1 g, protein: 0.2 g.

14. Cucumber chips

Preparation time: 15 minutes
Dehydration time: 6 hours
Servings: 4

Ingredients:

- 3 cucumber, sliced into rounds
- 1 tablespoon avocado oil
- 2 teaspoons apple cider vinegar
- Salt to taste

Direction:

1. Toss the cucumber slices in avocado oil and vinegar.
2. Season with the salt.
3. Add the cucumber slices to the cosori premium food dehydrator.
4. Dehydrate at 135 degrees f for 6 hours.
5. Storage suggestions: store in an airtight container.

Tip: you can use a mandoline slicer to slice the cucumbers thinly. Dry the cucumber slices with a paper towel before processing.

Nutrition: calories: 9, sodium: 0 mg, dietary fiber: 0 g, total fat: 0 g, total carbs: 2.1 g, protein: 0.2 g.

15. Dehydrated okra

Preparation time: 15 minutes
Dehydration time: 12 hours
Servings: 4

Ingredients:

- 12 okra, sliced

Direction:

1. Add the okra to the cosori premium food dehydrator.
2. Dry at 130 degrees f for 12 hours.
3. Storage suggestions: store in an airtight container.

Tip: sprinkle with powdered herb or spice for added flavor.

Nutrition: calories 70, fat 4, fiber 4, carbs 30, protein 2

16. Dried sweet potato

Preparation time: 10 minutes
Dehydration time: 12 hours
Servings: 4

Ingredients:

- 2 sweet potatoes
- 1 teaspoon onion powder

Direction:

1. Season the sweet potato slices with onion powder.
2. Arrange in a single layer in the cosori premium food dehydrator.
3. Set at 115 degrees f.
4. Process for 12 hours.
5. Storage suggestions: store in a sealable plastic bag.

Tip: use a mandolin slicer to prepare the sweet potatoes.

Nutrition: calories 70, fat 4, fiber 4, carbs 30, protein 2

CHAPTER 5: SIDE DISHES

17. Zucchini chips

Preparation time: 15 minutes
Dehydration time: 12 hours
Servings: 8

Ingredients:

- 4 cups zucchini, sliced thinly
- 2 tbsp. Balsamic vinegar
- 2 tbsp. Olive oil
- 2 tsp. Sea salt

Direction:

1. Add olive oil, balsamic vinegar, and sea salt to the large bowl and stir well.
2. Add sliced zucchini to the bowl and toss well.
3. Arrange zucchini slices on dehydrator trays and dehydrate at 135 f/ 58 c for 8-12 hours.
4. Store in air-tight container.

Nutrition: calories: 40 fat: 3.6g protein: 0.7g carbs: 1.9g

18. Eggplant slices

Preparation time: 10 minutes
Dehydration time: 4 hours
Servings: 4

Ingredients:

- 1 medium eggplant, cut into ¼ inch thick slices
- ¼ tsp. Onion powder
- ¼ tsp. Garlic powder
- 1 ½ tsp. Paprika

Directions:

1. Add all ingredients into the mixing bowl and toss well.
2. Arrange eggplant slices on dehydrator trays and dehydrate at 145 f/ 63 c for 4 hours or until crispy.
3. Store in air-tight container.

Nutrition: calories: 32 fat: 0.3g protein: 1.3g carbs: 7.4g

19. Tasty zucchini chips

Preparation time: 15 minutes
Dehydration time: 8 hours
Servings: 4

Ingredients:

- 2 medium zucchini wash and cut into ¼ inch slices
- 1/8 tsp. Cayenne pepper
- ½ tsp. Garlic powder
- 1 tsp. Olive oil
- 1/8 tsp. Sea salt

Direction:

1. Add all ingredients into the mixing bowl and toss well to coat.
2. Arrange zucchini slices on dehydrator trays and dehydrate at 135 f/ 58 c for 6-8 hours.
3. Store in air-tight container.

Nutrition: calories: 27 fat: 1.4g protein: 1.3g carbs: 3.6g

20. Brussels sprout chips

Preparation time: 15 minutes
Dehydration time: 6 hours
Servings: 4

Ingredients:

- 2 lbs. Brussels sprouts, wash, dry, cut the root and separate leaves
- 2 fresh lemon juice
- ½ cup water
- ¼ cup nutritional yeast
- 1 jalapeno pepper halved and remove seeds
- 1 cup cashews
- 2 bell peppers
- 1 tsp. Sea salt

Directions:

1. Add brussels sprouts leaves to the large bowl and set aside.
2. Add bell peppers, water, lemon juice, nutritional yeast, jalapeno, cashews, and salt to the blender and blend until smooth.
3. Pour blended mixture over brussels sprouts leaves and toss until well coated.
4. Arrange brussels sprouts on dehydrator trays and dehydrate at 125 f/ 52 c for 6 hours.
5. Allow to cool completely then store in air-tight container.

Nutrition: calories: 237 fat: 11.7g protein: 12.3g carbs: 27.7g

21. Bbq jerky strips

Preparation time: 15 minutes
Dehydration time: 6 hours
Servings: 4

Ingredients:

- 2 ½ pounds lean ground beef
- 2 tsp. Salt

- ½ tsp. Garlic powder
- ½ tsp. Onion powder
- 1 ½ tbsp. Brown sugar
- ¼ cup worcestershire sauce

½ cup barbecue sauce, slightly diluted with water

Direction:

6. Mix ground beef with dry ingredients until incorporated.
7. Combine liquids and coat beef strips with sauce.
8. Press strips into jerky gun. Squeeze onto dehydrator trays and dry at 145-155 degrees for 6-12 hours.

Nutrition: calories: 54, sodium: 329 mg, dietary fiber: 0 g, total fat: 1.2 g, total carbs: 4.6 g, protein: 5.8 g.

22. Bold beef jerky

Preparation time: 15 minutes
Dehydration time: 6 hours
Servings: 4

Ingredients:

- 2 pounds sliced lean meat
- ¼ cup soy sauce
- 1 tbsp. Worcestershire sauce
- 1 tsp. Hot sauce
- ¼ tsp. Pepper
- ¼ tsp. Garlic powder
- ¼ tsp. Onion powder
- ¼ tsp. Paprika
- 1 tsp. Liquid smoke

Direction:

1. Cut strips into ¼ inch thick slices.
2. Mix all ingredients and coat meat strips.
3. Cover and refrigerate overnight.
4. Place meat slices on dehydrator trays and dry at 145-155 degrees for 6-6 hours.

Nutrition: calories: 51, sodium: 27 mg, dietary fiber: 0 g, total fat: 1.7 g, total carbs: 0 g, protein: 8.3 g.

23. Orange flavored beef jerky

Preparation time: 15 minutes
Dehydration time: 6 hours
Servings: 4

Ingredients:

- 3 pounds lean beef, trimmed of all fat and sliced into strips 1/8 inches -3/8 inches thick
- 3 oranges, (2 peeled and juiced, and 1 zested)
- 3 tbsp. Soy sauce
- 3 tbsp. Rice vinegar
- 2 tbsp. Sugar
- 3 tbsp. Sesame oil
- 1 ½ tbsp. Toasted sesame oil
- 1 tsp. Asian chili-garlic paste
- 2 tbsp. Fresh ginger, grated

Direction:

1. Place all the ingredients, except for the beef, into a blender and process until smooth.
2. Pour marinade over meat and mix.
3. Keep marinated meat in refrigerator overnight.
4. Remove from refrigerator and let meat come to room temperature.
5. Lay meat on dehydrator sheets in a single layer.
6. Dehydrate at 145-160 degrees for 6-6 hours.

Nutrition: calories: 61, sodium: 16 mg, dietary fiber: 0 g, total fat: 1.6 g, total carbs: 4.3 g, protein: 7.3 g.

24. Pastrami jerky

Ingredients:

- 3 pounds lean beef, such as flank
- ½ cup soy sauce
- ¼ cup brown sugar
- ½ cup worcestershire sauce
- 1 tbsp. Lemon juice
- ½ tsp. Cayenne pepper
- 2 tbsp. Coarse pepper seeds
- 2 tbsp. Coriander seeds
- 1 tbsp. Mustard seeds

Direction:

1. Cut each slice of beef into ¼ inch thick strips.
2. Combine all ingredients except seeds. Pour ingredients over sliced meat and refrigerate overnight.
3. Remove from refrigerator and let meat come to room temperature.
4. Lay meat on dehydrator sheets and sprinkle with seeds.
5. Dehydrate at 145-155 degrees for 6-6 hours.

Nutrition: calories: 56, sodium: 50 mg, dietary fiber: 0 g, total fat: 1.4 g, total carbs: 4.2 g, protein: 6.1 g.

CHAPTER 6: MEAT

25. Pork jerky in chipotle sauce

Preparation time: 12 hours and 10 minutes
Dehydration time: 6 hours
Servings: 2

Ingredients:

- 1 tablespoon tomato paste
- 7 oz. Chipotle adobo sauce
- 1 teaspoon salt
- 1 teaspoon sugar
- 1 teaspoon garlic powder
- 1 lb. Pork tenderloin, sliced

Direction:

1. Mix the tomato paste, chipotle adobo sauce, salt, sugar and garlic powder in a bowl.
2. Transfer to a sealable plastic bag along with the pork tenderloin slices.
3. Seal and refrigerate for 12 hours.
4. Drain the marinade.
5. Add the pork slices to the cosori premium food dehydrator.
6. Process at 158 degrees f for 6 hours.
7. Storage suggestions: place in a glass jar with lid. Store in a cool dry place, away from sunlight.

Tip: pork tenderloin should be sliced at least 5 mm thick.

Nutrition: Calories 54 Fat 0.3 g Carbohydrates 11.3 g Protein 2.5 g

26. Paprika pork jerky

Preparation time: 12 hours and 10 minutes
Dehydration time: 6 hours
Servings: 2

Ingredients:

- 1 lb. Pork tenderloin, sliced
- ½ cup ketchup
- 1 teaspoon onion powder
- 1 teaspoon garlic powder
- 1 teaspoon smoked paprika
- 1 teaspoon ground mustard
- 1 teaspoon chili powder
- Salt and pepper to taste

Direction:

1. Add the ketchup to a bowl.
2. Stir in the onion powder, garlic powder, paprika, mustard, chili powder, salt and pepper.
3. Mix well.
4. Transfer the mixture to a sealable plastic bag.
5. Add the pork to the plastic bag.
6. Seal and refrigerate for 12 hours.
7. Remove the pork from the marinade.
8. Add to the cosori premium food dehydrator.
9. Dry at 158 degrees f for 6 hours.
10. Storage suggestions: store the pork jerky in a glass jar with lid. Store in a cool dry place for up to 2 weeks.

Tip: you can also use garlic salt in place of garlic powder and salt.

Nutrition: Calories 382 Fat 1.2 g Carbs 67.1 g Protein 26.1 g

27. Beef bulgogi jerky

Preparation time: 12 hours and 10 minutes
Dehydration time: 6 hours
Servings: 4

Ingredients:

- 2 lb. Beef round, sliced
- 4 tablespoons brown sugar
- 4 tablespoons soy sauce
- 1 tablespoon garlic powder
- 1 tablespoon sesame oil
- Sal to taste

Direction:

1. Place the beef inside a sealable plastic bag.
2. In a bowl, mix the remaining ingredients.
3. Add the mixture to the plastic bag.
4. Place the beef in the refrigerator for 12 hours.
5. Drain the marinade.
6. Add the beef to the cosori premium food dehydrator.
7. Set at 165 degrees f.
8. Process for 6 hours.
9. Storage suggestions: place in a glass jar with lid and store in a cool, dry place.

Tip: slice the beef across the grain. Each slice should be at least 5 mm thick.

Nutrition: Calories 382 Fat 1.2 g Carbs 67.1 g Protein 26.1 g

28. Mustard beef jerky with balsamic vinegar

Preparation time: 12 hours and 10 minutes
Dehydration time: 6 hours
Servings: 4

Ingredients:

- 2 lb. Beef round, sliced
- 2 tablespoons olive oil
- 1 tablespoon dijon mustard
- 1 cup balsamic vinegar
- 2 garlic cloves, crushed
- 1 teaspoon salt

Direction:

1. Add the beef to a sealable plastic bag.
2. Combine the rest of the ingredients in a bowl.
3. Mix well.
4. Pour the mixture into the plastic bag.
5. Place in the refrigerator for 12 hours.
6. Drain the marinade.
7. Add the beef slices to the cosori premium food dehydrator.
8. Set the dehydrator to 165 degrees f.
9. Dry for 6 hours.
10. Storage suggestions: keep the beef jerky slices in a glass container with lid. Store in an area away from sunlight.

Tip: you can dehydrate longer for up to 8 hours.

Nutrition: Calories 372 Fat 27.5 g Carbohydrates 9.6 g Protein 24 g

29. Buffalo jerky

Preparation time: 15 hours and 10 minutes
Dehydration time: 6 hours
Servings: 4

Ingredients:

- 2 lb. Beef round, sliced
- 1 teaspoon salt
- 1 cup buffalo sauce

Direction:

1. Season the beef slices with the salt.
2. Add the buffalo sauce to a bowl.
3. Stir in the seasoned beef.
4. Cover the bowl.
5. Refrigerate for 15 hours.
6. Drain the marinade.
7. Add the beef slices to the cosori premium food dehydrator.
8. Process at 165 degrees f for 6 hours.
9. Storage suggestions: place the beef jerky in a sealable glass container. Store for up to 2 weeks.

Tip: you can also add hot sauce to the marinade for extra zing.

Nutrition: Calories 372 Fat 27.5 g Carbohydrates 9.6 g Protein 24 g

30. Barbecue beef jerky

Preparation time: 12 hours and 10 minutes
Dehydration time: 6 hours
Servings: 4

Ingredients:

- 2 lb. Beef round, sliced
- Salt and pepper to taste
- 2 teaspoons dried oregano
- 2 teaspoons ground cumin
- 1 teaspoon onion powder
- 1 teaspoon ground coriander
- 4 cloves garlic, grated
- ½ cup olive oil
- ½ cup lime juice
- 1 teaspoon red pepper flakes

Direction:

1. Add the beef slices to a sealable plastic bag.
2. In a bowl, mix the salt, pepper, herbs, spices, garlic, olive oil, lime juice and red pepper flakes.
3. Pour mixture into the plastic bag.
4. Turn to coat beef slices evenly with the mixture.
5. Seal and marinate for 12 hours.
6. Drain the marinade.
7. Place the beef slices to the cosori food dehydrator dehydrator.
8. Set it to 165 degrees f and process for 6 hours.
9. Storage suggestions: keep the beef jerky in a vacuum sealed plastic bag.

Preparation & dehydration **Tip:** you can also use lemon juice instead of lime juice.

Nutrition: Calories 372 Fat 27.5 g Carbohydrates 9.6 g Protein 24 g

CHAPTER 7: FRUIT RECIPES

31. Raw fig balls

Preparation time: 15 minutes
Dehydration time: 6 hours
Servings: 4

Ingredients:

- 1 cup raw almonds
- 10 dried figs
- ½ cup raisins
- ½ tsp. Almond extract
- ½ tsp. Vanilla extract
- ¾ cup unsweetened coconut flakes

Direction:

1. Place the almonds in a food processor and pulse until they are ground. Add the figs, raisins and extracts and pulse until well combined.
2. Once the mixture is a dough-like consistency, roll into balls. Roll the balls in the coconut flakes.
3. Place balls on dehydrator trays and dry at 135 degrees for 4-6 hours.

Nutrition: calories: 141, sodium: 4 mg, dietary fiber: 3 g, total fat: 9.7 g, total carbs: 12.3 g, protein: 2.8 g.

32. Spiced apple chips

Preparation time: 15 minutes
Dehydration time: 6 hours
Servings: 4

Ingredients:

- 3-4 ripe apples (any variety)
- 1 tbsp. Ground cinnamon
- 1/8 tsp. Either nutmeg, cloves, allspice, ginger or cardamom
- 1 tbsp. Sugar

Direction:

1. Slice the apple into thin rounds, between 1/8 – 1/4 inch thick. Peels can be removed or left intact. Remove core and seeds.
2. Toss sliced apples with the cinnamon, nutmeg, cloves and sugar.
3. Arrange in a single line in your dehydrator and set temperature to 135. Allow apples to dehydrate for 6-8 hours.

Nutrition: calories: 36, sodium: 1 mg, dietary fiber: 2.7 g, total fat: 0.1 g, total carbs: 10.3 g, protein: 0.2 g.

33. Spicy strawberry fruit leather

Preparation time: 15 minutes
Dehydration time: 6 hours
Servings: 4

Ingredients:

- 1 lb strawberries, hulled and chopped
- 1/3 cup granulated sugar
- 1 tbsp. Lemon juice
- 1 jalapeno or serrano pepper, seeds removed

Direction:

1. Puree strawberries, sugar, lemon juice and pepper.
2. Pour mixture onto fruit leather sheet of your dehydrator.
3. Spread puree evenly, about 1/8 inch thick, onto drying tray.
4. Set the temperature to 140 degrees. Dry for 6-8 hours, or touch center of leather to determine dryness.

Nutrition: calories: 67, sodium: 0 mg, dietary fiber: 0 g, total fat: 0 g, total carbs: 17.9 g, protein: 0.1 g.

34. Blackberry tuile

Preparation time: 10 minutes
Dehydration time: 3 hours
Servings: 4

Ingredients:

- 1 ½ lb. Blackberries
- 2 tablespoons white sugar

Direction:

1. Process the blackberries and sugar in a blender.
2. Strain the mixture to remove the seeds.
3. Add the mixture to the blender.
4. Process on high speed.
5. Pour the fruit liquid into a fruit roll sheet.
6. Place these in the cosori premium food dehydrator.
7. Dehydrate at 165 degrees f for 3 hours.
8. Storage suggestions: store in a food container with lid, away from direct sunlight.

Tip: you can also slice the blackberries first and remove the seeds so you only have to blend it once.

35. Fruit leather

Preparation time: 30 minutes
Dehydration time: 8 hours
Servings: 4

Ingredients:

- 3 peaches, sliced
- 3 apricots, sliced
- 1 tablespoon sugar

Direction:

1. Put the peaches and apricots in a pot over medium low heat.
2. Sprinkle with sugar.
3. Mix well.
4. Cook for 10 minutes.
5. Let cool.
6. Transfer to a blender.
7. Blend on low speed until pureed.
8. Pour the mixture into a fruit roll sheet.
9. Place the roll sheet in the cosori premium food dehydrator.
10. Dehydrate at 165 degrees f or 8 hours.
11. Storage suggestions: arrange the solidified fruits on a baking tray and let it sit for a few minutes before storing in a food container.

Tip: you can also dehydrate for up to 12 hours to obtain drier results.

36. Vanilla-apricot slices

Preparation time: 15 minutes
Dehydration time: 6 hours
Servings: 4

Ingredients:

- 6-9 medium sized apricots, pitted
- 1 ½ tsp. Honey
- 4 tbsp. Warm water
- Seeds from one vanilla bean, scraped out

Direction:

1. In a bowl, mix honey and vanilla seeds. Add the water and mix well. Combine until vanilla seeds are well separated.
2. Slice apricots into thin slices. Place apricot slices onto dehydrator tray and brush on a thin layer of vanilla mixture. It is not necessary for all the vanilla seeds to stick to the fruit.
3. Dehydrate for 9-12 hours at 135 degrees.

Nutrition: calories: 17, sodium: 0 mg, dietary fiber: 0.5 g, total fat: 0.2 g, total carbs: 4.1 g, protein: 0.3 g.

37. Watermelon candy slices

Preparation time: 15 minutes
Dehydration time: 6 hours
Servings: 4

Ingredients:

- 1 watermelon
- Fleur de sel

Direction:

1. Cut the watermelon into slices and remove the rinds. Slices should be approximately ¼ inch thick.
2. Lay watermelon slices on trays.
3. Sprinkle fleur de sel on top of the watermelon.
4. Place sheets in dehydrator at 135 degrees for 18 hours.

Nutrition: calories: 9, sodium: 0 mg, dietary fiber: 0 g, total fat: 0 g, total carbs: 2.1 g, protein: 0.2 g.

38. Honey peaches with bourbon

Preparation time: 4 hours and 10 minutes
Dehydration time: 16 hours
Servings: 1

Ingredients:

- 1 peach, cored and sliced
- ¼ cup honey
- ¼ cup hot water
- 3 tablespoons bourbon

Direction:

1. Add the slices to a sealable plastic bag.
2. In a glass bowl, mix the honey and hot water.
3. Mix until the honey has been dissolved.
4. Pour in the bourbon.
5. Let cool.
6. Once cool, add this to the plastic bag.
7. Marinate for 4 hours.
8. Drain the marinade.
9. Add these to the cosori premium food dehydrator.
10. Dehydrate at 145 degrees f for 16 hours.
11. Storage suggestions: pack in a sealable plastic bag for up to 10 days.

Tip: you can also skip the bourbon and marinate in honey only.

Nutrition: Calories 389 Fat 6.4 g Carbs 22.9 g Protein 49.3 g

CHAPTER 8: GRAINS, NUTS AND SEEDS RECIPES

39. Almond cranberry cookies

Preparation time: 15 minutes
Dehydration time: 6 hours
Servings: 4

Ingredients:

- Wet pulp from almond milk
- 1 banana
- 2 tbsp. Coconut oil
- ¾ cup shredded coconut flakes
- ½ cup dried cranberries
- 1 tbsp. Honey
- ½ cup almonds, coarsely chopped

Direction:

1. Place almond pulp, banana and coconut oil in food processor.
2. Mix remainder of ingredients and add to the almond pulp mixture.
3. Place a small scoop of dough on dehydrator sheets and flatten into a cookie.
4. Set temperature to 105 degrees and dehydrate for 6 hours or more.
5. Set temperature to 105 degrees and dehydrate for 6 hours or more.

Nutrition: calories: 91, sodium: 2 mg, dietary fiber: 2.3 g, total fat: 7.6 g, total carbs: 4.8 g, protein: 2 g.

40. Apple and nut "raw" cereal

Preparation time: 15 minutes
Dehydration time: 6 hours
Servings: 4

Ingredients:

- 1 apple, peeled, cored and diced
- 1 cup sprouted wheat berries
- ½ cup flax seeds, ground
- ½ cup diced raw walnuts
- ½ cup millet flour
- 1 cup sunflower seeds
- 1 tsp. Cinnamon
- ¼ tsp. Salt
- ¼ cup coconut oil, melted
- ¼ cup maple syrup
- 3 tbsp. Apple juice

Direction:

1. Combine apple, wheat berries, flax seeds, walnuts, flour, seeds, cinnamon and salt.
2. Blend coconut oil, maple syrup and apple juice with a whisk.
3. Add dry ingredients to wet ingredients and stir thoroughly.
4. Dehydrate at 115 degrees for 18-24 hours. When crispy, break into large pieces.

Nutrition: calories: 120, sodium: 19 mg, dietary fiber: 2.5 g, total fat: 7.6 g, total carbs: 9.9 g, protein: 4.2 g.

41. Apple cinnamon graham cookies

Preparation time: 15 minutes
Dehydration time: 6 hours
Servings: 4

Ingredients:

- 1 cup cashews, soaked for 1 hour
- 1 cup pecans, soaked for 1 hour
- 6 cups ground almonds
- 2 apples, peeled, cored and chopped
- 1 pear, peeled, cored and chopped
- 1 cup almond butter
- 1 ½ cups flax seed
- ½ cup honey
- 1 tbsp. Cinnamon
- ½ tsp. Nutmeg
- Pinch of salt

Direction:

1. After nuts have been soaked, drain and rinse them.
2. Pulse cashews and pecans in food processor until small crumbs form. Add the ground almonds and place in a bowl.
3. In the food processor, combine apples, pear, almond butter, flax seed, honey, cinnamon, nutmeg and salt. Add the ground nuts.
4. Spread mixture on dehydrator trays, about ¼ inch thick, to the edges.
5. Dehydrate 6-8 hours at 115 degrees. Flip over and cut into squares. Continue dehydrating for 6-8 hours or until crunchy.

Nutrition: calories: 160, sodium: 2 mg, dietary fiber: 3.5 g, total fat: 13.3 g, total carbs: 6.8 g, protein: 5.1 g.

42. Asian-inspired nuts

Preparation time: 15 minutes
Dehydration time: 6 hours
Servings: 4

Ingredients:

- 16 ounce jar of roasted peanuts
- 1/3 cup soy sauce
- ¼ cup water
- 1 ½ tsp. Sesame oil
- ½ tsp. Five spice powder
- ¼ tsp. Ground ginger

Direction:

1. Place nuts in a bowl. Combine all other ingredients and whisk together.
2. Pour over nuts. Marinate nuts at least 8 hours or overnight.
3. Drain liquid and place nuts on dehydrator tray. Dehydrate for 5 hours at 135 degrees.

Nutrition: calories: 152, sodium: 5 mg, dietary fiber: 2.3 g, total fat: 13.1 g, total carbs: 4.4 g, protein: 6.9 g.

43. Banana breakfast crepes

Preparation time: 15 minutes
Dehydration time: 6 hours
Servings: 4

Ingredients:

- 2 medium size ripe bananas
- 1 tsp. Ground flax seed
- 1 tsp. Almond meal
- 1 tsp. Almond milk
- Dash of cinnamon

Direction:

1. Place all ingredients in a food processor and blend into a liquid.
2. Line 2 dehydrator sheets and pour mixture onto them. Liquid should only be about 1/8 inches in thickness. Spread with a spatula.
3. Dehydrate at 115 degrees for 3 hours. Crepes should be totally smooth. Do not remove crepes early or they will not hold their shape. Cut into crepe-sized circles.

Nutrition: calories: 48, sodium: 1 mg, dietary fiber: 1.6 g, total fat: 2 g, total carbs: 6.6 g, protein: 1.2 g.

44. Basic "soaked nuts"

Preparation time: 15 minutes
Dehydration time: 6 hours
Servings: 4

Ingredients:

- Nuts, in any quantity and variety
- Sea salt, approximately 1 tbsp. Per every 4 cups of nuts
- Filtered water (to cover the nuts)

Direction:

1. Combine nuts, sea salt and water in a glass bowl. Cover with a lid or plate and place in a warm location for 12 hours.
2. Remove lid and rinse nuts in a colander.
3. Spread nuts in a single layer on dehydrator trays for 12-24 hours at 105-150 degrees.

45. Flax seed crackers

Preparation time: 15 minutes
Dehydration time: 6 hours
Servings: 4

Ingredients:

- 2 cups flaxseeds
- 2 cups water
- ¼ cup low sodium soy sauce
- 2 tbsp. Sesame seeds
- Sea salt and black pepper, to taste
- 1 ½ tbsp. Fresh lime juice

Direction:

1. Cover flax seeds with water and soak for 1-2 hours. Mixture should be gooey, but not too thin. Add more water to achieve this texture.
2. Stir in the remainder of the ingredients.
3. Spread the mixture about 1/8 inch thick on dehydrator sheets.
4. Set the temperature to 105-115 degrees and dehydrate 4-6 hours. Flip over mixture and dehydrate another 4-6 hours. Break crackers into large pieces after dehydrating.

Nutrition: calories: 133, sodium: 7 mg, dietary fiber: 6.5 g, total fat: 8.2 g, total carbs: 7.1 g, protein: 4.6 g.

CHAPTER 9: HERBS & POWDER

46. Dried basil powder

Preparation time: 10 minutes
Dehydration time: 15 hours
Serving: 5

Ingredients:

- 3 cups basil leaves

Direction:

1. Add the basil leaves to the cosori premium food dehydrator.
2. Dry at 105 degrees for 15 hours.
3. Grind the dried basil in a spice grinder or food processor.
4. Storage suggestions: store in an empty spice jar.

Tip: use only fresh basil leaves.

Nutrition: calories 198, fat12, carbs 16, protein 8

47. Dried herb mix

Preparation time: 15 minutes
Dehydration time: 8 hours
Serving: 5

Ingredients:

- ½ cup thyme leaves
- ½ cup rosemary leaves
- 2 teaspoons lemon zest
- 6 cloves garlic, peeled

Direction:

1. Combine all the ingredients in a food processor.
2. Pulse until smooth.
3. Spread the mixture in the cosori premium food dehydrator.
4. Dehydrate at 135 degrees f for 8 hours.
5. Storage suggestions: store in an empty spice bottle.

Tip: you can also add other herbs into the mix such as oregano or thyme.

Nutrition: calories 98, fat12, carbs 16 , protein 8

48. Onion powder

Preparation time: 10 minutes
Dehydration time: 8 hours
Serving: 5

Ingredients:

- 5 onions, sliced

Direction:

1. Arrange the onion slices in a single layer in the cosori premium food dehydrator.
2. Dehydrate at 145 degrees f for 8 hours.
3. Transfer the dried onion to a food processor.
4. Pulse until powdery.
5. Storage suggestions: store the onion powder in a mason jar.

Nutrition: calories 76, fat 5 , fiber 3 , carbs 5 , protein 3

156. Tomato powder

Preparation time: 15 minutes
Dehydration time: 12 hours
Serving: 5

Ingredients:

- Skins from 10 tomatoes

Direction:

1. Add the tomato skins to a cosori premium food dehydrator.
2. Dry at 135 degrees f for 12 hours.
3. Transfer the dried tomatoes to a coffee grinder.
4. Grind until the mixture turns to powder.
5. Storage suggestions: store in a glass jar with lid.

Tip: you can also make tomato flakes from this recipe.

Nutrition: calories 243, fat 14, fiber 3 , carbs25 , protein 14

49. Leek powder

Preparation time: 5 minutes
Dehydration time: 12 hours
Serving: 5

Ingredients:

- 4 cups leeks, sliced

Direction:

1. Place the leeks in the cosori premium food dehydrator.
2. Dehydrate at 135 degrees f for 4 hours.
3. Put the dried leeks in a spice grinder.
4. Grind until powdery.
5. Storage suggestions: store in a tightly sealed food or spice container.

Tip: do not use any browned parts of leeks.

Nutrition: calories 23, fat 14, fiber 3 , carbs2 , protein 4

50. Dried parsley, basil & oregano powder

Preparation time: 15 minutes
Dehydration time: 8 hours
Servings: 5

Ingredients:

- 2 tablespoons parsley leaves
- 2 tablespoons basil leaves
- 2 tablespoons oregano leaves
- 2 tablespoons brown sugar
- 2 tablespoons salt

Direction:

1. Add the herb leaves to the cosori premium food dehydrator.
2. Dehydrate at 135 degrees f for 8 hours.
3. Transfer the dried leaves to a food processor.
4. Stir in the sugar and salt.
5. Storage suggestions: store in a mason jar with lid.

Tip: you can also skip the sugar and salt, and simply mix the dried herbs.

Nutrition: calories 98, fat12, carbs 16 , protein 8

51. Garlic powder

Preparation time: 15 minutes
Dehydration time: 12 hours
Servings: 2

Ingredients:

- 6 heads garlic, cloves separated, peeled and sliced

Direction:

1. Spread the garlic slices in the cosori premium food dehydrator.
2. Dry at 125 degrees f for 12 hours.
3. Transfer the dried garlic into a blender or spice grinder.
4. Storage suggestions: sift the mixture before storing. Store the garlic powder in an airtight spice jar. Keep it in a cool and dry area.

Tip: you can also use a coffee grinder to grind the dried garlic.

Nutrition: calories 98, fat2, carbs 16 , protein 8

52. Powdered ginger

Preparation time: 15 minutes
Dehydration time: 8 hours
Serving: 5

Ingredients:

- 5 pieces ginger, sliced

Direction:

1. Put the ginger in the cosori premium food dehydrator.
2. Dry at 95 degrees f for 8 hours.
3. Transfer the dried ginger to a food processor or spice grinder.
4. Grind the dried ginger into powder.
5. Storage suggestions: store in a mason jar.

Tip: use a mandoliner slicer to slice the ginger.

Nutrition: calories 75, fat 3, fiber 4, carbs5, protein 10

53. Onion & garlic powder mix

Preparation time: 20 minutes
Dehydration time: 12 hours
Servings:

Ingredients:

- 5 cloves garlic, peeled and sliced
- 1 onion, sliced

Direction:

1. Place the garlic and onion slices in the cosori premium food dehydrator.
2. Dehydrate at 135 degrees f for 12 hours.
3. Transfer to a spice grinder.
4. Grind until powdery.
5. Storage suggestions: store in a mason jar.

Tip: slice the onion and garlic thinly before dehydrating.

Nutrition: calories 75, fat 3, fiber 4, carbs5, protein 10

54. Kimchi powder

Preparation time: 5 minutes
Dehydration time: 12 hours
Servings: 5

Ingredients:

- 2 cups kimchi

Direction:

1. Add the kimchi to the cosori premium food dehydrator.
2. Dehydrate at 155 degrees f for 12 hours.
3. Add the dried kimchi to a spice grinder, blender or food processor.
4. Process until powdery.
5. Storage suggestions: store the powder in an empty spice jar.

Tip: dehydrate longer if there is still moisture after 12 hours.

Nutrition: calories 76, fat 5 , fiber 3 , carbs 5 , protein 3

CONCLUSION

Dehydrating has the potential to be a great solution for many people who are trying to find a cheaper and healthier way to eat, store, and preserve their foods. After the initial investment that comes in the form of buying Dehaydrating supplies, canning your own food in the comfort of your kitchen can be a rewarding – and economic – experience. For beginners who are just trying to figure out whether they'd like to take Dehaydrating up as for the long-term, you do not have to go all out and buy all the supplies. There are many alternatives to the standard Dehaydrating supplies that you can purchase – they tend to be cheaper and just as effective as the original canning supplies.

You do need to know, though, that there are different methods for different foods. Some methods involve boiling water; other methods involve pressure cookers and other tools. With every method, there are different sets of supplies needed. If you are a beginner, you will struggle with finding the appropriate tools and selecting the right methods for canning and preserving your foods.

When food comes out of the dehydrator, it looks vastly different from its original state. Hummus and soups can look as cracked and parched as a desert floor. Food can come off the trays in thin sheets, which you can break into smaller pieces. Properly dried pieces of fruit bend but don't break, and they do not feel moist when you squeeze them. Other foods—vegetables, grains, and legumes—should be hard and dry.

It is possible to burn food in a dehydrator, so pay attention to both the temperature and timing recommendations given in the recipes. Also, when you're learning how to dehydrate food, be sure to check the food every few hours. You may need to rotate the trays to ensure that the food dries evenly, and if you find that part of your recipe is dry before the rest, remove that part and store it while the rest of the recipe continues to dry. There is often one ingredient in each recipe that takes longer to dry than the rest, and that ingredient will be called out in the recipe as the barometer for when the food is dry. In the **Red Curry Vegetable Stir-Fry**, for example, that ingredient is the red bell pepper, which has a very high-water content.

Storing dried food is a crucial step to ensure the most extended shelf life. If not stored well, moisture, heat and oxygen decreases the shelf life and turn them bad sooner than expected. Store you dehydrated bounties in a cool and dry place, or in zip lock bags in the freezer to ensure longer shelf life. You can increase it by vacuum sealing the bags and then store them in the freezer.

The moral of the book is that before you get too enthusiastic about dehydrating batches upon batches of dried foods and pilling your pantry up with all your favourite foods, you need to look and practice all the rules of dehydration and have an idea for the space you have for storing; it will be of no use if you are drying more than the available space unless you intend to sell or gift them.

Remember, different foods have different timings and pre-treatments, so you must follow each step accordingly. Thoroughly drying the food is the key to successful dehydration. The presence of liquid in the dehydrated food turn it fetid and prone to many harmful bacteria such as E. coli. Also, selecting the best quality food ensures a healthy and perfect dried food. Always prefer farmer's market for selecting fruits and vegetables as they provide the freshest food.

When you start to head off with your creative ideas for dehydration, try to limit it to one or two new ingredients. Occasionally what appears to be a great idea, can muddle the flavours or emphasise the taste of the original fruit, vegetable or meat. Limiting the ingredients to one or two possible suspects will enable you to distinguish the culprit quickly.

FREEZE-DRYING
GUIDEBOOK FOR PREPPERS

How to Freeze-Dry and Preserve Nutrient Dense Food

Safely at Home to Be Prepared for the Incoming Crisis.

1800 Days of Tasty Recipes and Log Book Included

Tyler Gordon

INTRODUCTION

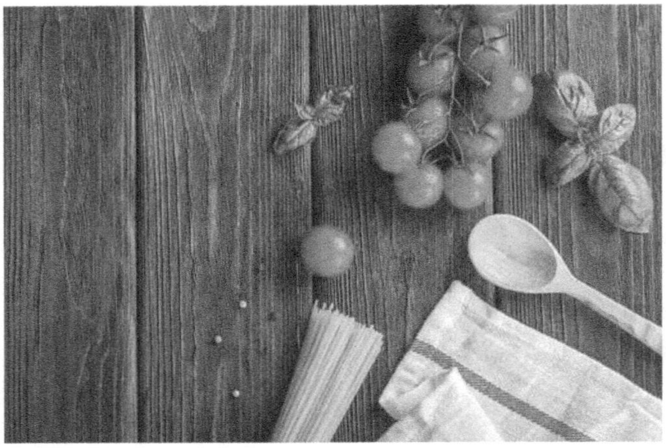

We can't deny the importance of food for survival. Healthy food helps us develop and grow, which plays a vital role in the body's healthy functioning, like working, playing, and thinking. We can't even imagine a healthy lifestyle without having a balanced diet. The nutrients in our food, like vitamins, proteins, fats, and carbohydrates, help our mental and physical growth.

The process is used to treat and handle the food in such a way as to stop and slow down the process of food spoilage and to prevent foodborne illnesses along with maintaining its nutritional values, texture, and taste. The few of the oldest methods of preservation of food are drying, fermentation and refrigeration. The modern techniques used nowadays are freezing, pasteurization, irradiation, and caning. We can enjoy various food throughout the year using all these methods.

In the current era, the amount of food wasted yearly is beyond imagination. According to research, Japan totaled approximately 8 million tons of food wastes, the USA spoiled 40 million tons, and Canada wasted 35.5 million tons of food. It is not the situation of the 1 or 3 countries. Every developed or developing country is facing these challenges. If these numbers made you think, you must find the reason for preserving the food. Food preservation can help every developing country prevent and deal with the crisis.

Here are the following benefits of the preservation of food:

- The preservation of food helps to prevent nutrient loss by preventing microbial spoilage. Freezer drying and other controlled preserving techniques can retain nutrients better.
- It helps you get a life longer shelf full of various seasonal food.
- It helps you to save money. Instead of wasting the food, you can preserve it for future use.

This book is based on the preservation method known as Freeze-Drying.

Start reading this book, and you will be able to master this method and feel a sense of accomplishment. Let's start the journey toward learning the Freeze-Drying Method.

CHAPTER 1: FREEZE-DRYING BASICS

The other name that we use for freeze-drying is lyophilization. In this procedure, a frozen sample is placed in the vacuum to remove water and other solvents from the food, allowing ice to convert from a solid to a vapor state without going into liquid form.

A Brief History

This preservation method was first applied to food products after the Second World War without the need for a refrigerator. Freeze-dried food is an essential component of astronaut and military rations. It began as a tubed meal and freeze-dried snacks that were difficult to rehydrate. Astronauts transformed these foods into hot meals by improving the rehydration process in which the freeze-dried food is transferred into a hot meal with water. When the technology and food processing improved, NASA searched for ways to provide a complete nutrient profile by reducing the amounts of crumbs and bacteria causing diseases and toxins. The complete profile was made by adding algae like vegetable oil. Unsaturated fatty acids are very profitable in vision and mental development because they are stable in space travel. Then crumb problem was solved by adding gelatin coating to the food to prevent crumbs. The disease-producing bacteria were reduced by quality control. This is done to evaluate food material before, during, and after the processing. After these three innovations, NASA provided them with safe food to their crews from the dried meals.

The ration for the Military comes in the same way. Allocations were used based on acceptance, nutrition, producibility, and sanitation. The life for rations was a minimum of three years, which was deliverable by airs, was consumable in the environment, and will provide a complete nutritional profile. The freeze-dried coffee was also replaced with dried coffee in the meal.

Coffee was the first frozen product produced, but herbs, vegetables, fruits, fish, and dairy products can be successfully freeze-dried. This procedure is called sublimation, as minimal heat input is required for its long-term food preservation properties. Freeze-drying can be achieved in different volumes, from a small freeze dryer to a large production scale.

The Goal of Freeze-Drying

The freeze-drying process can accomplish many things. Its primary goal is to protect a sample's biological and chemical structure with the help of sublimation. Once the procedure completes, we can use the model for long-term preservation of the food that needs to be eaten. There are limitless applications present in the laboratory.

The Equipment Required for Freeze-Drying

You must meet particular requirements if you want to freeze-dry a sample successfully. First, the freeze dryer's collector coil should be 15 to 20 degrees colder than the freezing point of the food you want to store to trap the released water vapors. Secondly, you need a vacuum pump that will reach a minimum of 0.020mBar. This deep vacuum creates a negative pressure that forces the free-flowing water molecules left during sublimation to release the oxygen from the environment and travel to the collector coil. Thirdly, you need a drying accessory like a chamber or tray dryer, manifold, and glassware to contain your sample. Lastly, a detection system that makes the freeze-drying process easier by informing us that the piece has been finished drying.

Included with Purchase

Vacuum Pump

- Oil filter
- Stainless Steel Trays
- Freeze drying Guide
- 50-count Miller Bag
- 50 packets of oxygen absorber
- Impulse sealer

A few items are essential, while others are desirable depending upon the position of the freeze dryer in our homes.

Essential Items

- **Designated Spot** for the freeze drier away from the main traffic flow in the home. There are certain rooms in houses where you can place the freeze dryer. Some might put it somewhere in the garage. The weight table, cart, or countertop must handle a weight of nearly 110-120lbs.
- **A designated electrical outlet** is significant for sufficient electrical power to turn a freeze dryer. A 20-amp circuit is required for a large-size outlet, while 110-volt will work fine for small industries. Don't use a power surge or extension.
- **A Vacuum Pump** is also required for the process of freeze-drying. You can use an oil pump or oil less pump. You will get the former along with each purchase.
- **Bucket** to contain extracted water from the food that will turn to ice in food processing. The ice that will melt will go into the bucket.

Nice to Have

- **A heavy-duty cart** with wheels will be friendly, depending on where the freeze dryer will be stored or used. For example, you want to move the freeze dryer from one place to another, the cart will be helpful.
- **Extra sets of Trays** will benefit those who want a large quantity of freeze-dried food. The additional trays can be filled and frozen, so we put them into the dryer.
- **Silicon Mats** offer protection for the stainless-steel trays and make it easier to remove some food that has a juicy texture due to which food stick to the metal trays.
- **Mylar bags** help make packets for the fam

- idly or individual snacks.
- **Oxygen absorber packets** help to remove any remaining oxygen from the sealed pack. A 300CC absorber packet will be enough for the 1-gallon Mylar or plastic self-seal bag. This will be good for anyone who doesn't keep a vacuum sealer.
- **A Vacuum Sealer** could be optional when an oxygen absorber is present. Impulse sealer will create a sealed seam for the Mylar bags. This sealer will not help to remove any oxygen. A vacuum sealer can be used to suction out the oxygen so that we can quickly seal the packet. In comparison, you can add an oxygen absorber to remove the oxygen from the pack.

Equipment and Types of Freeze Dryers

There are a lot of freeze dryers available, although most of them contain specific essential components including a vacuum chamber, shelves, refrigeration, and a control system.

The Function of Essential Components

Chamber

- It is a highly polished and insulated internal surface. It is consisted of stainless steel and is based on several shelves that hold the product. The electric and hydraulic motor ensures the vacuum is tight when we close it.

Process Condenser

- It is based on the refrigerated coils or plates placed on the chamber's internal or external surface. During the process of drying, water is trapped by the condenser. During the primary drying, the temperature of the condenser should be less than the temperature of the product. It should have a defrosting mechanism that ensures the maximum number of vapors is condensed in the air.

Shelf Fluid

- An external heat exchanger source regulates the heat energy needed during the primary and secondary phases. By using a pump, silicone oil is circulated in the entire system.

Refrigeration System

- This system helps us cool shelves and aid in the processing of the condenser with the help of the compressor and liquid nitrogen. This will supply the energy that is necessary for the product to freeze.

Vacuum System

- In the process of drying, a vacuum of 50-100 m is applied with the vacuum system's help to remove the solvent. A two-stage rotary vacuum pump is usually used, but if the chamber is large enough, a large number of pumps will be needed.
-

Control System

- The control system sets up values for the temperature of the shelf, pressure, and time duration that will depend upon the product and the process. The freeze dryer can run for several hours or days, depending on the product.

Types of Freeze Dryers

Contact Freeze Dryers

These freeze dryers use the conduction of the food with the heating element to transfer the sublimation energy. This freeze dryer is used for sample analysis. The one-way contact freeze dryer heat is shelf-like platforms that contact the sample. During freeze-drying, the shelves play a significant role as they behave like a heat exchanger. These dryers are linked with a silicone oil system that will remove the heat energy during the freezing process and provide it during drying times. The shelf-fluid system provides particular temperatures in the shelves in the drying process by pumping fluid at low pressure.

The drawback to this type of freeze dryer is that the heat will transfer from the heating system to the sample side and touch the heater. The problem can be lessened by increasing the sample's surface area and connecting a ribbed tray. It will compress the piece between the two plates. They will be crammed with heated mesh from above and below the surface.

Radiant Freeze Dryers

These freeze dryers heat the sample in the tray using infrared radiation. This heating lets flat trays as an infrared source that will lead the heat toward the downward direction of the product. It has a low capacity to penetrate the radiation, so it is used with very shallow trays.

Microwave-Assisted Freeze Dryers

This kind of freeze dryer uses microwaves for the deeper penetration of the radiations to increase the sublimation speed. This is a complicated method to set up and run because microwaves can create an electrical field that will cause gases in the chamber to become plasma. This plasma can burn the sample. The sublimation rate in a product could affect the microwave impedance. In this, the microwave power will be changed accordingly.

The Food Freeze-Drying Process

In the procedure of freeze-drying food, we lowered the temperature to below freezing point, and after this, we applied a high-pressure vacuum to remove the water in the form of vapors. All the vapors unite on the condenser, turn back to the ice, and are removed. When the temperature rises gradually, all the moisture is released from the food. In this way, the physical structure of the food remains the same and is then preserved for rehydration later. In the following chapters, we will study these procedures in detail.

The Characteristics of the Freeze-Drying Process

There are six main physical phenomena that can noticeably influence the whole freeze-drying process. These six properties are as follows:

- The transition of water into ice.
- Then, the transition of ice into vapors.
- Then, the removal of water molecules from material structures so that we can obtain low pressure.
- Re-sublimation of the water vapors on the surface of the container.
- The main characteristic of freeze-drying that separates it from vacuum drying is the necessity to keep water frozen. It is a complex problem in freeze drying.
- It is a mass exchange process. They need heat transport.

The amount of heat in sublimation should be 2885kg. If the heat supply is too low, the process will be slow, increasing the heat. If it is high, the heat will accumulate in the material, and its temperature will rise. This resultantly leads to the appearance of liquid water. So, we need to maintain a balance between the amount of heat that is supplied and that is used. This can be achieved by measuring the amount of heat provided. Maintaining a constant low temperature during the sublimation process proves that the balance between the amount of heat given and the heat used for it is held.

CHAPTER 2: SCIENCE BEHIND FREEZE-DRYING

FDA states lyophilization is a process in which we remove water from the product after freezing it and then place it under a vacuum that allows ice to change from a solid to a vapor state without going into a liquid phase. This whole process consists of three strategies:

1. Freezing
2. Sublimation
3. Desorption

The freeze-drying process follows the principle of sublimation that changes a solid to a gas as it removes ice from the frozen food as water vapors. Due to the sublimation operation, the original food maintains its texture and flavor when rehydrated. The complete freeze-drying process is divided into two steps:

- Freezing
- Vacuum Drying

First, the food is frozen below 0°F . The colder it is, the easier the following stage will be. After freezing, the food is subjected to vacuum drying. The air and water vapors are removed from the food processor chamber with the help of a vacuum pump. It means we need to remove the water vapor inside the food. When the two steps have been adequately completed, the food is dry enough to be safe at room temperature.

Is Freeze-Drying Food Safe?

Yes, the food is safe if:

1. The first condition for the safety of the food is that the two processes, freezing and vacuum drying, should be done perfectly.
2. The freezing process should be fast, and the vacuum chamber should leave just residual moisture. For example, at 41°F, the food will chill safely for 1-4 hours. If the food is pre-refrigerated or pre-frozen, we can place a freeze dryer to minimize this concern.
3. Safe drying food is defined as the safe residue moisture level.
4. For food to be safe, it should be dried to a crisp or breakable texture. However, food with high sugar levels may be flexible but will not be sticky when appropriately dried.
5. Good food handling techniques should be used to prepare the food before freeze-drying, as this process doesn't kill bacteria.

Where Do the Microorganisms Go During Freeze-Drying Process?

They will go nowhere but inactive under the extreme conditions of freeze-drying. In other words, scientists use laboratory versions of freeze-drying to preserve the microorganisms for future studies because they can be rehydrated. When we freeze-dry the raw food, the organisms are present in that food but activate upon rehydration. The food items that we cook before eating should also be cooked as freeze-dried food, like all the raw food such as meat, eggs and foods that contain these essential ingredients.

Can Freeze-Dried Foods Be Safely Vacuum-Packaged?

Yes, freeze-dried food can be safely vacuum-packaged. However, vacuum packaging is not part of the food safety process itself. Even removing oxygen from the package might make it more prone to bacterial decay in a moist environment. Luckily in the absence of moisture, the botulism bacteria will not be able to grow. Therefore, it is necessary to place properly dried food in vacuum packages or containers that are oxygen absorbent.

CHAPTER 3: FREEZE-DRYING WITH A FREEZE-DRYER MACHINE

What is a Freeze Dryer?

A freeze dryer removes water from the food to preserve it and prolong its shelf life, making it convenient for transport. In the freeze-dryer, we freeze the material, reduce the pressure and add heat to change the frozen material into vapors.

A freeze dryer consists of three phases:

1. Freezing
2. Primary Drying (Sublimation)
3. Secondary Drying (Adsorption)

Phase 1: Freezing Phase

This is the very critical phase. In the freeze dryer, we use different methods to freeze a product.

- First, freezing can be done in a freezer or on the shelf of the its dryer.
- The freeze-dry cools the material and allows sublimation rather than melting. It saves the physical form of the food.
- A freeze dryer dries large ice crystals produced by slow freezing.
- In biological methods, crystals are very large. They may break the cell wall. This leads to less-than-ideal freeze-drying results. This is the reason that freezing is done rapidly.

Phase 2: Primary Drying (Sublimation)

- The second phase is primary drying and sublimation. In this phase, the pressure of the liquid is lowered, and heat is added to the material for water to sublimate.
- The vacuum speed of the freeze dryer hustles up the sublimation. The cold condenser of the freeze dryer provides a surface for the water vapor to adhere and solidify. The condenser protects the vacuum pump from the water vapors.
- 95% of the water is removed in this phase.
- Excessive heat can alter the structure of the material.

Phase 3: Secondary Drying (Adsorption)

- Water molecules are removed in the final phase of the freeze dryer, also known as adsorption.
- The bonds between water molecules are broken by raising the temperature compared to the primary drying phase.
- The freeze-dried material keeps a porous structure.
- When the freeze-drying process is complete, the vacuum can be broken down into an inert gas even if the material is sealed.
- Most materials can be dried to 1-5% moisture.

Freeze Dryer Problems to Avoid:

- If we heat the product at too high temperature, it can melt back or the product can collapse.
- The condenser becomes overloaded when too much vapor hits the condenser.
- Vapor creation is too much.
- The surface area is too much.
- The condenser area is too small.
- Insufficient refrigeration.

The vapors are produced faster than through the vapor port, the port between the condenser and product chamber that leads toward increased chamber pressure.

CHAPTER 4: PREPARATION OF FREEZE-DRIED FOOD

In the process of freeze-drying, the fruits and vegetables become dry. They can be airy, dry, crispy, and brittle. They taste crunchy in their freeze-dried state. Due to this reason, we need to rehydrate them for regular use in our meals.

Are Freeze-Dried Foods Healthy?

Freeze-dried food is a healthy choice. It is the most intensively used method of dehydration as it has a lot of benefits. It is the best way to preserve plants and vegetables by keeping their color, structure, and flavor alive. This is also why it is widely used to produce high-value food products.

Other studies have shown that the freeze-drying method is a fantastic method of preserving anti-oxidants. Anti-oxidants are beneficial compounds that help fight the damaging effect of oxidative stress in your body. It also increases the fruit's phytochemical concentration. Due to the lack of water activity, the lesser will be the growth of the bacteria and yeasts. In this way, by removing the water content, freeze-drying helps prolong a food life. Freeze drying is essential for fresh plant-based foods that we cannot find throughout the year. It will make it easier to handle and store for longer time.

Can Freeze-Dried Foods Be Rehydrated?

Yes, we can rehydrate the freeze-dried food as the food can absorb the moisture that it had lost during the freeze-drying process. For this, we can add hot water to regain its consistency.

Rehydrate Freeze-Dried Foods?

Rehydrating freeze-dried food is an easy job that might not require a lot of effort. Due to their airy texture, they can easily absorb water in a wet environment. Just open the container, place all the contents in the warm water, and let them soak until you get the consistency you want. You can also use cold water in the absence of a hot one.

Rehydrate Freeze-Dried Vegetables?

The process of rehydrating dried vegetables is just similar to that of fruits. In the case of the vegetables, you only need to soak them in hot water for 5-10 minutes, and they will go into their initial state. When you are using this food in the soups, we don't need to rehydrate them as they will cook with the food.

How Long Will It Take to Rehydrate Freeze-Dried Foods and Vegetables?

Rehydrating freeze-drying food will not take longer, depending on the fruit or vegetable you want to rehydrate. You need to have hot water in the bowl. Let the vegetables and fruits soak in the water, and they will get fresh.

What Happens After Rehydration?

After soaking them in warm water, the food will regain its fresh texture and shape that you can enjoy as if you had just bought it from the market.

Conclusion

This way, you can prepare your freeze-dried food, and it will be ready to eat.

CHAPTER 5: USING A MACHINE TO FREEZE-DRY

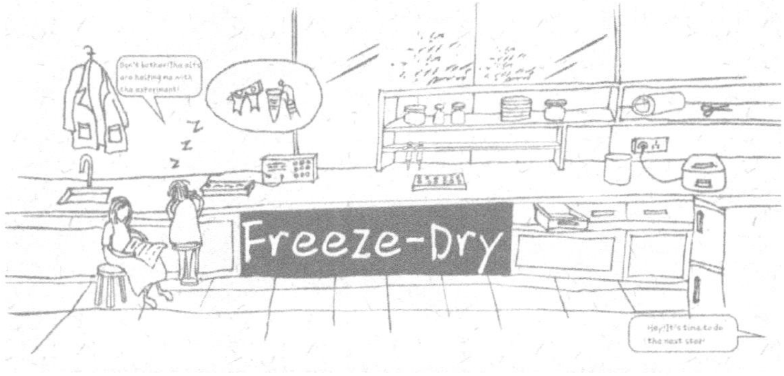

The basic principle in freeze-drying is sublimation. In this process, the solid converts into a gas without entering the liquid phase. This process is similar to evaporation when the molecules get enough energy to break free from the molecules around them.

Factors

Heat and atmospheric pressure are the two factors determining which phase a product will take: solid, liquid, or gas. The different temperature and pressure ranges will determine which configuration they will become.

Explanation

The water will take a liquid form if the temperature is between the sea level freezing and boiling point. In the second case, if the temperature increases above 32°F while the atmospheric pressure is below 0.06atm, the water will not remain in the liquid state. It will convert into the form of vapors, and will become a gas. This is happening in the freeze-drying machine. This machine consists of a freeze-drying chamber with shelves attached to the heating units. There is a freezing coil that is connected to the compressor of the refrigerator and a vacuum pump.

In most machines, we place the unfrozen material on the shelves. After this, we seal the chamber and start the process. The machine starts running the compressor and lowers its temperature in the room. This way, the material becomes frozen and separates the water around it. After this, the machine switches on the vacuum pump to push the air out of the chamber and lower its atmospheric pressure below 0.06atm. The heating units that are present apply a small amount of heat to the shelves, which causes the ice to change its phase. Due to the low atmospheric pressure, ice turns directly into water vapor. These water vapors go out of the freeze-drying chamber and past the freezing coil. The water vapors condense in the form of ice. In the same way, water frosts on colder days. This process continues for many hours, and the material gradually dies out.

This also takes significant time because overheating the material can significantly change its composition and structure. Apart from this, accelerating the sublimation process produces more water vapors in a time. Then, pumping systems will be removed from the chamber. This way, the material will rehydrate, although its quality will somehow be degrading.

After the material is dried, it will be sealed in a moisture-free package that is oxygen-absorbent. The package will be secure until it is on the shelf for years without degrading and is safe from moisture; otherwise, it will eventually spoil. The material will go through the complete process almost unscathed if everything goes fine.

CHAPTER 6: FREEZE-DRYING WITHOUT A MACHINE

Are you the one who wants to make freeze-dried food at home without a machine?

Yes, this is possible, but it comes with a few precautions.

This is shocking news for many, but you don't need fancy machines to have freeze-dried food. However, making them will take some time and effort. Also, as professionally dried foods are, you can't store them for a more extended period. It will be better to eat it as soon as possible.

Freeze-Drying Food - The Home Freezer Method

Freeze Drying Food Without a Machine

Freeze drying is a great way to store food for longer terms. Luckily, there is no need to worry if you don't have a machine for this process. It will take a longer duration of time to get the results like a freeze dryer. Either you are camping or want to store the food for the future, freeze-dried food can be used for a longer duration of time.

Using a Freezer

1. **Lower the temperature of your freezer a day before freeze-drying.** The temperature of your freeze dryer should be around -34°C. If you have a home freezer, keep its temperature to 10°F. Most are set to 0°F. If the freezer does not go lower than that, then it will not be a problem. It will take more prolonged duration of time to dry the food. Pick a freezer thermometer to test the freezer's temperature if it doesn't have a dial.
2. **Pick a food that you want to freeze dry.** The vegetables and fruits which have high water content are easy to freeze dry.
   - So, start freezing the fruits like apples, potatoes and other vegetables. You can also freeze-dry cooked pasta, meat and noodles.
   - We can freeze-dry the dairy products, but they will not have the same creamy taste and texture.
   - The meat should be cooked before freeze-drying. You can freeze-dry it on the same day, but you can also store it in the refrigerator for longer.
   - The other foods that can be freeze-dried at home are steak, ground beef, fish, herbs and instant coffee.
3. **Wash and dry the product before freeze-drying.** Rinse the fruits and vegetables you want to dry in the cool running water. Then let them dry with a paper towel or clean cloth. It will save you time. You can also use a vegetable brush to remove the dirt from the products.
4. **Cut them into pieces.** When you cut them, it will be easier to get freeze-dried. Try to make pieces of equal sizes, so they will all freeze-dry at the same rate. If you are trying to freeze small dry fruits like blackberries or raspberries, you don't need to cut them into pieces. Meanwhile, if you want to freeze dry meat, cook it first and cut it into slices. You can also cut them in the form of strips and pieces.
5. **Place a baking sheet with parchment paper.** Cut down the parchment paper to cover the complete baking sheet with overhanging edges on the sides. This will save the headache of battling to remove every piece that is frozen on the baking sheet. You can also use plastic wrap or wax paper instead.
6. **Place the pieces with free space,** and arrange the details on the baking sheet by keeping a distance between each of them. This can be done to free them from getting stuck with each other.
7. **Making a single layer** will create ease for you. So, try not to overlap them. If you are freeze-drying two different foods, you need to place them on other parchment papers because they both have different rates for freeze-drying.
8. **Now place the baking tray in the freezer for 10 days.** Place that tray on the shelf and don't disturb it for 7-10 days.
9. **Test it after 7 Days.** Take a piece out of the freezer and place it at room temperature for a few hours. There will be no change in color. If the fruit's color turns black, it will show that the fruits need more time in the freezer.

- When it's time to test the meat, take it out, wait for it to warm for 10 minutes, and bend it in half. If you find moisture in the meat, then it needs more time for freeze-drying. You can again place it in the fridge and check it for 2 days.
- The temperature of your freezer will describe how long it will take for 1 week.

10. **Remove the tray and place it in the freezer bag.**
    - Lift both ends of the parchment paper to loosen the pieces. Then add the pieces into a freezing bag, remove air from it, and seal it.
    - You can use a rolling pin to remove air from the bag.
11. **Storing the Bag.** Store these freeze-dried bags or camping bags. Just make sure that the loads are not exposed to direct sunlight or moisture. You can use this freeze-dried food and rehydrate them by placing the pieces in a small amount of water.

Freeze Drying with Dry Ice

1. **Wash the product you want to Freeze-Dry**. First, wash fruits and vegetables in cool water before drying them with a paper towel. If you are drying the beef or fish, make sure that you cook them first.
2. **Make slices of the larger pieces into shorter ones.** Pick a sharp knife to cut the larger fruits and vegetables into smaller chunks. When you are freeze-drying cooked meat, slice it into slivers. Make pieces of the same sizes so that they can dry at the same time.
3. **Place food chunks in the bag and seal them**. Now, add sliced chunks into the freezer bags. Try to put 1 type of food in the bag at once rather than mixing all of them. After this, remove the air from the bags with the help of your hands, or a rolling pin. It will ensure that no ice crystals will form on the food.
4. **Choose a large storage box.** A large size water container will work nicely. Always remember that the box should fit in your freezer. You can also have freeze-dried small quantities. Pick a plastic container that you are not using for other purposes, and make holes in the lid.
5. **Pour dry ice into the bottom of the box.** Put leather or work gloves over your hand to put dry ice into the bottom of the box till it forms an even layer. The dry ice you are using is equal to the weight of the food. So, if you are freezing 5 pounds of food, you must have 5 pounds of dry ice. If it is not covering the entire box, add another 1 pound to it until it does.
    - Five pounds of dry ice will be enough for up to 4 layers of food.
    - Don't touch the dry ice with your hands- it might burn your skin.
    - You can use oven mitts if you don't have heavy-duty leather gloves.

    Make a layer of food bags between ice sheets, and then pour 1 to 2 pounds of dry ice to cover the bags. Don't place two bags on top of each other. You might need to rearrange the pieces of dry ice. So that the bags are fully covered, try to make sure that each bag is as flat, and that there is no overlapping.
6. **Add dry ice to the top of the bag.** Depending on the box size and the number of bags, you must make alternating layers of dry ice and food bags. Each food layer should have a dry ice on top and below it.
7. **Make holes in the lid.** Use a box cutter or sharp knife to make holes on top of the box. These holes help moisture and gas to escape from them. That is necessary for the dry ice and the food to fully dry.
8. **Poking too many holes in the lid.** The idea behind this is to escape at a comparatively slow rate.
9. **Keep the box in the freezer for 24 hours.** We can detect that dry ice has been done once it disappears. The time you take to freeze-dry the food will depend upon the quantity you are freeze-drying. Use gloves to remove the lid and look into the container.

    Suppose the dry ice will have gone on the bottom and top too. Then the food is ready for storage. But in case you will see the dry ice chunks, reinsert the box into the freezer and wait for 3-6 hours before checking again.
10. **Store freeze-dried foods in freezer bags.** As the foods are already in freezer bags, you can take them out and use them at room temperature. The freeze-dried food will stay good for 25 years. You can rehydrate them whenever the need arises.

Conclusion

If you are the one who was looking to freeze-dry food at home, the above-provided methods are the best for you without investing in expensive equipment. Now, sit at your home, enjoy healthy food, and become more self-reliant.

CHAPTER 7: FREEZE-DRYING USING LIQUID NITROGEN

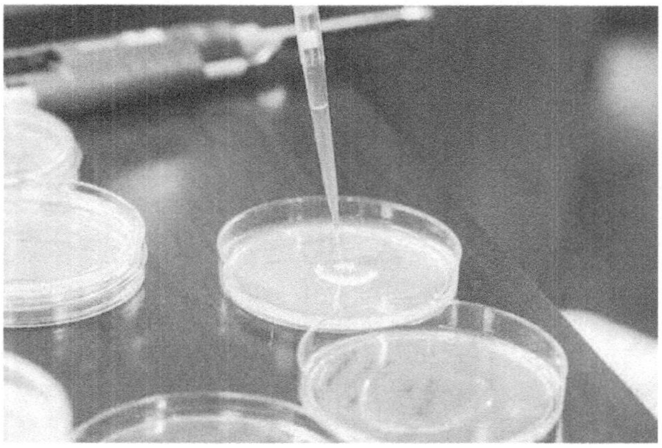

At -196°C, liquid nitrogen freezes food very quickly. When we freeze-dry food with the help of a conventional freezer, it can form large crystals in the products that might damage their integrity and nutritional content. The ice crystal size is created when we do flash freezing with the help of nitrogen, which keeps the food intact. The low temperature effectively kills any parasite that is present in the food.

Preparation

Get liquid nitrogen from a laboratory supplier or a welding supply company. The quantity of nitrogen that is required depends upon the amount of food. Start preparing the food and arranging all the items in a particular order.

If you want to prepare a freeze-dried fruit, peel it, cut it to the desired size, remove the seeds, and store it in an airtight container until you need it. Place these food items near the working place so you can use them when needed. If you are working from left to right, firstly place the gloves and goggles, then food items, then nitrogen and stainless-steel bowl, and at the end, freeze dryer. Keeping all the things and equipment in one place will reduce the risk of an accidental spill and enhance efficiency. Keep the food items in a stainless-steel bowl. Start wearing gloves and goggles with care. Slowly, put this liquid nitrogen over the food. Then, wait until the rest of the nitrogen has evaporated.

Drying

First, check the chamber to make sure that the machine is clean and dry. After this, place the frozen food in the chamber and carefully close the lid. Now, activate the freeze-drying device. Then, a vacuum pump will lower the atmospheric pressure inside the chamber to below 0.06atm. The refrigeration coil will lower the temperature to -50°C. The device will slowly heat the food, purify the ice crystal, and begin the drying process. It will take a few hours to several days. It will depend upon the size and quantity of the food. Some devices allow for the removal of an item in the drying phase that determines product readiness, while others use an indicator light for signal completion.

Now, place the freeze-dried food in the plastic bags explicitly used for the vacuum sealing. Keep this bag in the vacuum sealing device, shut down the closure, and activate it. When the air is finished from the pack, the machine will seal it and show the process' end with the help of the indicator light. This oxygen-free environment of a vacuum-sealed bag will help achieve the maximum benefits of using nitrogen.

Precautions

- Never allow liquid nitrogen to come in contact with your skin.
- Always wear insulated gloves.
- Always wear safety goggles when dispensing liquid nitrogen.
- Don't place liquid nitrogen in a sealed container that will lead toward the entrapment of the gas.

When you have direct contact with liquid nitrogen, it will cause severe cold burns.

CHAPTER 8: INSTRUCTIONS FOR STORING FREEZE-DRIED FOOD

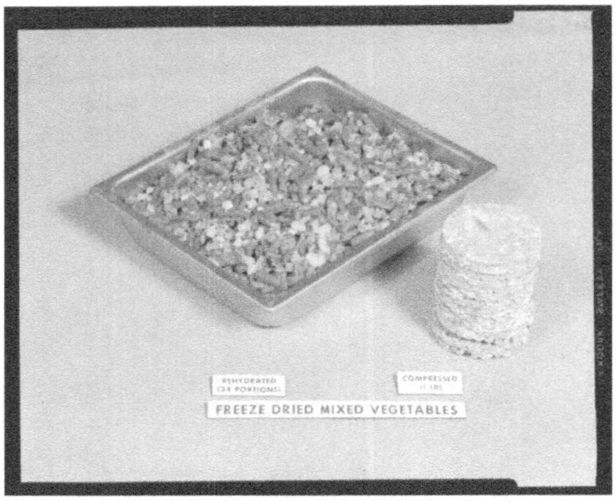

We can store freeze-dried food for up to 25 years. The duration of how long it will remain depends on how you keep it. Here are the best ways to freeze-dry food so you can use it when needed.

Make Sure It's Dry.

First, when you remove the food from the freeze dryer, break the large pieces of food into small ones to check whether the ice particles are cold or not. If it is not, it is dry. Freeze-drying works from the outer side of the food to the inner side. But if you find it cold in the central portion, you can put it back into the freeze dryer for a dry cycle of a shorter duration. The freeze dryer will ask you for more drying time if it does not dry.

Seal It.

First of all, place freeze-dried food in an air-tight container. If you will not do this, it will reabsorb the moisture from the air and will spoil.

- If you want to store it for 25 years, the shelf life of Mylar bags will be the easiest and the less expensive option.
- Use an oxygen absorbent material to ensure there is no oxygen in your bag that will destroy the food over time.
- After this, seal the bag with an impulse sealer or a flat iron.
- You can also store food for long-term purposes in cans.
- Another good option for storing food is vacuum-sealed bags. You can store food except for meats or other high-protein food.

Air-tight jars can also work well for snacks such as vegetables, fruits, cheesecake, and ice cream. We can use these jars for a few months. Seal the jar tightly after you grab your perks.

CHAPTER 9: ADVANTAGES AND DISADVANTAGES OF FREEZE-DRYING

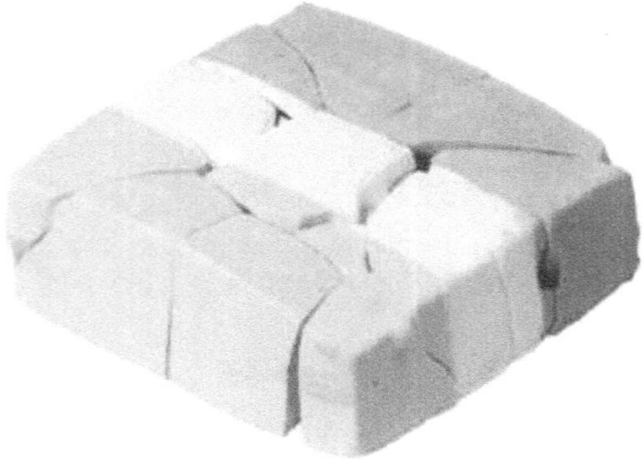

Advantages of Freeze-Drying

Freeze-Drying is the Most Reliable Method of Food Preservation.

As we have read earlier, for food preservation, we need to remove the moisture through a process called sublimation. If we do not remove this moisture, it will lead to food decomposition and mold growth. Freeze-drying removes about 98-99% of the moisture content. The lesser the humidity, the more the shelf life would be.

Freeze-Dried Foods Can Be Stored For a Long Duration.

Freeze-dried vegetables and fruits have a longer average shelf life of nearly 25-30 years. We can store freeze-dried food at many temperatures without affecting the food or packaging. The food will remain fresh for many years.

Freeze-Drying Retains the Fresh Product's Nutritional Value, Flavor, and Color.

Freeze-drying is similar to keeping the food in a state of suspended animation. So once rehydrated, the food will be fresh and nutritious as it was at the moment of freezing. This way, freeze-drying will retain the new product's nutritional value, flavor, and color.

Freeze-Drying Makes Food More Appetizing.

When you put the food in your mouth after it has been freeze-dried, it will appear fresh and soft.

Freeze-Drying Significantly Reduces the Weight of Food.

The lyophilization removes about 98% of the water from the food, leading to a lesser weight of the food by 90%. This is an amazing benefit for those who carry their food for months and days.

Cheaper in Cost

The foods that are home freeze-dried are cheaper than commercially freeze-dried food. By preservation of food, the cost of the meal will be lesser as we will be able to save more of the food.

Disadvantages of Freeze-Drying

Cost

The first downside of freeze drying is the cost. The equipment that requires shallow temperatures for freeze-drying is costly. This procedure is carried out under a vacuum that allows ice to change directly into vapor from solid.

Food Selection

Not every food can be freeze-dried. It is selective for specific fruits and meats. Any food that is difficult to tolerate can be damaging during the initial freezing process. It preserves the food's color properties, which is not right in every case. The number of foods can be pretreated, so they are not subject to color loss.

Storing

Food storage can be another disadvantage of freeze-drying foods. While storing the freeze-dried food, it should maintain the shape, size, and color of the food. Due to this reason, they might need some extra storage space compared to other food that is preserved. If the dried food will not be stored correctly or will be subject to humidity, it will deteriorate or spoil quickly. These foods require airtight storage, moisture-tight containers, cans, and bags.

Microbial Growth

The less water there is in the product, the slower the micro bacteria grow. The microorganism-causing disease in raw food remains present during storage. That might lead to food-borne illnesses. Therefore, a particular food needs to be cooked before the freeze-drying process.

Silicone Oil Leakage

The standard fluid is to heat or cool down shelves in the freeze dryer. The continuous heat cycle can lead to the leakage of the silicon oil in the weak areas that will connect the hose and the shelf. This will contaminate the food and will lead to the losses of the major food products. To prevent this thing from happening, we used a spectrometer to identify the vapors that are released by silicon oil to prevent the contamination of the product.

Higher Level of Oxidation

Although the food is preserved, antioxidant content and the pores in the freeze-dried product allow easy access to oxygen that might lead to increased oxidation. They will degrade the bioactive compounds that are present in the food.

CHAPTER 10: COMMON PROBLEMS OF FREEZE-DRYING AND HOW TO SOLVE THEM

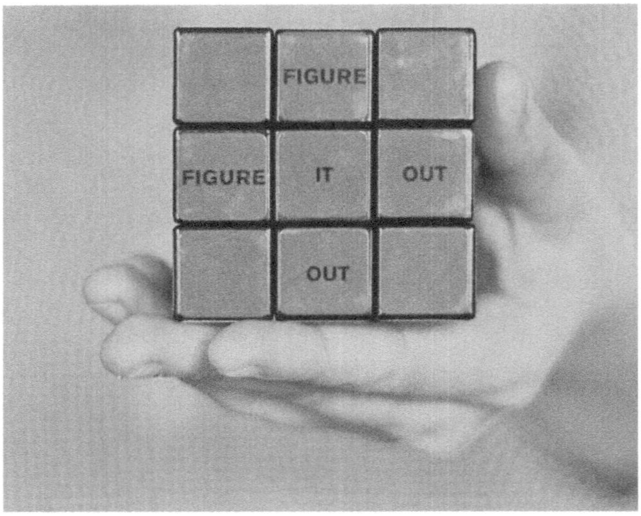

Mixing Raw Meat with Other Foods

Scientists use freeze-drying to save bacteria samples. It means the chances of bacteria are high in raw meat. During the freeze-drying process, water vapor moves around the drying chamber. Please never mix the fruits and vegetables that are supposed to be eaten raw with meat. Try to incorporate the food on the kitchen cutting board. Don't try to mix them in a freeze-drying chamber.

Mixing Foods with Dissimilar Flavors

There are a certain number of foods you can mix and match in the vacuum chamber, provided you will put the intensely flavored food on the top of the shelves. These combinations might have a strange taste, but when we freeze-dried green beans and bananas in the same food, we will end up with green bean-flavored bananas. The flavor was elusive, and it was there. Try to be careful about sweet and savory food separation with good results.

Freeze-Dry High Sugar Foods

Some of the foods with high sugar content, like fruits, jams, or jellies, do not dry freeze fully. No matter how long you leave them in the container, in the end, they will still be sticky. This is because sugar binds with free water molecules that restrain them from escaping the food. This trait is beneficial for the preservation of food. When the binding is free, it will slow down the bacteria and help mold growth. This is because these organisms need water for their survival. Unluckily, it results in a less-than-ideal freeze-dried product. Most plain fruits work very well, but the sweeter fruits require a longer drying cycle. The fruit that took a very long time was the pear.

Trying to Dry High Fat Foods

During the freeze-drying method, we should know how much fat is considered too much. So, I tried some frozen breakfast patties and pre-cooked food. Try to remove that excess fat as much as before freeze-drying. Usually, grease also smells bad like other food items. Therefore, meat or dairy products with a high-fat level should be best used within five years.

Freeze-Drying Large Pieces of Meat

Large pieces of meat don't rehydrate well, so try to have a short piece of meat. Even the sausage patties were chewy, too. If you want the best results, in the end, try to have meat that is grounded, diced, and shredded. It would be good if we had served it in a sauce soup or even better. If you want to make a tastier meal, rehydrate it with plenty of water and provide a large surface area so it can soak the maximum of water. When you have a small piece of meat, it can make tempting snacks. Try to have plenty of liquid along with you. Just don't eat too many dried pieces of meat.

Not Using a Liner in the Pans

Whenever you load the freeze dryer, use liners for the pans as they are stainless steel, food grade, and non-reactive. If you let them set around, the pans will warm up, and there are chances that they will start absorbing moisture from the environment and get soggy. So, try to invest in the liners and save yourself from many headaches. You can also use parchment paper or a reusable one.

Expecting Quick Drying in Hot Weather

The hotter your freeze dryer is, the harder it has to work. The higher the temperature, the more time it will take to dry. If you live in an area where the temperature is hot, try putting the freeze dryer in an air-conditioned space. Don't try to put the temperature below 0°C because there is water in the compressor, but below the 0-degree temperature, it will freeze and destroy the compressor.

Freeze-Drying Fruit with Tough Skins Whole

Fruits with hard skin, like grapes, cherries, and tomatoes, can save hours of freeze-drying time. The grapes, cherry, and tomatoes should be sliced half lengthwise. For cranberries and blueberries, you can freeze them on a baking sheet before drying them and then give them a brief spin in a food processor. This goal is to cut the skin so slightly that water can escape and leave the fruit intact.

Filling the Trays with Liquid Before Placing Them in the Unit

It is the simplest thing, but we often miss it: the liquid could spill. So, if you want to load a tray of soup and milk, be cautious about how far the liquid should travel. Place the tray in the freeze dryer and then put a drink. Or you can load it next to the freeze dryer and transport its inches instead of feet. Each tray should hold a quarter.

Filling the Freeze-Dryer Too Full

The HRFD (Harvest Right Freeze-dryer) works by pulling the water out of the food and then freezing that water inside the vacuum chamber, forming a layer of ice. If there is too much food, then it will be too much ice, and the machine will not be able to finish the drying cycle. Many complain that they must empty the unit, place the food in the freezer, defrost the team, and start the process again. It is a big hassle. Load the unit the first time and save yourself from trouble. At one time, freeze-dry no more than 10 pounds. If the food is high in moisture, 6 pounds will be enough.

Mixing Food Sizes and Stacking the Food Unevenly on the Trays

The other problem is that people combine food of different shapes and sizes and then stack them unevenly on the trays. This way, big chunks will be cold from the middle after the small bits have been finished. For this purpose, try to chop your food thin to have the fastest drying time. Then spread it evenly on the tray to avoid having cold spots.

CHAPTER 11: WHAT CANNOT BE FREEZE-DRIED AND WHAT CAN BE

Suppose you are looking to buy a freeze dryer to preserve your food. Then, the most important thing you should know is which foods you can freeze-dry and which cannot. In this chapter, you will find the answer to this question. Here is the list of foods that can or cannot be frozen dry.

Foods We Can Freeze-Dry

We can freeze-dry foods, including vegetables, fruits, meats, dairy, eggs, desserts, pet food, etc. As mentioned earlier, freeze-drying removes moisture from the food, so we can't freeze-dry oil-based foods like butter, honey, and jam.

- Fruits
- Vegetables
- Meats
- Dairy
- Eggs
- Full Meals
- Deserts, Snacks, and Candy
- Drinks
- Herbs and Spices

Fruits

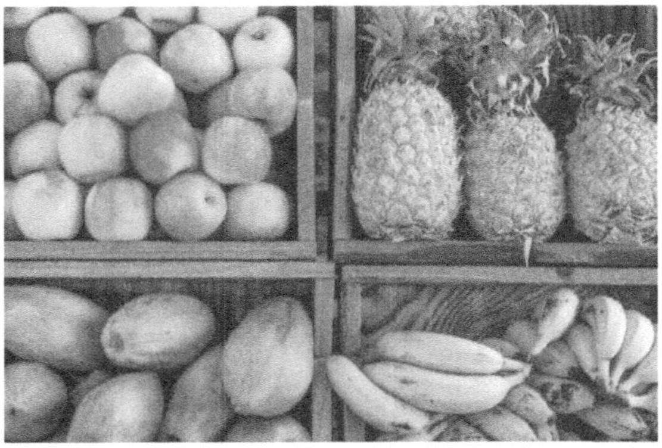

Fruits that can be freeze-dried are:

- Apple Slices
- Apricots
- Bananas
- Blackberries
- Blue Berries
- Cantaloupe
- Coconut
- Cherries
- Grapes
- Kiwis
- Lemons
- Mango
- Oranges
- Pineapple
- Raspberries
- Strawberries
- Watermelon

Vegetables

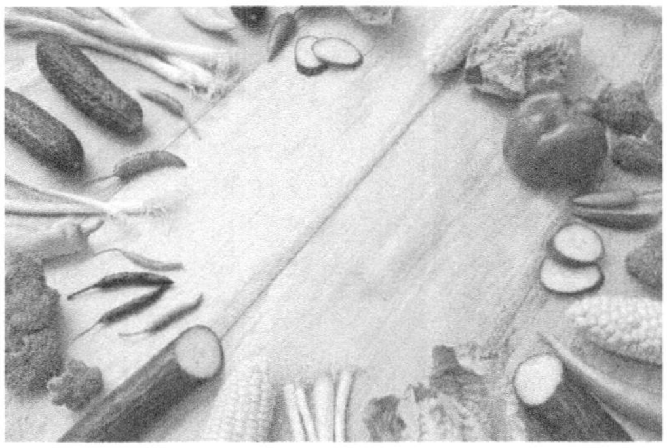

Vegetables that can be freeze-dried are:

- Beans
- Carrots
- Corn
- Eggplant
- Kale
- Mushroom
- Peas
- Onions
- Peppers
- Pumpkin
- Spinach
- Swiss Chard
- Tomatoes
- Potatoes
- Yam
- Zucchini

You need to remember that freeze-drying never kills bacteria, so try to use healthy fruits and vegetables. Clean it before putting it into a batch. Then, peel and cut the fruits and vegetables into evenly sized portions, and make an even layer in a tray. Cutting the fruits is essential because that makes the membranes thick, making it challenging for them to release water. This is because they have a high amount of sugar.

Meat

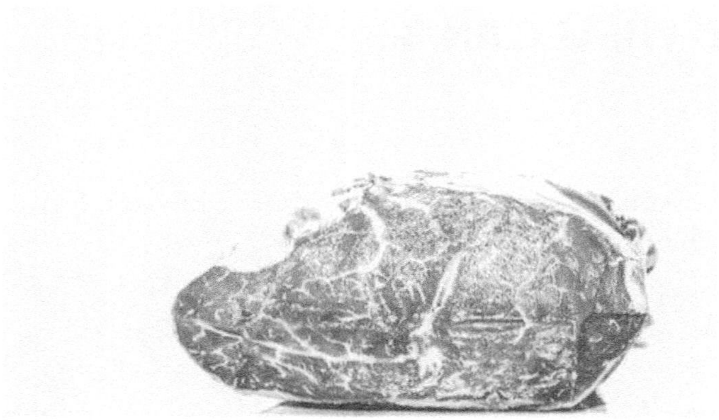

Meats that can be freeze dried include:

- Chicken
- Ham
- Turkey
- Roast Beef
- Sausage
- Fish
- Steak

Raw meat can be freeze-dried and stored in Mylar bags if they have oxygen absorbers for 10-15 years. After this, the natural, freeze-dried beef is submerged in water for a few minutes. Then dried, with a paper towel, grilled, baked, or fried as if it was fresh raw meat.

How to Freeze-Dry Meat

To freeze raw meat:

- First of all, dice it into large pieces, remembering to remove as much fat as possible.
- Secondly, place the pieces of meat on trays and freeze them dry.

- Thirdly, when the freeze-drying process is complete, break one of the most significant pieces in half and ensure no ice crystals are present in the middle of the meat. If there are ice crystals, add more time until you can be sure there is no ice left in the most prominent piece of meat.
- Lastly, store the meat in an airtight container and make sure that there should be an oxygen absorber. Along with it, mark the contents of the containers and record the date they were freeze-dried. If the meat is frozen and dried, you can use it for 10-15 years.

Dairy and Eggs

Dairy and Eggs that can be freeze-dried include:

- Cottage Cheese
- Cream Cheese
- Cheese
- Yogurt
- Eggs
- Ice Cream
- Butter Milk
- Milk
- Cheez Whiz
- Sour Cream

There are many ways you can freeze-dry the dairy product. You can spread it on the tray or you can fold it into molds and save it on the tray. Dairy product like yogurt can be placed into small individual clumps. During the preparation of ice-cream, try to buy high quality brands. Some ice-creams has air into it and will crystallize in the freeze dryer. The fat can not be freeze-dried due to its high fat content.

Full Meals

- Casseroles
- Chicken Parmesan
- Chili
- Fajitas
- Chow Mein
- Enchiladas
- Ham Fried Rice
- Jambalaya
- Hash Browns
- Lasagna
- Pasta
- Macaroni & Cheese
- Mashed Potatoes
- Pizza
- Meat Loaf
- Meatballs
- Pasta
- Roast Turkey Dinner
- Rice
- Scrambled Eggs
- Roast Beef Dinner
- Soup
- Stew

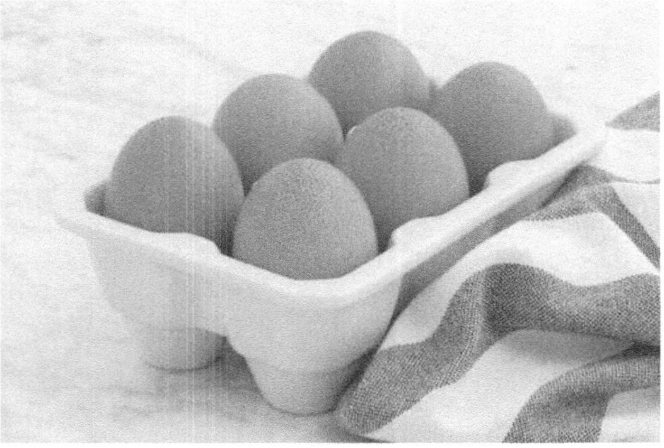

Snacks and Candy

- Cookies
- Gummy Bears
- Jell-O
- Junior Mints
- Marshmallows
- Lemon Bars
- Pie
- Pudding
- Saltwater Taffy
- Salsa
- Skittles

Can You Freeze-Dry Cookies?

Yes, any kind of cookies can be freeze-dried and stored for years in Mylar bag provided there is an oxygen absorber. The cookies will be crunchy and flavor will be preserved so well. This taste will remain good even years later.

<u>Drinks that Can Be Freeze-Dried</u>

- Coffee
- Orange Juice
- Smoothies

Freeze-drying orange juice is very simple and works well to store in Mylar bags so that it can easily be mixed with water later. Pour orange juice in the freeze dryer trays about 2/3 to the top and carefully slide the tray in the freeze dryer. After it is finished, you can break up the dried orange juice and store in a Mylar bag with an oxygen absorber.

Herbs and Spices

- Basil
- Chives
- Garlic
- Ginger
- Horseradish
- Jalapeño
- Lavender
- Mint
- Oregano
- Sage
- Thyme

Foods We Cannot Freeze-Dry

Foods that don't freeze-dry well include:

- Butter
- Jam
- Honey
- Peanut Butter
- Mayonnaise
- Syrup
- Pure Chocolate

The foods described above can't freeze-dry well as they secrete oil. The process of sublimation can't work with oily products.

Treats that Don't Change a Lot By Freeze-Drying

These foods can be freeze-dried but don't change much. This is because they don't have enough moisture for freeze-drying.

- Pop-Tarts
- Peppermint Patty
- Twizzlers Licorice
- Oreos

Ultimately What Should You Freeze-Dry?

In a nutshell, it is safe to freeze different dry foods. Experiment with other foods to find out which meal is best for your family. Once you find your freeze-dried food, dry a lot of it and take it wherever you want in any emergency situation. It is satisfying to freeze-dry your food and store it for 25 years.

FREEZE-DRYING
COOKBOOK FOR PREPPERS

How to Freeze-Dry and Preserve Nutrient Dense Food

Safely at Home to Be Prepared for the Incoming Crisis.

1800 Days of Tasty Recipes and Log Book Included

Tyler Gordon

CHAPTER 12: FREEZE-DRY RECIPES

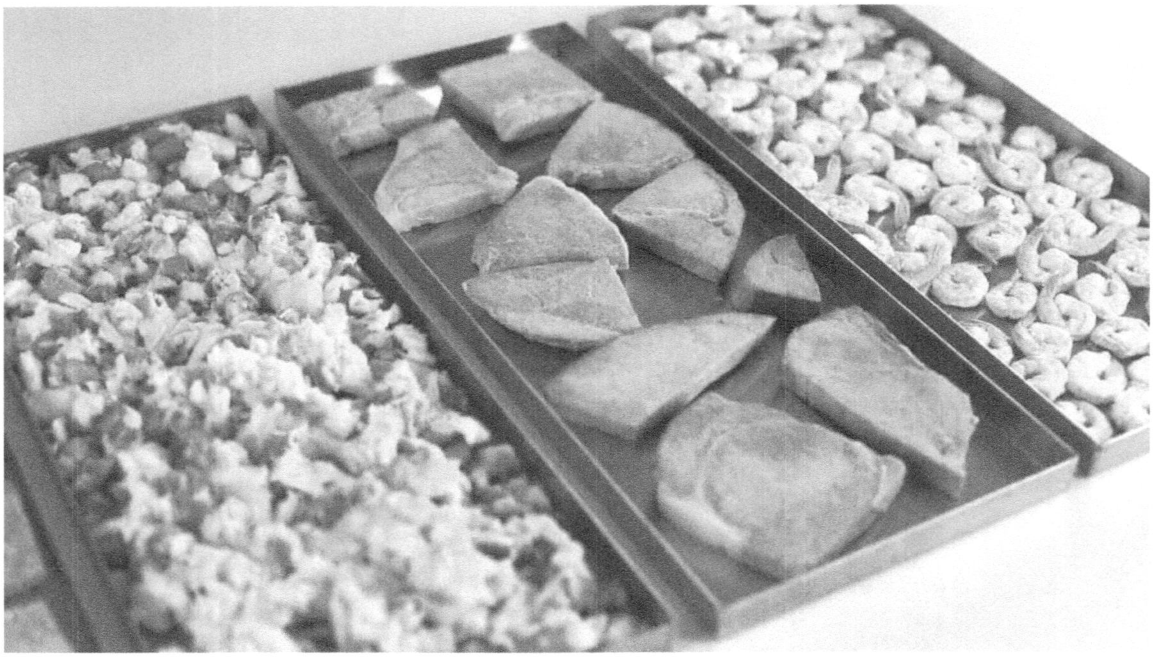

1. Freeze Dried Strawberries

Preparation time: 10 min
Servings: 3

Ingredients:

- Half-quarter strawberries

Directions:

1. First of all, wash all the strawberries, and then dry them.
2. Slice these strawberries thinly. You will get five slices from each strawberry after cutting them thinly.
3. Then, place them on the sheets of the freeze dryer. Place all of the strawberries until all the plates are occupied. You can line up the strawberries or put them in an overlapping way.
4. Place that plate into the freeze dryer and turn on the machine.
5. Press the button "Not Frozen" and let the machine do its work.
6. Once the freeze-dried strawberries are done, remove them from the freeze dryer, and keep them in a Mylar bag and an oxygen absorber.

Nutritional Facts: Calories 1 kcal, Fat (grams): 0.01 g, Carbs (grams): 0.31g, Fiber (grams): 0.1g, Sugar (grams): 0.2g, Protein (grams): 0.9

2. Freeze-Dried Raspberries

Preparation time: 10 min
Cooking time: 24 hours
Servings: 20

Ingredients:

- 20 cups raspberries
- Water

Directions:

1. First, wash your raspberries, remove any stems, and let them dry.
2. Fill the freeze dryer tray with raspberries.
3. Make a single layer with little overlap. You can also get the puree from the freeze dryer and freeze-dry it.
4. As a precaution, don't put more fruits on the tray than your machine's size.
5. After this, freeze the berries overnight. Place the tray in the freeze dryer and turn on the machine.
6. Choose "Frozen" and let the machine work for the rest.
7. When it is done, you can check it with the moisture meter.
8. You can add more time as needed.
9. In the end, you can pack them in a Mylar bag or grind them in the form of powder.

Nutritional Facts: Calories 233kcal, Fat (grams): 0.31g, Carbs (grams): 59.8g, Fiber (grams): 8.4g, Sugar (grams): 51.35 g, Protein (grams): 2.12 g

3. Freeze-Dried Plum Bites

Preparation time: 12 hours
Total time: 1 day, 8 hours
Servings: 4

Ingredients:

- 2 lbs. fresh plums (weighed after pits are removed)
- 1/4 cup honey

Directions:

1. First of all, wash the plums to remove any dirt and debris. Remove all of the stems and leaves from the plums.
2. Then, cut down the plums and remove the pits. Discard the pits.
3. Add all the pitted plums in the food processor and honey into it. Close the lid and process it until it becomes soupy.
4. It will not be perfectly blended, but little pieces of the skin will be visible but don't have to leave any fruit remaining.
5. Pour its puree into the ice cube tray. After pouring it into its place, please wait for it to be hard and then place it in the freezer.
6. Place parchment paper on the freeze dryer plate. Then place pre-frozen cubes on the lined tray. Just remember they shouldn't touch one another.
7. Place trays in the freeze dryer and run on the standard cycle.
8. If drying full-size cubes, add about 5-7 hours to the dry cycle.
9. When the cycle is completed, check that the cubes are dried. Store it in an airtight container at room temperature.

Nutritional Facts: Calories 266 kcal, Fat: 0.23 g; Carbohydrates 70.18 g; Fiber: 2.1g; Protein: 0.88 g; Sodium 44 mg

4. Homemade Muesli Bars

Preparation time: 10 min
Cooking time: 15 min
Servings: 4

Ingredients:

- 4 tbsp. butter
- 2 cup oats
- 2 cups dried coconut
- 1/2 cup unsalted sesame seeds
- 1/2 cup wheat germ
- 1/4 cup unsalted pumpkin seeds
- 1/4 cup unsalted sunflower seeds
- 1 cup unsweetened dried cranberries
- 1 cup flaxseeds
- 1/2 cup honey
- 1/2 cup packed sugar

Directions:

1. Collect the ingredients.
2. Place parchment paper on the baking pan. Set it aside.
3. Pick a large skillet and place it over low to medium heat. Then toast the rolled oats, dried coconuts, sesame, and pumpkin seeds. Stir it occasionally till it becomes golden, and be careful not to burn the mixture.
4. Place all the stuff in the metal bowl, set it aside, and cool it down.

1. When the mixture calms down, stir it and mix unsweetened cranberries and flax seeds.
2. Keep a small saucepan over medium heat and cook butter, honey, and brown sugar.
3. Stir it continuously until all of the sugar is dissolved.
4. Let it boil, reduce the heat to low, and don't stir it for 5 minutes.
5. Then add the hot butter mixture to these dry ingredients. Stir them until they are combined.
6. Add this mixture to the baking pan.
7. Press the mixture with the backside of the spoon
8. Let it cool, and then cut it into pieces.

Nutritional Facts: Calories 960 kcal, Fat (grams): 54.36 g, Carbs (grams): 120.08g, Fiber (grams): 26.1g, Sugar (grams): 60.86g, Protein (grams): 27.93g

5. Puffed Millet Oats

Preparation time: 15
Cooking time: 30
Servings: 6

Ingredients:

- 1 cup puffed millet
- 1 cup gluten-free rolled oats
- ½ cup freeze-dried apples
- 1 tbsp. milled flax seeds
- 2 tbsp. hulled hemp seeds
- ½ cup unsweetened apple sauce
- 1 tbsp. cinnamon
- ½ pure bourbon vanilla extract
- ½ tsp. nutmeg
- 3 drops of liquid stevia

Directions:

1. Heat the oven to 325°F.
2. Then pick a large bowl and add all the oats, millet, cinnamon, and hemp. Stir it.
3. Pick a baking sheet with foil and wipe some oil on a non-stick pan.
4. After this, spread the granola on the sheet for equal baking.
5. Bake it for 30 minutes and then stir it after every 10 minutes.
6. Let it cool and then store it in an airtight container.

Nutritional Facts: Calories 202 kcal, Fat (grams): 4.9 g, Carbs (grams): 38.47g, Fiber (grams): 6.9g, Sugar (grams): 1.23g, Protein (grams): 7.8g

6. Strawberry Shortcake Oreo Balls

Preparation time: 10 min
Cooking time: 25 min
Servings: 10

Ingredients:

- 18 Golden Oreos
- 4 oz. of whipped cream cheese
- 1-2 oz. vanilla candy coating
- 3 tbsp. French vanilla instant pudding mix
- 3 tbsp. strawberry gelatin mix
- 1 tbsp. freeze-dried strawberries

Directions:

1. Pre-heat the oven to 350 degrees and place parchment paper on the baking sheet.
2. Now run 18 Oreos with the help of the food processor. Mix Oreo crumbs in a small mixing bowl. Then add the rest of them to a larger one.
3. Pick a large spoon and stir it in the cream cheese along with the Oreo crumbles in a large bowl. I patted it, stirred and then repeat it until it was thoroughly mixed.
4. Line this baking sheet with wax paper and spray generously with a non-stick pan.
5. Please place them in your freezer and chill for 15 minutes.
6. Recover your small bowl of Oreo crumbles.
7. After this, add 3 tbsp. of vanilla pudding mix and strawberry, gelatin mix and stir them well.
8. Spread it on the baking sheet for 6 to 7 minutes. Let it cool.
9. Then run your freeze-dried strawberries in your food processor and add them to the crumble mix.
10. Heat and melt your vanilla coating in a double boiler. If it looks thick, you can add more and more spoons to it. Heat it again and stir it well.
11. Use a fork and dip your Oreo balls one at a time in the vanilla coating and then dip them into the Oreo crumbles, gelatin, and pudding mix right after.
12. Set the dipped Oreo balls on the wax paper and continue this process until all are dipped.
13. Let it set for 10-20 minutes in the refrigerator and then serve.

Nutritional Facts: Calories 254 kcal, Fat (grams): 8.1 g, Carbs (grams): 43.55 g, Fiber (grams): 7.3 g, Sugar (grams): 32.58 g, Protein (grams): 1.87 g

7. Eton Mess with Strawberry Meringues

Preparation time: 10 min
Cooking time: 10 min
Servings: 3

Ingredients:

- Half cup whipping cream
- Half cup Greek yogurt
- Half tbsp. rose water
- ½ cup powdered sugar
- 1 cup strawberries
- 2 tbsp. freeze-dried strawberries
- 1 tbsp. rose petals for garnishing
- Mint leaves

Directions:

1. Pick a large bowl and whisk the cream until it thickens.
2. Take a separate bowl and whisk the yogurt until it smoothens. Then, fold it through the whipped cream, vanilla bean seeds, icing, and rose water.
3. Chop the strawberries and keep a few of them for garnishing.
4. After this, break up the meringues, and start making layers of cream and berries in a bowl.
5. Make the layers and garnish them with strawberries, freeze-dried berries, mint, and rose petals.

Nutritional facts: Calories 182 kcal, Fat (grams): 7.25 g, Carbs (grams): 26.7 g, Fiber (grams): 1 g, Sugar (grams): 24.05 g, Protein (grams): 3.82 g

8. Cheesy Chili Mac in a Jar Recipe

Preparation time: 10 min
Cooking time: 10 min
Servings: 3

Ingredients:

- 1 ½ cup elbow macaroni
- ½ cup freeze-dried protein
- 1/3 cup cheese powder
- 1.5 tbsp. butter powder
- 2 tbsp. non-fat dry milk
- ½ cup taco seasoning mix
- ½ tsp. white pepper
- ½ tsp. salt
- ½ cup vegetable powder

Directions:

1. Boil three cups of water to rehydrate protein and pasta.
2. Allow pasta to soak when you are preparing the sauce
3. Then add 1.5 cups of water to dry the ingredients.
4. Mix it thoroughly and allow it to sit and rehydrate while the pasta is rehydrating
5. Mix it with pasta and serve it.
6. First of all, place pasta and protein into the bottom layer of a quart jar

7. Enter ingredients into a zip-top bag and keep it on top of the pasta mixture
8. Close the pot with a vacuum seal.
9. You can store it for 2 or 4 years
10. Use a vacuum seal for the best result

Nutritional Facts: Calories 639 kcal, Fat (grams): 40.51 g, Carbs (grams): 56.61g, Fiber (grams): 5 g, Sugar (grams): 5 g, Protein (grams): 10.77 g

9. Freeze Peppers, Both Hot & Sweet

Preparation time: 10 min
Cooking time: 10 min
Servings: 3

Ingredients:

- 2 to 4 bell peppers or hot peppers

Directions:

1. First of all, you need to wash all the peppers.
2. Then you can slice or chop the peppers. Always wear gloves when you are working with hot ones. This is because milder peppers can sting.
3. Spread all of the cookies on a layer. Place them in the freezer and let it stay there for about 10 to 20 hours.
4. When the peppers are frozen, you can use and place them in the container you want to store and put them in the freezer.

Nutritional Facts: Calories 20 kcal, Fat (grams): 0.98 g, Carbs (grams): 22.87 g, Fiber (grams): 0.5 g, Sugar (grams): 1.55 g, Protein (grams): 0.61 g

10. Apple Crumb Cake

Preparation time: 20 min
Cooking time: 20 min
Servings: 3

Ingredients:

- 2 cup flour
- ½ scrambled eggs
- 1 tbsp. baking powder
- 1 cup water
- 1 cup sugar
- 1 tsp. salt
- 1 cup chopped apple slices
- ½ cup brown sugar
- 1 tsp. cinnamon
- ½ cup butter powder

Directions:

1. Pick a bowl and blend all of the ingredients in it.
2. Pour them into a greased baking dish.
3. Mix all the ingredients well with a fork until they are crumbly.
4. Sprinkle these crumb topping on top of the cake.
5. Lastly, bake it at 375°F for 20 to 25 minutes.

Nutritional Facts: Calories 696 kcal, Fat (grams): 2.88 g, Carbs (grams): 159.35 g, Fiber (grams): 4.2 g, Sugar (grams): 79.33 g, Protein (grams): 10.58 g

11. Freeze-Dry Eggs

Preparation time: 10 min
Cooking time: 15 hours
Servings: 5

Ingredients:

- 24 Medium sized eggs

Directions:

1. Push the start button of the freezer. It will prompt the vacuum chamber to cool down for 15 minutes. Along with it, make sure the valve is closed.
2. Crack the eggs and place them in a blender. Blend them well until they become smooth. You can also use a whisk for this. You can blend dozens of eggs at a time.
3. Pour all of the eggs into the freeze dryer pan.
4. Keep them in the freezer until they become solid.
5. Add the trays into a freeze dryer, close the door and seal them.
6. Now, wait for the magic of the freeze dryer.
7. It will take 15 to 20 hours. It only depends upon the number of eggs you want to freeze-dry.
8. After turning off the freeze dryer, check the eggs. If you feel them wet again, put them in the freeze dryer and repeat the process. Click on the more time button.
9. Remove the eggs from the tray and shift them into jars or Mylar bags for long-term storage.

Nutritional Facts: Calories 302 kcal, Fat (grams): 20.09 g, Carbs (grams): 1.52 g, Fiber (grams): 0 g, Sugar (grams): 0.78 g, Protein (grams): 26.53 g

12. Freeze-Dry Cheese

Preparation time: 10 min
Cooking time: 20 hours
Servings: 80

Ingredients:

- 5 lbs. of cheese (sliced/ shredded)

Directions:

1. Pre-freeze the cheese in your freeze dryer. If the cheese is sliced or shredded, you can skip this step. It will extend the drying time.
2. Place your tray in the freeze dryer machine when it is ready to begin.
3. Let the machine do the rest of the things. When this happens, the cheese should be warm. They will be crispy and dry. If it is not, let it freeze-dry.
4. Pack it into a Mylar bag along with an oxygen absorber.

Nutritional Facts: Calories 82 kcal, Fat (grams): 6.02 g, Carbs (grams): 2.47 g, Fiber (grams): 0 g, Sugar (grams): 2.08 g, Protein (grams): 4.65 g

13. Freeze-Dried Candy

Preparation time: 10 min
Cooking time: 10 min
Servings: 3

Ingredients:

- 1 cup freeze-dried candy
- 1 tbsp. your favorite flavor

Directions:

1. It depends on your flavors, the cooking method, the type of dish, and the food.
2. Try to ensure that the recipe you choose will elevate the food's original flavor.
3. Do experimentation with different recipes.

Nutritional Facts: Calories 301 kcal, Fat (grams): 16.61 g, Carbs (grams): 33.47 g, Fiber (grams): 1.9 g, Sugar (grams): 29.02 g, Protein (grams): 4.41 g

14. Oatmeal Freeze-Dried Cookies

Preparation time: 10 min
Cooking time: 8 hours
Servings: 10

Ingredients:

- 2-4 medium apples (sliced)
- 2 cup milk
- 2 tbsp. honey, sugar
- 1 tbsp. butter
- 1 tbsp. salt
- 1 tsp. cinnamon
- 1 cup rolled oats

Directions:

1. Chop up the apples and make a layer on the bottom of the crockpot.
2. Add the rest of the ingredients to the milk
3. You can cook it for 6 hours or can warm it overnight.
4. Add these trays to the freeze dryer and freeze them overnight
5. Place it in the freeze dryer with the proper setting.

Nutritional Facts: Calories 105 kcal, Fat (grams): 3.5 g, Carbs (grams): 19.77 g, Fiber (grams): 2.9 g, Sugar (grams): 11.73 g, Protein (grams): 3.34 g

15. Freeze-Dried Sweet Corn

Preparation time: 2 hours
Cooking time: 40 hours
Servings: 5

Ingredients:

- 5-lb. sweet corn

Directions:

1. Pick the sweet corn that you want to freeze-dry.
2. Remove dust from the corn by shucking it.
3. Blanch the corn thrice.
4. Now blanch the corn in ice water. Once you feel the water is getting less cold, you can change it and place another bowl of cold water in it.
5. When the corn has been blenched, drain the water off.
6. Now cover the freeze dryer plate with parchment paper.
7. Spread the corn on the freeze dryer in a single layer.
8. Now place the plate in the freeze dryer.
9. Start the freeze dryer on the regular cycle.
10. It will lead to the mid-drying cycle that will take the most extended time.
11. When the sensors detect that the food is ready, it will lead to the final cycle.
12. When the freeze dryer shuts off, the food will need some extra time for drying.
13. Once the food is ready, immediately put it into a Mylar bag, or you can use a jar for storage along with an oxygen absorber.

Nutritional Facts: Calories 327 kcal, Fat (grams): 1.91 g, Carbs (grams): 82.24 g, Fiber (grams): 5.4 g, Sugar (grams): 14.65 g, Protein (grams): 7.89 g

16. Freeze-Dried Cherries

Preparation time: 10 min
Cooking time: 10 hours
Servings: 2

Ingredients:

- 2 cups pitted cherries

Directions:

1. First of all, turn on your freeze dryer.
2. Pick a tray and fill it with pitted cherries.
3. Place the tray in the freeze dryer.
4. Turn on the freeze dryer for a day and a half until all the cherries dry.
5. Store in an airtight container.

Nutritional Facts: Calories 88 kcal, Fat (grams): 0.24 g, Carbs (grams): 21.81 g, Fiber (grams): 2.7 g, Sugar (grams): 18.54 g, Protein (grams): 1.88 g

17. Cook & Freeze-Dried Beans

Preparation time: 5 min
Cooking time: 1 hour 30 min
Servings: 8

Ingredients:

- Half-pound dried beans
- 3 cups water

Directions:

1. Place the dried beans in a stock pot.
2. Add one cup of beans to 3 cups of water.

3. Boil it over a high flame. Then lower the flame and let them soak. After some time, check if they are soft enough to eat. Don't let the beans be so soft.
4. Place these beans in a strainer and rinse them with cold water.
5. Divide them into the freezer container and keep a space between them.
6. Fill it with cold fresh water above the beans. Allow space between these layers so that they can expand on freezing.
7. Seal and label it with a type of bean.
8. Place it in the freezer and store it for 5 to 8 months.

Nutritional Facts: Calories 12 kcal, Fat (grams): 0.26 g, Carbs (grams): 2.45 g, Fiber (grams): 1.1 g, Sugar (grams): 0.44 g, Protein (grams): 0.64 g

18. Freeze-Dried Apples

Preparation time: 15 min
Cooking time: 10 hours & 15 min
Servings: 4

Ingredients:

- Eight apples

Directions:

1. Cut down the apples in half and then into pieces. I can get 14 cuts per apple. If you slice them too large, they will take a long time to freeze-dry.
2. Place the apple slices on the freeze dryer sheets. After this, line them up in a single layer. The apples can touch the tray.
3. Place the freeze dryer tray into the Harvest Right Freeze-Dryer. Press "Not Frozen" and start the machine. I added two extra drying hours.
4. Remove the freeze-dried apple chips from the machine and package them in a Mylar bag. Add an O2 absorber for longer storage.

Nutritional Facts: Calories 189 kcal, Fat (grams): 0.62 g, Carbs (grams): 50.27 g, Fiber (grams): 8.7g, Sugar (grams): 37.82g, Protein (grams): 0.95 g

19. Vegetable Soup in a Jar

Preparation time: 10 mins
Cook Time: 10 mins
Total Time: 10 mins
Servings: 5

Ingredients:

- Half cup sliced potatoes
- Half cup dehydrated sliced onion
- 1 cup dehydrated sliced potatoes
- ¼ cup sliced tomatoes
- ½ dehydrated summer squash
- ¼ sliced carrots
- ¼ shredded cabbage
- ¼ cup dehydrated sliced zucchini
- ½ cup dehydrated vegetable stock

Directions:

1. Make a layer of the dehydrated ingredients in a jar. It should be fully occupied. It will be alright to push the ingredients down to fill them more.
2. You can also pack the soup ingredients in a vacuum-sealed bag.
3. Make labels on the jars with different contents and dates. Save it from direct sunlight.
4. To make the soup, combine all the soup mixtures in 10 cups of water, boil it, and then simmer. Let the soup thicken.
5. You can also combine a soup mixture in a cooker and cook it for 5 hours.

Nutritional Facts: Calories 245 kcal, Fat (grams): 21.89 g, Carbs (grams): 12.95 g, Fiber (grams): 1.8 g, Sugar (grams): 1.6 g, Protein (grams): 1.54 g

20. No-Churn Freeze-Dried Fruit Ice Cream

Preparation time: 30 min
Servings: 6

Ingredients:

- 2 oz. egg whites
- 1/4 oz. sugar
- 1/2 tsp. (heaping) kosher salt
- 1/2 tsp. cream of tartar
- 6 oz. heavy cream
- 1/3 oz. freeze-dried fruits

Directions:

1. Fill a pot with inches of water. Bring it to a boil. After this, let it simmer to get a steady supply of steam. Place a thick ring into the water. It will act as a booster seat.
2. Then, combine all the egg whites, salt, sugar, and lemon juice in the bowl of a stand mixer. Place it over the water bath so it can sit on the ring of the foil. The bowl should not touch the sides of the pot. Cook and stir it continuously with a spatula. It will not take longer than 5 minutes in stainless steel.
3. Transfer this bowl to a stand mixer when the mixture boils. Whisk it at high speed. However, the time that it will take varies.
4. Once the meringue is thick and stiff, whip this heavy cream and add dried fruits to it.
5. Don't do this process in the food processor. You can use it in an open whisk until the mixture is thoroughly combined. Add salt as much as needed.
6. Scrape ice cream into a large container and cover it with a layer of plastic wrap, pressing it directly against the surface of the ice cream.
7. To protect the ice cream from freezer odors, cover it with a sheet of foil if the container does not have a lid.
8. Freeze it until it becomes ready to scoop. Serve and enjoy.

Nutritional Facts: Calories 109 kcal, Fat (grams): 10.56 g, Carbs (grams): 2.3 g, Fiber (grams): 0.5g, Sugar (grams): 0.86 g, Protein (grams): 1.97g

PICKLING AND FERMENTING

GUIDEBOOK FOR PREPPERS

1000 Days of Recipes to Preserve Fruits, Vegetables, Meat, and Fish Before the Food Riot Starts.

Tyler Gordon

INTRODUCTION

Foods and beverages that have undergone fermentation can require some getting used to. Words like "aged" and "cured" on food containers will be a helpful indicator while searching for fermented foods.

Making fermented food at home is simple. This book teaches you how to ferment proteins, legumes, vegetables, fruits, dairy products, sourdough, alcoholic and nonalcoholic beverages, and even your own vinegar.

You don't need to consume a whole meal of fermented foods to reap their health advantages and enjoy their flavors. Simply adding some sauerkraut to your sausage enhances the flavor while providing health benefits. The same is true for eating some miso soup beforehand or adding some pickles to a sandwich.

Your health will improve more quickly as you consume and prepare fermented foods. Naturally, sharing what you know with others would only be fair if you've begun to appreciate the benefits of such foods. Encourage your friends to learn more about fermented foods by letting them sample the healthy foods you made yourself.

Due to its health advantages, fermentation is experiencing a rebirth in the modern world. Probiotics are abundant in fermented foods and beverages and aid in improving gut health. You might wish to start fermenting your own food for a variety of additional reasons as well. Beyond the benefits to health and food preservation, fermented food simply tastes fantastic!

In the past, pickling and other preservation methods were essential, even lifesaving. Only recently have people been able to keep food for lengthy periods using temperature control reliably; in the past, they had to come up with inventive ways to prevent rotting. Pickles have been a staple of ancient trip fare for millennia, nourishing many families during the lean winter months. Fermented pickles have a distinct flavor and scent that cannot be replicated using vinegar-brine procedures. Fermented pickles are also the healthiest sort of pickled food because they contain living bacteria and probiotics that are created during the fermenting process.

Don't worry if you've never fermented anything before. This book will teach you the fundamental methods and instructions you need to master the fermentation process. After you have mastered these methods, you can graduate to more complicated projects. We'll cover the fundamentals of hygienically and adequately fermenting food, what kinds of foods you can ferment, and how to do it. So, whether you're an experienced fermenter or new to the process, this guide has something for you.

This guide covers you, so don't worry!

CHAPTER 1: INTRODUCTION TO PICKLING AND FERMENTING

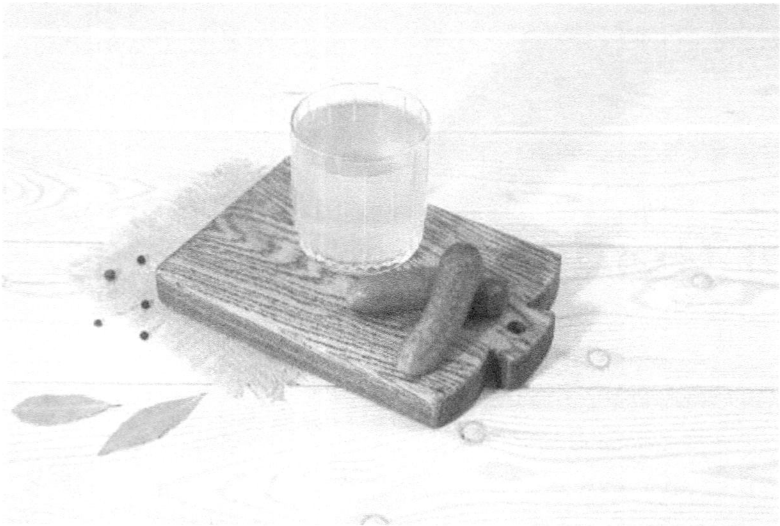

Food that has undergone biochemical changes due to the activity of enzymes or microbes, resulting in significant modifications to the food, is referred to as fermented food.

However, according to microbiologists, fermentation is a type of energy-producing microbial metabolism in which an organic or carbohydrate substrate undergoes incomplete oxidation while acting as an electron acceptor. This indicates that fermentation includes the procedures involved in the lactic acid bacteria or yeasts that manufacture ethanol from organic acids.

Regardless of these classifications, food that lactic acid-producing microbes have impacted is considered to be fermented food. To put it more plainly, food is considered to be fermented if it has aged with yeast and/or bacteria.

Many people may be unaware that the most typical foods they eat are fermented. For instance, fermented grapes are used to make wine, fermented milk is used to make cheese and yogurt, fermented soybeans are used to make miso and tempeh, and fermented grains are used to make most bread and beer. In addition, countless other delicious and healthy foods and beverages are fermented.

Ancient civilizations used fermentation as their primary means of food preservation, even after a culture had passed away. It follows that people in ancient times could eat fermented food even after several months or years. Additionally, it has been shown that the fermentation process not only preserved the nutritional value of food but also unlocked a wide range of textures and flavors that enhance the enjoyment of the dish.

Many ancient people's fermented foods have been improved with health benefits, opening the door for other people and businesses to improve their fermentation techniques. They also recorded the causes and results of their fermentation processes simultaneously. They were aware that the effectiveness of the fermentation process depends on how effectively the food is fermented in response to the process. A range of amino acids, minerals, and vitamins are among the many nutrients produced and released throughout time by fermentation.

It is a process in which bacteria, yeast, and other microbes manufacture enzymes that cause organic molecules to be chemically changed into simpler chemicals. The enzymes break down complex chemical molecules into simpler substances and nutrients. Food that has undergone fermentation has a particular texture, taste, and flavor that enhances the original product and makes it easier for humans to digest. Typically, in groups or individually, yeasts, molds, or bacteria trigger fermentation processes.

All bacteria have specialized metabolic genes that produce enzymes that can digest particular subtypes of sugar compounds. Different types of microorganisms are present during the fermentation process in varying concentrations. Together, they produce the desired fermented byproduct for you. The type and quantity of bacteria utilized in the fermentation process will affect the flavor of specific fermented foods.

Different Forms of Fermentation

Alcohol Fermentation

Alcohol is produced when yeasts break down the pyruvate molecules found in carbohydrates. Alcoholic fermentation is the most well-known type of fermentation. Humans have long savored the byproducts of wine, beer, and other beverages.

Acetic Fermentation

Sour vinegar and other condiments are created from fruit or grain sugars. When the fermentation of alcohol is finished, this procedure begins. The most frequent result of acetic acid production is vinegar. Because of this, apple cider and apple cider vinegar are different products.

Lactic Acid Fermentation

Lactic acid is formed as a result of the digestion of sugars or carbohydrates. This fermenting technique is said to be the earliest. Most civilizations worldwide use fermented milk products consumed for generations.

You must remember that food fermentation is a form of controlled degradation when you start working on it. Fermentation produces potent smells and odors that may appeal to certain people but not others. These dishes are not fresh, but they are also not bad. By consuming fermented foods, you can enhance your body's digestion of other foods and prevent harmful bacteria from flourishing inside you. Your taste will determine the type of fermented food you consume. Try a few different fermentations using this method to see which ones best fit your taste. They're a great way to improve your health and reduce food waste.

Benefits of Fermentation

Foods that have undergone fermentation have many advantages. Compared to their unfermented counterparts, most foods are more nutrient-rich when fermented. Let's examine some of these meals' benefits.

Enhanced Gut Health

Probiotics are added to food during fermentation, increasing their quantity. These bacteria can treat stomach aches and digestive issues as well as balance the microbiota in the gut. According to studies, probiotics can help with some IBS or irritable bowel syndrome symptoms. Most people worldwide with this illness exhibit either modest or severe symptoms. Fermented foods, like cheese and yogurt, for example, can lessen symptoms like bloating, according to research by Guyonnet D et al. on adults.

Additionally, they might increase stool frequency, which reduces constipation. Further, fermented foods can lessen the intensity of gas and diarrhea. You should consider including fermented foods in your diet if you have digestive troubles or stomach problems.

Enhanced Immunity

Your immune system and intestinal health are closely intertwined. You have a lower chance of getting illnesses like the common cold, the flu, fever, etc., thanks to the bacteria in your gut. Additionally, these nutrients boost immunity. Fermented foods boost your immunity since they include a lot of probiotics. Consuming probiotic foods can also help you recover from infections more quickly. Most fermented foods are high in iron, zinc, and vitamin C. Your immune system is known to be strengthened by these foods.

Enhanced Digestion

Foods are easier for the body to digest because fermentation breaks down different meal components. For instance, lactose, a natural sugar in milk, is converted into galactose and glucose during fermentation. These latter are basic sugars that are simple for your body to process. You can eat fermented foods, including cheese, yogurt, and kefir, if you have lactose sensitivity. Additionally, the process of fermentation aids in the destruction or breakdown of chemical compounds like lectins and phytates into smaller and more palatable ones. These are frequently located in grains, legumes, nuts, and seeds. As a result, your body has no trouble digesting meals like tempeh, made from fermented legumes or beans.

Loss of Weight

Additionally, studies indicate a connection between particular probiotic strains and weight loss. Lactobacillus gasseri and Lactobacillus rhamnosus are two of these strains that have a reputation for lowering abdominal fat.

How Does Pickling Work, and What is It?

Although this question initially looks straightforward, clarifying the processes you want to take place is crucial. This contrasts with merely hoping for the best and tossing some vegetables in a jar. You can confidently follow a recipe if you understand the pickling procedure. Or, even better, you can develop the confidence to disregard a recipe and create your own peculiar, fascinating, and, most importantly, palatable inventions.

The method of pickling involves immersing the edible product you're trying to preserve in an acidic solution. Usually, vinegar is used for this, although brine—a salt solution—is occasionally applied. The solution is edible to humans, but the most crucial component is unfriendly to microbes. Since you probably intend to eat this item, using an inedible solution defeats the point.

The term "pickling" typically relates to the use of this solution to preserve fresh plants; however, there are some exceptions, including pickled eggs. Meat can also be preserved similarly, which is known as curing. We'll concentrate on fresh produce.

The vinegar method is easy to use and understand, which is why it's so well-liked. Because vinegar is so acidic, it takes care of your preserving job. Since vinegar typically has a pH of 2 or 3, it generates a climate unfriendly to dangerous germs.

Of course, pickling can be done with acidic liquids other than vinegar. The most popular acid used is simply vinegar. For instance, using a technique we'll discuss later, limes and lemons can be pickled in their acidic juice.

Things may get weird when it comes to the brine solution approach. Salt is not acidic. So how do we define pickling in this context? The brine helps a fermentation process that results in the production of lactic acid rather than immediately pickling the food. The lactic acid preserves the food.

Meals that have been pickled have the obvious advantage of not spoiling as quickly as fresh foods. Pickling alters the flavor, consistency, and even nutritional value of food and preserving it.

You don't have to pickle everything, so don't stress. However, you might be tempted to once you see how simple and helpful it is.

Health Advantages of Pickling

Given the minimum work required for pickling, the health advantages are enormous. Pickles are made from plants, rich in healthy nutrients like vitamins and minerals, and have little fat and calories.

Let's take a moment to consider the lowly dill pickle. This is the classic pickle that we are all accustomed to. Additionally, it pairs amazingly well with your preferred sandwich. In its most basic form, a dill pickle is a cucumber that has been pickled with dill.

According to an analysis of its nutritional value, one whole dill pickle has 23% of the necessary daily quantity of vitamin K. You need this vitamin to thrive since it is vital. It is used by the body to aid in blood clotting and stop excessive bleeding. It has also been connected to healthy bones.

Vitamin A intake should be between 21% and 24% of the daily recommended value. The immune system is strengthened by vitamin A, which also benefits and protects the eyes and the skin. Retinol, another name for it, is frequently found in vitamin supplements and is occasionally used in skin treatments.

7% of adults should consume calcium daily for strong bones, teeth, and nerves.

Potassium, a mineral and an electrolyte, accounts for 5% of the daily recommended intake. Potassium is a multi-tasking mineral that supports the health of your heart rhythm, muscles, nerves, blood pressure, and even your body's natural pH balance.

Vitamin C preserves cells and keeps them healthy, promotes wound healing, and maintains the health of the skin, blood vessels, bones, and cartilage, in 3-4% of the daily recommended allowance.

Pickles are the tastiest option if you have to choose between eating a few of them daily or popping a multivitamin. Dill pickles include a lot of beta-carotene, crucial for lowering your risk of heart disease, stroke, cancer, respiratory disorders, other diseases, and all of these vitamins and minerals. Additionally, they are loaded with antioxidants, which aid in lessening the adverse effects of free radicals on the body. These consequences include a variety of unpleasant chronic diseases, heart disease, cancer, and inflammation. Simply said, consuming more antioxidants will benefit your overall health.

Enhancing the Flavor of Pickles

Discovering just how wonderful pickled food can be is one of the most thrilling aspects of pickling at home. Pickles might sometimes be overlooked as a tiny component of your diet, serving only as a condiment for a certain sandwich or meal. People frequently find it challenging to come up with ideas for what to do with all of the pickles, especially now that alternative food preservation techniques are available.

However, this does not have to be the case. There are no restrictions on how to use pickles or what foods to serve them. Instead, consider them a flavor enhancer that can be added to nearly anything.

Cooking involves many different aspects, but one of them is the idea of balancing various flavors. These flavors include acid and salt. Many savory recipes contain acid, such as vinegar or lemon juice. Even tomatoes contribute a small amount of acid to the dish. Acidity contrasts with other flavors and helps food to be balanced. Since salt is a flavor enhancer, it draws attention to other flavors. A typical tip is adding a tiny touch of salt to something sweet to highlight the sweetness without overdoing the salt to give it a salty flavor.

Why Have We Been Discussing Flavor Theory?

Pickles are usually acidic and salty. You can rely on those two; however, the recipe may require additional tastes. As a result, you can add some pickle to almost any dish and, in addition to bringing the flavors together, elevate the dish to new heights by adding a layer of complexity. For this reason, pickles are frequently used in meals across many cultures as an ingredient or a side dish.

Even if you don't want to use the pickle itself, vinegar can be substituted in a recipe with pickling brine. Additionally, you may use pickling brine in marinades to give the food you're marinating incredible, nuanced flavors. Making your own pickles enables you to experiment with cooking much more, and experimenting is where things can get a lot more delicious and enjoyable.

The type of vinegar used alters the pickled food's texture and flavor, whether it be cucumbers, onions, or something else entirely. You see, the acid in the vinegar affects your meals in several ways. The fact that it makes the environment within the jar uninhabitable for microorganisms is the most visible of these effects. But the lovely process of osmosis also turns the vegetable itself acidic. As a result, the water inside the vegetable is pulled into the acidic pickling solution, while the acid in the solution is absorbed into the vegetable. This occurs because the vegetable is significantly less acidic than the vinegar. This increases the acidity of the vegetable, keeping harmful germs from destroying your product while decreasing the acidity of the solution. The veggie becomes crisper since it contains less moisture. Despite logic stating that a watery vegetable preserved in liquid should be squishy and mushy, dill pickles remain crisp rather than soggy. They give sharpness to your dish that might not otherwise be present, which is another reason they are so enjoyable to eat.

You may read about how wonderful home pickling is, but the only way to believe it is to do it yourself. So, let's go over the details of the pickling procedure before trying out a few international recipes.

Everything You Should Know Before Pickling

The art of pickling dates back over 4,000 years. It was rumored that pickles were a component of Cleopatra's beauty regimen. Even Julius Caesar's soldiers received pickles as a source of energy. The average American consumes 9 pounds of pickles annually, making pickles a vital component of the national identity. While neither Cleopatra nor Napoleon's claims are strongly supported by science, pickled foods are a healthy, economical, and enjoyable way to enjoy the flavor of fresh food all year round.

What Exactly is Pickling?

Pickling is the anaerobic fermentation process used to preserve food in brine or vinegar, which can hold perishables for months. The two methods of pickling that are most frequently used are the water bath canning process, which involves preserving vegetables in a vinegar-brine, or wild fermentation, which calls for fermentation tools like a pickling crock or a fermentation kit like the Perfect Pickler.

Beginners may find it intimidating to begin the pickling process at home, but with a few inexpensive tools and ingredients, we can all quickly pickle like masters in no time.

Before Pickling

Although it's understandable if you want to start immediately, pickling requires some preparation. Equipment must be obtained, ingredients must be located, and safety regulations must be followed.

Safety comes first because it will determine the tools and components that are required:

- Check it before you consume it, just like you should with everything you intend to eat. Throw away your pickle if you notice that it smells bad, is discolored, or has mold developing on it. Although it is regrettable to have to discard anything like this, food poisoning is a much worse condition.
- Before utilizing it, make sure everything is clean. Jars and lids, in particular, fall under this. Before usage, run a load through the dishwasher or wash in hot, soapy water. Jars can also be sterilized by baking them for around fifteen minutes at 320–350°F (160–180°C).
- Pickle brine shouldn't be reused because it would have been diluted, making it harder to measure a healthy brine. Pickling liquid should always be acidic enough to kill any microorganisms.
- Different pickling procedures used in various recipes have an impact on storage. Always keep quick pickles in the refrigerator. Other pickles should be sealed, kept in a cool, dark location, and ideally kept in the refrigerator once they are opened.

PICKLING AND FERMENTING

COOKBOOK FOR PREPPERS

1000 Days of Recipes to Preserve Fruits, Vegetables, Meat, and Fish Before the Food Riot Starts.

Tyler Gordon

CHAPTER 2: FRUITS RECIPES

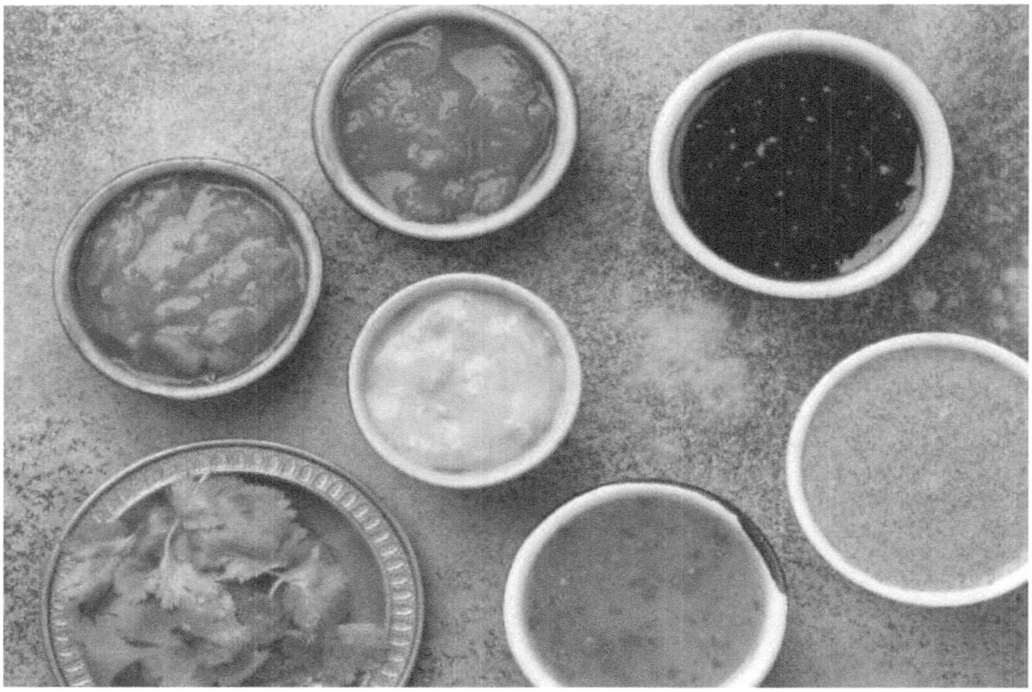

1. Five Spice Apple Chutney

Preparation time: 10 minutes
Fermentation time: 3 days
Servings: 4

Ingredients:

- 3 c. cored, coarsely chopped apples
- ½ c. chopped pecans
- ¼ c. lemon juice
- ½ c. pure water
- ½ c. raisins
- ½ tsp. sea salt
- 2 – 4 tbsp. whey liquid
- 2 tbsp. sucanat or rapadura or any other natural sweetener of your choice
- 2 tsp. five spice blend

Directions:

1. Add apples, pecans, lemon juice, water, raisins, salt, whey, sweetener, and five spice. Blend into the mixing bowl and mix well.
2. Spoon the mixture into the jar. Tighten the lids and place them on your countertop for two to three days.
3. Stir daily. Remove any mold that may appear on top.
4. Chill until ready to use. Use within 2 – 3 weeks.
5. Make sure to put the name and date on the jar.

Nutritional values:

Calories: 138
Carbohydrates: 32.2 g
Protein: 3.8 g
Fat: 0.4 g
Fiber: 7.4 g
Sugar: 14.6 g

2. Spicy Pear Chutney

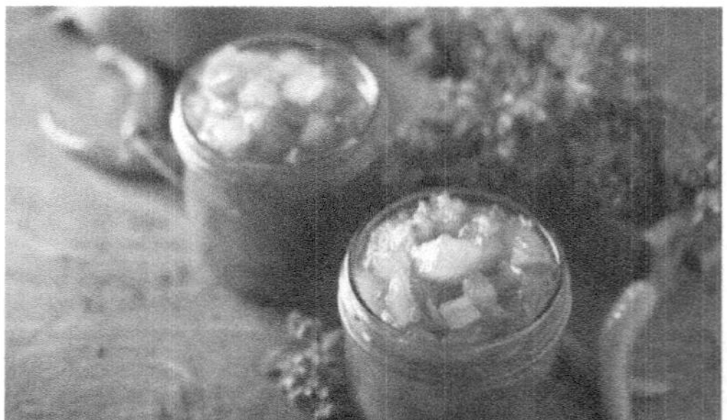

Preparation time: 15 minutes
Fermentation time: 3 days
Servings: 1 quart

Ingredients:

- 1 ½ to 2 pears, cored, chopped
- ¼ c. chopped cashews or pecans

- Juice of ½ to 1 lemon
- ½ tbsp. grated ginger
- ¼ c. filtered water
- 1 hot chili pepper, fresh or dried, chopped

Directions:

1. Add pears, cashews, lemon juice, ginger, water, raisins, salt, onion, and chili pepper into a bowl and stir well.
2. Spoon the mixture into the jar. Press the fruits down so that the water comes up. Tighten the lids and place them on your countertop for two to three days.
3. Stir daily. Remove any mold that may appear on top.
4. Chill until ready to use. It can last for two to three weeks.
5. Make sure to put the name and date on the jar.

Nutritional values:

Calories: 302
Fat: 7 g
Carbs: 26 g

Protein 35

3. Curried Mango Ginger Chutney

Preparation time: 15 minutes
Fermentation time: 2 – 3 days

Ingredients:

- 6 c. peeled, diced ripe mango
- 4 cloves of garlic, minced
- ½ c. minced fresh cilantro
- 4 tsp. curry powder
- 6 tbsp. whey liquid
- 1 tsp. red pepper flakes or crushed peppercorns
- 5 tsp. minced fresh ginger
- 1 sweet red onion, minced
- 4 tbsp. lemon juice
- 2 tsp. sea salt
- 4 basil leaves, chopped

Directions:

1. Add mango, garlic, cilantro, curry powder, red pepper flakes, onion, lemon juice, ginger, salt, and basil into a bowl and stir well.
2. Spoon the mixture into the jars. Tighten the lids and place them on your countertop for 2 – 3 days.
3. Stir daily. Remove any mold that may appear on top.
4. Chill until ready to use. Use within 2 – 3 weeks.
5. Make sure to put the name and date on the jar.

Nutritional values:
Calories: 302
Fat: 7 g
Carbs: 26 g
Protein 35

4. Brandied Fruit

Preparation time: 60 minutes
Fermentation time: 40 days
Servings: About 1 quart

Ingredients:

- 4 ½ c. diced fruits (use any one type of fruit or mixture of fruits) of your choice
- 2 ½ c. firmly packed light brown sugar
- 2 ½ c. sugar
- 2 c. brandy

Directions:

1. Add fruits, brown sugar, and sugar into a bowl and mix well. Cover the bowl and place it on your countertop for an hour. Toss the fruit mixture after every 15 minutes.
2. Transfer the mixture into the jar. Add brandy and stir. The fruits should be covered in brandy. Fasten the lid.
3. Place the jar in a dry, cool area for about 40 days.
4. This jar is to be placed at room temperature. It can last for four months.
5. Add more fruits to replace the used ones when you use some fruits. If you add a cup of fruit, add ¼ cup of white sugar and ¼ cup of brown sugar and some brandy to cover the fruits.

Nutritional values:

Calories: 138
Carbohydrates: 32.2 g
Protein: 3.8 g
Fat: 0.4 g
Fiber: 7.4 g
Sugar: 14.6 g

5. Figs with Onions & Cardamom Ferment

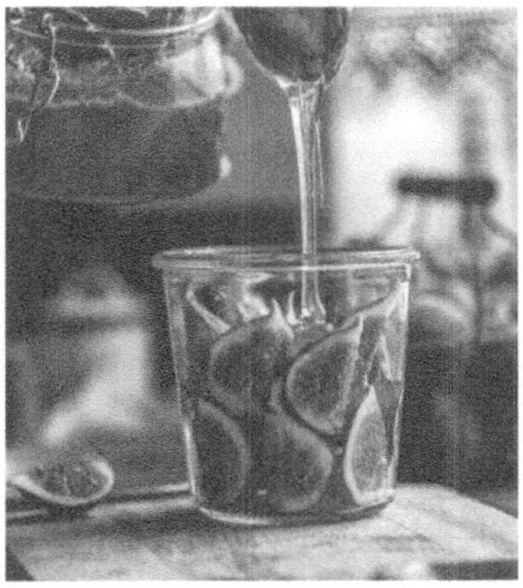

Preparation time: 10 minutes
Fermentation time: 6 days
Servings: 2 quarts

Ingredients:

- 4 tbsp. sea salt
- 16 to 20 whole, firm figs
- 2 sticks cinnamon
- 10 to 12 cardamom pods, slightly crushed

- 1 tbsp. organic green tea leaves
- 7 c. boiled water
- 1 small shallot or red onion, thinly sliced

Directions:

1. Combine salt and boiling water in a bowl.
2. Add onion, green tea leaves, and spices into the jar. Place the figs in the jar. There should be enough figs to fill the jar up to the top, leaving 2 inches of headspace.
3. Place the fermentation lid on the jar without using the spring. Fasten the moat and mason ring. The moat is to be filled and the cap placed on the bottle.
4. Set aside the jar on your countertop for 5 to 6 days. Now remove the fermentation lid and place the original lid of the jar.
5. Place the jar in the refrigerator for 2 to 3 days.
6. The figs are ready to use now.
7. Keep the jar refrigerated. It can last for about a month.

Nutritional values:

Calories: 199
Fats: 27 g
Carbs: 10.8 g
Protein: 27 g
Fiber: 10 g

6. Mixed Fruit Chutney

Preparation time: 15 minutes
Fermentation time: 3 days
Servings: 4

Ingredients:

- 2 c. chopped mixed fruit of your choice
- ½ red pepper, chopped
- 2 small cloves of garlic, minced
- ¼ c. raisins
- Juice of a lemon
- Zest of a lemon, grated
- ½ tsp. mustard seeds
- Salt to taste
- ½ c. chopped red onion
- ½ jalapeño, minced (optional)
- 1 tbsp. minced fresh ginger
- 2 tbsp. ginger bug
- ¼ tsp. ground cinnamon
- ½ tbsp. sugar

Directions:

1. Add fruits, onion, sugar, ginger, garlic, mustard, ginger bug, salt, red pepper, cinnamon, lemon juice, and zest into a bowl. Mix until well combined. Add more seasonings if required.
2. Transfer into a jar.
3. If there isn't sufficient liquid in the jar (the liquid in the jar should cover the fruits), pour three to four tablespoons of water into the jar.
4. Tighten the lids and place them on your countertop for 2 – 3 days.
5. Stir daily. Remove any mold that may appear on top.
6. Chill until ready to use. Use within 2 – 3 weeks.
7. Make sure to put the name and date on the jar.

Nutritional values:

Calories: 199
Fats: 27 g
Carbs: 10.8 g
Protein: 27 g
Fiber: 10 g

7. Peach Chutney

Preparation time: 15 minutes
Fermentation time: 2 – 3 days
Servings: 2 quarts

Ingredients:

- 8 peaches, pitted, chopped
- 1 c. chopped pecans
- ½ c. lemon juice (about 5 lemons)
- 1 c. raisins
- 1 ¼ tbsp. sea salt or to taste
- 2 onions, chopped
- 2 hot peppers, sliced
- 2 tbsp. grated fresh ginger
- 2 c. water

Directions:

1. Add peaches, pecans, lemon juice, raisins, onion, hot pepper, and ¼ tablespoon of salt and ginger into the mixing bowl and mix well.
2. Spoon the mixture into the jar. Tighten the lids and shake the jar.
3. Add water and one tablespoon of salt into a bowl and stir until salt dissolves completely.
4. Pour the brine into the jar, all over the mixture. Press the vegetables with a spoon so that the liquid comes up. Place the jar someplace warm, without sunlight falling on it.
5. Taste it after two days and decide if you want to ferment it for a couple more days.
6. If you are happy with the fermentation, place the jar in the refrigerator until use. Use within 2 – 3 weeks.
7. Make sure to label the bottles with their name and date.

Nutritional values:

Calories: 138

Carbohydrates

32.2 g

Protein: 3.8 g
Fat: 0.4 g
Fiber: 7.4 g
Sugar: 14.6 g

8. Rumtopf

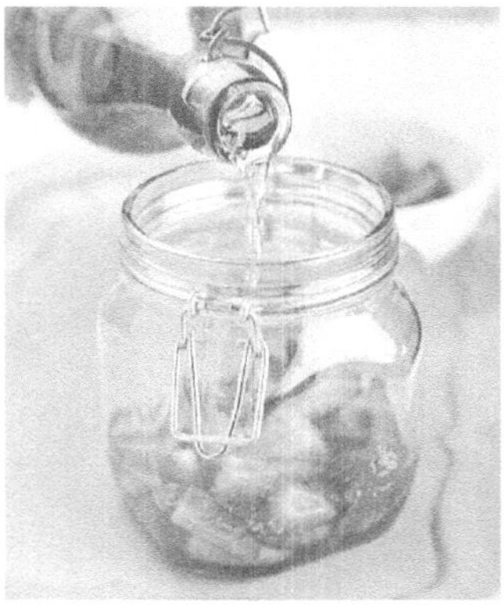

Preparation time: 30 minutes
Fermentation time: 6 months
Servings: 6 quarts

Ingredients:

To start Rumtopf:

- 1 lb. mixture of soft fruits like cherries, raspberries, plums, berries, peaches, red and black currants
- 4 c. strong dark rum
- 6 oz. sugar

To add later:

- Dark rum, if required
- ½ lb. seasonal fruit of your choice (to be added every month for 4 – 5 months)
- 3 oz. sugar (to be added each time ½ lb. fruit is added)

Directions:

1. Start making this recipe 4 – 6 months before Christmas.
2. If the fruits you use have pits or stones, remove them, and add them to a bowl.
3. Add sugar and toss well. Stir in the rum.
4. Once well combined, cover and set aside for 8 – 9 hours.
5. Transfer the fruit mixture into the jar.
6. Place fermentation weights in the jar. Fasten the lid. Place the jar in a dry, cool place.
7. Add seasonal fruit and sugar every 3 – 4 weeks and mix well. Add rum if necessary to cover the fruits. Place fermentation weights in the jar. Fasten the lid. You mustn't forget to place the jar someplace cool and dry each time.

Nutritional values:
Calories: 199
Fats: 27 g
Carbs: 10.8 g
Protein: 27 g
Fiber: 10 g

9. Spiced Pickled Cherries

Preparation time: 20 minutes
Fermentation time: 30 days
Servings: 2 quarts

Ingredients:

- 2 lb. cherries, discard stems, rinsed, pat dried
- 2 c. water
- 4 tsp. black peppercorns
- 1 tsp. red pepper flakes (optional)
- 2 c. cider vinegar
- ⅔ c. sugar
- 2 tsp. coriander seeds
- 1 stick of cinnamon, broken into 4 pieces
- 4 – 6 whole cloves
- 4 pods cardamom

Directions:

1. Pour vinegar and water into a saucepan. Add sugar and spices and place the saucepan over medium flame.
2. When it begins to boil, lower the flame and simmer for 10 – 12 minutes.
3. Meanwhile, make sure that the cherries are well dried. Remove the pit from the cherries. It can be done easily with a cherry pitter.
4. Add the cherries along with the juice into the jars. Add equal quantities in each jar.
5. Drizzle equal amounts of the vinegar mixture into the jars, ensuring a piece of cinnamon, cardamom, and a clove in each jar.
6. Fasten the lid and place the jar on your countertop to cool completely.
7. Place the jar in the refrigerator for 1 -4 weeks, depending on how you like it.
8. It can last for 2 – 3 months.

Nutritional values:

Calories: 183
Fats: 23 g
Carbs: 21 g
Protein: 23 g
Fiber: 3 g

10. Umeboshi (Pickled Ume Plum)

Preparation time: 15 minutes
Fermentation time: 60 days
Servings: 2 quarts

Ingredients:

- 2 lb. unripe ume plums or apricots, remove stems
- ½ c. neutral alcohol like vodka
- 4 oz. salt
- 10 – 20 red shiso or perilla leaves (optional)

Directions:

1. Add plums into a large bowl. Pour enough water to cover the plums. Let it soak for 9 – 10 hours.
2. Place a layer of plums in the jar. Sprinkle a little salt over it. Repeat this layering of plums and salt until all of it is added.
3. Fasten the lid and place the jar on your countertop. Let it ferment for three weeks.
4. Now take out the plums from the jar and retain the liquid from the jar.
5. Place the plums on a screen, without overlapping, in the sun during the day. Take it back to your countertop during the night. Do this (drying in the sun) for three days.
6. By the end of 3 days, the plums would have shrunk, and salt will be visible on the plums.
7. Now add the plums back into the jar. Add the red shiso leaves as well and mix.
8. Fasten the jar's lid and place it at room temperature for 1 – 2 months.
9. It is now ready to use.

Nutritional values:

Calories: 183
Fats: 23 g
Carbs: 21 g
Protein: 23 g
Fiber: 3 g

11. Lacto-Fermented Raspberry Preserves

Preparation time: 10 minutes
Fermentation time: 2 days
Servings: 3 quarts

Ingredients:

- 12 c. fresh raspberries
- 3 tsp. sea salt
- 6 tsp. Pomona's pectin
- ¾ c. palm sugar or Rapadura
- 12 tbsp. whey liquid
- 6 tsp. calcium water (which comes along with the pectin)

Directions:

1. Add raspberries, salt, pectin, sugar, whey liquid, and calcium water into a bowl and mash with the potato masher until raspberries are crushed. Let a few remain chunky.
2. Transfer into the jar. Ensure that there is at least an inch of headspace on top.
3. Fasten the lid and place the jar at room temperature for several days.
4. You might find some scum on top. Remove it if it is there.
5. When active fermentation stops, place the jar in the refrigerator.
6. It can last for two months. To make it last longer, transfer the berries into a freezer-safe container and freeze. It can last for 6 – 8 months.
7. Make sure to put the name and date on the jar.

Nutritional values:

Calories: 138
Carbohydrates: 32.2 g
Protein: 3.8 g
Fat: 0.4 g
Fiber: 7.4 g
Sugar: 14.6 g

12. Fermented Strawberry Preserves

Preparation time: 20 minutes
Fermentation time: 3 days
Servings: 2 quarts

Ingredients:

- 8 c. sliced strawberries
- 2 small green apples, grated
- Juice of a lemon
- 1 c. honey
- 1 tsp. Himalayan pink salt
- 4 tbsp. whey liquid

Directions:

1. Add strawberries, apples, lemon juice, and honey into the pot and mix well, mashing slightly with the back of a spoon.
2. Cook over low heat. Do this until the sauce thickens. Then, take the pot away from the heat and set aside to completely cool.
3. Add whey and salt and mix well.
4. Fasten the fermentation lid and place the jar at room temperature for 2 – 3 days or until you are satisfied with the fermentation.
5. Remove this lid, place the jar's original lid, and fix it tightly.
6. Chill until ready to use.
7. Make sure to put the name and date on the jar.

Nutrition values:

Calories: 361
Total Fat: 16.3 g
Saturated Fat: 4.9 g
Cholesterol: 114 mg
Sodium: 515 mg
Total Carbs: 19.3 g
Fiber: 0.1 g
Sugar: 18.2 g
Protein: 33.3 g

13. Strawberry Chia Jam

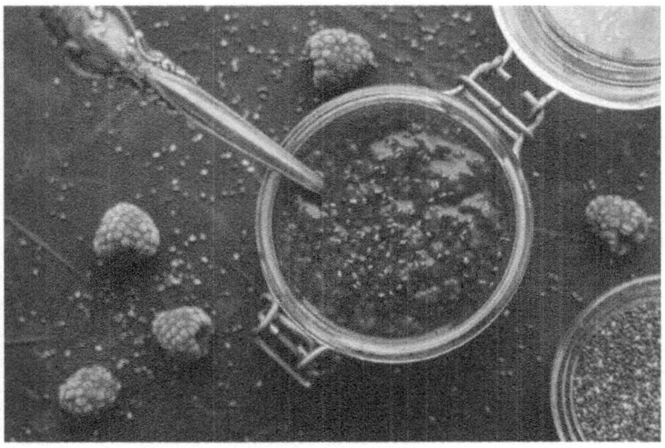

Preparation time: 15 minutes
Fermentation time: 2 days

Ingredients:

- 4 c. organic strawberries
- 4 tbsp. chia seeds
- ½ c. kombucha or whey liquid or water kefir
- 4 tbsp. sugar or honey
- 4 tsp. sea salt

Directions:

1. Add strawberries into a bowl. Scatter sugar and salt over it. Chill overnight.
2. Transfer the strawberries to the pan. Place the pan over medium flame. Stir constantly until sugar dissolves.
3. Turn up the heat and bring it to a rapid boil. Allow it to boil for 5 minutes. Turn off the heat and set aside for 10 to 12 minutes to cool.
4. Stir in chia seeds and kombucha. Let it cool for another 10 minutes.
5. Spoon the mixture into jam jars. Tighten the lids and place them on your countertop for two days. Open the jar on the second day to remove any built-up gasses.
6. Refrigerate the jam until use. It can last for two months.
7. Make sure to label the jars with their name and date.

Nutrition values:
Calories: 350
Total Fats: 24 g
Carbs: 6 g
Protein: 26 g
Fiber: 2 g

14. Chia Plum Jam

Preparation time: 20 minutes
Fermentation time: 3 days
Servings: 5 ounces

Ingredients:

- 1 lb. red, ripe, firm plums, pitted, chopped
- ½ tbsp. Kombucha or whey liquid or sauerkraut juice
- ¼ c. chia seeds + 1 – 2 tbsp. extra if required
- 2 – 4 mint sprigs
- ¼ c. raw honey
- ¼ tsp. salt
- A tiny pinch of ground cardamom (optional)
- A tiny pinch of ground cloves (optional)

Directions:

1. Combine plum, salt, honey, kombucha, mint, and ¼ cup of chia seeds into a bowl.
2. Add spices if used and mix well.
3. Spoon the mixture into jam jars. Tighten the lids and place them in a cool, dark area for three days. Open the jar on the second and third day and stir the jam. Do this at least twice daily.
4. Discard the mint sprigs.
5. If you think the jam is not thick enough, add 1 – 2 tablespoons of chia seeds and mix well. Tighten the lid of the jar.
6. Refrigerate the jam until use. It can last for two months.
7. Make sure to label the jars with their name and date.

Nutrition values:
Calories: 350
Total Fats: 24 g
Carbs: 6 g
Protein: 26 g
Fiber: 2 g

15. Blueberry Jam

Preparation time: 10 minutes
Fermentation time: 2 days
Servings: About 2 cups

Ingredients:

- 1 lb. blueberries
- ½ tsp. sea salt
- 6 tbsp. honey or sucanat
- 3 tbsp. whey or water kefir

Directions:

1. Add strawberries, salt, and honey into the saucepan and mix well, mashing slightly with the back of a spoon.
2. Cook for 5 minutes on low heat in a saucepan. Remove from the heat and set aside to cool completely.
3. Add whey and mix well.
4. Spoon the mixture into jam jars. Tighten the lids and place them on your countertop for two days. Open the jar on the second day to remove any built-up gasses.
5. Refrigerate the jam until use. It can last for two months.
6. Make sure to label the jars with their name and date.

Nutrition values:
Calories: 170
Total Fats: 19.2 g
Carbs: 0.5 g
Protein: 35 g
Fiber: 0 g

CHAPTER 3: VEGETABLE RECIPES

52. Cabbage Sauerkraut

Preparation time: 15 minutes
Fermentation time: 3 days
Servings: 4 quarts

Ingredients:

- 2 medium heads of green cabbage (about 3 lb. each), thinly sliced into ribbons
- 2 tbsp. caraway seeds (optional)
- 3 tbsp. kosher salt
- 3 tbsp. dill (optional)

Equipment:

- Bowl
- 2 Masons jars (1 ½ quart each)
- Fermentation weights
- Rubber band
- Cotton cloth

Directions:

1. Add salt and cabbage into a bowl and toss well. Massage the cabbage using your hands for about 8 – 10 minutes. In a while, the cabbage will become softer and will release water.
2. Add caraway seeds and dill and stir well. Transfer the cabbage into the jar. Place one large cabbage leaf on top of the sliced cabbage and place the fermentation weight on the cabbage leaf.
3. Keep the jar covered with cloth and fasten it with a rubber band. Set aside the jar for 24 hours.
4. Press the cabbage every 2 hours or so. The cabbage should sink in the liquid.
5. Once 24 hours have passed, check for the liquid in the jar; if it is not over the cabbage, combine two cups of water and two teaspoons of salt in a bowl and pour as much as required to keep the cabbage below the water level.
6. Cover it with the cloth again and place it at room temperature for 3 – 10 days. Make sure that there is no sunlight falling on the jar.
7. Taste the sauerkraut daily, from the 3rd day. When you are happy with the fermentation, remove the fermentation weights. Place the original lid of the jar and fasten the lid.
8. Transfer the jar to the refrigerator. It can last for 4 – 5 months.
9. If you see any scum or mold floating, remove it.

Nutrition values:

Calories: 213
Total Fat: 7.5 g
Saturated Fat: 1.1 g
Cholesterol: 20 mg
Sodium: 297 mg
Total Carbs: 10.4 g
Fiber: 0.2 g
Sugar: 0.1 g
Protein: 13.1 g

53. Vegetable Sauerkraut

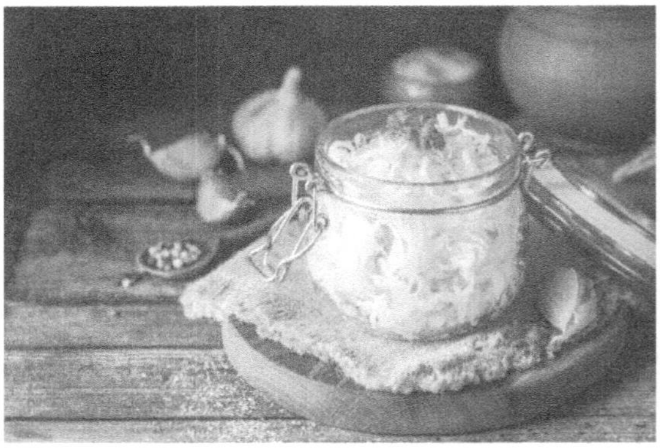

Preparation time: 15 minutes
Servings: 1 quart

Ingredients:

- 4 c. finely grated or chopped red or green cabbage
- ½ medium beet, finely shredded
- 1 ½ tbsp. grated ginger
- 2 medium carrots, finely shredded
- 2 cloves of garlic, minced
- 1 ½ tbsp. grated, fresh turmeric
- 1 tsp. Sea salt or more to taste

Equipment:

- Bowl
- 1 Masons jar (1 ½ qt. size)
- Fermentation weights
- Rubber band
- Cotton cloth

Directions:

1. Add salt and cabbage into a bowl and toss well. Massage the cabbage using your hands for about 8 – 10 minutes. In a while, the cabbage will become softer and will release water.
2. Add beets, ginger, garlic, turmeric, and carrots and stir well. Massage the vegetables once again.

3. Transfer the vegetables into the jar. Place one large cabbage leaf on top of the vegetables and the fermentation weight on the cabbage leaf.
4. Keep the jar covered with cloth and fasten it with a rubber band. Set aside the jar for 24 hours.
5. Press the mixture every 2 hours or so. The vegetable mixture should sink into the liquid.
6. Once 24 hours have passed, check for the liquid in the jar; if it is not over the mixture, combine two cups of water and two teaspoons of salt in a bowl and pour as much as required to keep the mixture below the water level.
7. Cover it with the cloth again and place it at room temperature for 3 – 10 days. Make sure that there is no sunlight falling on the jar.
8. Taste the sauerkraut daily, from the 3rd day. When you are happy with the fermentation, remove the fermentation weights. Place the original lid of the jar and fasten the lid.
9. Transfer the jar to the refrigerator. It can last for 4 – 5 months.
10. If you see any scum or mold floating, remove it.

Nutrition values:

Calories: 100
Total Fats: 9 g
Carbs: 75 g
Protein: 7 g
Fiber: 1 g

4. Transfer the mixture into the jar. Place one large cabbage leaf on top of the mixture and place the fermentation weight on the cabbage leaf.
5. Keep the jar covered with cloth and fasten it with a rubber band. Set aside the jar for 24 hours.
6. Press the mixture with a wooden spoon every 2 hours or so. The mixture should sink into the liquid.
7. After 24 hours, check for the liquid in the jar; if it is not over the mixture, combine two cups of water and two teaspoons of salt in a bowl and pour as much as required to keep the mixture below the water level.
8. Cover it with the cloth again and place it at room temperature for 3 – 15 days. Make sure that there is no sunlight falling on the jar.
9. Taste the sauerkraut daily, from the 3rd day. When you are happy with the fermentation, remove the fermentation weights, and fasten the original lid of the jar.
10. Transfer the jar to the refrigerator. Let it remain in the refrigerator for at least a week before serving. It can last for 4 – 5 months.
11. If you see any scum or mold floating, remove it.

Nutrition values:

Calories: 321
Total Fats: 11 g
Carbs: 28 g
Protein: 31 g
Fiber: 1 g

54. Apple & Daikon Radish Sauerkraut

Preparation time: 15 minutes
Fermentation time: 3 days
Servings: 4 quarts

Ingredients:

- One head of green cabbage, cut into thin ribbons
- 4 medium daikon radishes with some of its greens, cut into matchsticks
- 2 firm apples, cored, cut into matchsticks
- 4 tbsp. pickling spice blend
- 2 tbsp. Himalayan pink salt

Equipment:

- Bowl
- 2 Masons jars (1 ½ quart each)
- Fermentation weights
- Rubber band
- Cotton cloth

Directions:

1. Add radish, apple, salt, and cabbage into a bowl and toss well. Sprinkle the pickling spice, blend over the mixture, and toss well.
2. Massage the mixture using your hands for about 8 – 10 minutes. In a while, the mixture will become softer and will release water.
3. Pound the mixture with a pestle until well-mashed.

55. Easy Fermented Vegetables

Preparation time: 15 minutes
Fermentation time: 5 days
Servings: 4 quarts

Ingredients:

- 2 tbsp. Himalayan Sea salt or pickling salt
- 5 c. small cauliflower florets
- 2 carrots, cut into strips
- 20 cloves of garlic, peeled
- 2 tbsp. black peppercorns
- 2 qt. water
- 12 radishes, quartered
- 2 c. green beans, trimmed, cut into 2-inch pieces
- 10 whole green chilies

Equipment:

- Bowl
- 1 Masons jar (2 ½ qt. size)

Directions:

1. Add salt and water into a bowl and mix well until salt dissolves completely.
2. Add all the vegetables and black peppercorns into the jar. Pour brine over the vegetables in the jar. The vegetables should be covered in water so add more water if required.

3. Fasten the lid of the jar and place it on your countertop for 2 to 3 days. Transfer the jar into the refrigerator when you are happy with the fermentation. Let it remain in the refrigerator for at least a few days before serving. It can last for about one month.
4. If you see any scum or mold floating, remove it.

Nutrition values:

Calories: 321
Total Fats: 11 g
Carbs: 28 g
Protein: 31 g
Fiber: 1 g

56. Basil Leaves

Preparation time: 15 minutes
Fermentation time: 3 days
Servings: 4 quarts

Ingredients:

- Basil, whole leaves
- Salt, non-iodizing

Directions:

1. Mix basil leaves with salt and massage lightly. A brown juice will come out, and leaves will shrink, which is expected.
2. Put leaves in the jar and squeeze out bubbles as much as possible.
3. Cover with a weight to keep basil under the brine. Add water as needed.
4. Throw the lid on (not too tight) and let ferment at room temperature for 1-2 weeks.
5. Once the preferred taste is achieved, tighten the lid, and put it in the fridge.

Nutrition values:

Calories: 182
Total Fats: 9 g
Carbs: 10 g
Protein: 27 g
Fiber: 0.2 g

57. Fermented Carrots with Galangal and Lime

Preparation time: 15 minutes
Fermentation time: 5 days
Servings: 4 quarts

Ingredients:

- 2 lb. carrots, cut into ¼-inch thick slices
- 2 tbsp. grated lime zest
- 2 tbsp. thinly sliced galangal or ginger
- 4 tsp. pickling salt

Equipment: 1 Masons jar (2 ½ qt. size)

Directions:

1. Add pickling salt and water into the saucepan. Place the saucepan over medium flame and mix well until salt dissolves completely. Turn off the flame and let the solution cool completely.
2. Add all the vegetables and black peppercorns into the jar. Pour brine over the vegetables in the jar. The vegetables should be covered in water so add more water if required.
3. Fasten the lid of the jar and place it on your countertop for 2 to 3 days. Transfer the jar into the refrigerator when you are happy with the fermentation. Let it remain in the refrigerator for at least a few days before serving. It can last for about one month.
4. If you see any scum or mold floating, remove it.

Nutrition values:

Calories: 213
Total Fat: 7.5 g
Saturated Fat: 1.1 g
Cholesterol: 20 mg
Sodium: 297 mg
Total Carbs: 10.4 g
Fiber: 0.2 g
Sugar: 0.1 g
Protein: 13.1 g

58. Green Beans

Preparation time: 15 minutes
Fermentation time: 3 days
Servings: 5 quarts

Ingredients:

- 1 tsp. non-iodized salt
- 2 cloves of garlic, crushed
- ½ tsp. red chili flakes
- ½ tsp. mustard seeds
- 2 lb. green beans

Directions:

1. Add mustard seeds and red chili flakes to the jar.
2. Pack in green beans and add crushed garlic halfway through.
3. Add in the remaining green beans, leaving 2 inches of headspace.
4. Add brine (one cup of water to one teaspoon of salt) until beans are covered.
5. Place the weight on the beans to keep them submerged. Then, seal the jar with a lid.
6. Set on the kitchen counter to ferment at room temperature. For half a gallon jar, it takes ten days to ferment.
7. Unseal jars to release the gas buildup every day before sealing again.
8. The beans are ready when the brine becomes foggy and then clear up again. Store in fridge.

Nutrition values:

Calories: 182
Total Fats: 9 g
Carbs: 10 g
Protein: 27 g
Fiber: 0.2 g

59. Lacto-Fermented Dill Pickled Cucumbers

Preparation time: 15 minutes
Fermentation time: 3 days
Servings: 4 quarts

Ingredients:

- 2 tbsp. mustard seeds
- 2-3 tbsp. pickling spices
- 1-2 tsp. dried thyme
- 1 white onion, chopped
- 8 garlic cloves
- Salt, non-iodized
- 3 lb. small cucumbers

Directions:

1. Clean and trim ends of cucumbers.
2. In a big pot, add water and salt, and bring to a boil. Each quart of water needs 2 tbsp of salt. Make sure the salt completely dissolves.
3. When water starts boiling, remove from pot and let cool.
4. Place dill on the bottom of the jar, add some onion, a couple of garlic cloves, a few mustard seeds, thyme, and pickling spices.
5. Add cucumbers to the bowl, leaving 2 inches of headspace. Add more garlic and onions on top, then dill.
6. Pour brine over, submerging everything.
7. Seal the jars and place them outside at a warm temperature. You should see bubbles after a few days and unseal them a bit to let the gas out before sealing again.
8. Allow fermenting for about six days. The liquid should become cloudy. After the third day, do a taste test.
9. Throw in the fridge when at the right texture and taste.

Nutrition values:

Calories: 100
Total Fats: 9 g
Carbs: 75 g
Protein: 7 g
Fiber: 1 g

60. Lacto-Fermented Lettuce

Preparation time: 15 minutes
Fermentation time: 3 days
Servings: 4 quarts

Ingredients:

- Lettuce
- Sea salt
- Water

Directions:

1. Wash lettuce and discard any brown leaves.
2. Layer lettuce in a large vessel, sprinkle lightly with salt, and add another layer. For every quart of lettuce, use 2 tbsp salt. Mix and salt all layers and add more salt until you can taste the saltiness.
3. Weigh down the veggies in an open bowl or crock.
4. The brine will begin to form, and the lettuce should be covered in brine after 24 hours. If not, add some brine (one-quart water to one tablespoon of salt). Lettuce should be 2 inches below the brine.
5. Ferment for several days until the right texture and taste are achieved, then move to jars and cold storage.

Nutrition values:

Calories: 210
Total Fats: 21 g
Carbs: 9.3 g
Protein: 18 g
Fiber: 0 g

61. Pickled Onions

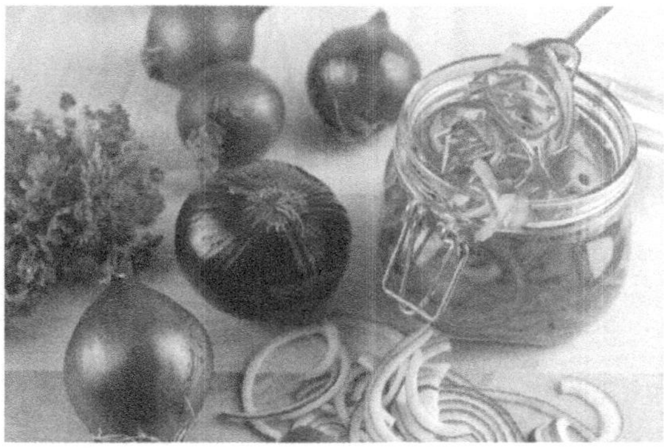

Preparation time: 15 minutes
Fermentation time: 3 days
Servings: 4 quarts

Ingredients:

- 3 c. onions, peeled
- 2 tbsp. salt
- 4 c. water

Directions:

1. Prepare the onions and add them to the jar, leaving 1-inch headspace.
2. Combine salt and water and pour into the jar.
3. Seal jar with lid and store in a dark place. Open once a day to release gas before sealing again.
4. Repeat for 3-4 weeks until there are no more bubbles.
5. Store in fridge.

Nutrition values:

Calories: 210
Total Fats: 21 g
Carbs: 9.3 g
Protein: 18 g
Fiber: 0 g

62. Pickled Zucchini

Preparation time: 15 minutes
Fermentation time: 3 – 5 days
Servings: 4 quarts

Ingredients:

- 5 sterilized canning jars with lids and rings
- 1 extra-large sliced zucchini, peeled and cut into thirds
- 1 sliced onion
- 1 sliced carrot
- 5 peeled and sliced garlic cloves
- 1 bunch of fresh dill, chopped
- 15 whole allspice berries
- 5 bay leaves
- 15 whole black peppercorns
- ½ oz. mustard seed

For the Brine:

- 32 oz. water
- 8 oz. white vinegar
- 1 oz. salt
- 10 oz. superfine sugar

Directions:

1. Remove seeds from the zucchini and slice into thin strips
2. Sterilize jars following the canning method.
3. Evenly distribute onion, carrot, garlic, and dill between the jars. Add zucchini to the jars and pack vertically.
4. Evenly distribute peppercorns, berries, mustard, and bay leaves in the jars.
5. Pour brine ingredients into a pan and bring to a boil. Stir for 1-2 minutes until sugar and salt dissolve.
6. Remove brine from heat and spoon into jars, leaving ¼" of space at the top.
7. Seal jars according to the method for canning

Nutrition values:

Calories: 100
Total Fats: 9 g
Carbs: 75 g
Protein: 7 g
Fiber: 1 g

63. Refrigerator Rainbow Carrot Pickles

Preparation time: 15 minutes
Fermentation time: 3 – 5 days
Servings: 4 quarts

Ingredients:

- 32 oz. Multi-colored carrots, scrubbed but not peeled
- ⅓ oz. White sugar
- ⅔ oz. pickling salt, divided
- ½ tsp. whole cloves
- 8 oz. water
- 12 oz. white wine vinegar
- 4 oz. honey

Directions:

1. Rinse carrots and drain. Slice carrots in ⅛" thick medallions and discard the tops.
2. Place carrots in a colander placed in a large bowl. Pour sugar and one teaspoon of salt into the carrots and toss. Let the mixture sit for 1 hour, rinse and drain.
3. Place cloves in a non-reactive 96-ounce pot on medium heat. Shake the pan for 1 minute until cloves are fragrant.
4. Slowly pour water into the pot. Add vinegar, honey, and the rest of the salt to the mixture and stir. Bring to a boil.
5. Add carrots and cook for 8 minutes, often stirring, until mixture returns to a simmer.
6. Scoop carrots into sterilized jars and pack them into the jars. Pour brine over the carrots, leaving ½" of space on the top of the jar. Apply and seal lids.
7. Place in the refrigerator for 24-48 hours before serving.
8. Stores for one month in the refrigerator.

Nutrition values:

Calories: 188
Total Fat: 8.5 g
Saturated Fat: 3 g
Cholesterol: 102 mg
Sodium: 115 mg
Total Carbs: 20.2 g
Fiber: 2.1 g
Sugar: 14.9 g
Protein: 32.7 g

64. Spicy Dill Avocado Pickles

Preparation time: 15 minutes
Fermentation time: 3 – 5 days
Servings: 4 quarts

Ingredients:

- 10 oz. distilled white vinegar
- 8 oz. filtered water
- 4 oz. white sugar
- 1 tsp. brown mustard seeds
- 1 tsp. rock salt
- 1 tsp. fresh dill, chopped
- ½ tsp. habanero pepper flakes
- ½ tsp. whole black peppercorns
- 2 habanero peppers
- 1 smashed garlic clove, cut in half
- 2 peeled unripe avocados, sliced into eighths

Directions:

1. Mix vinegar and water in a pan.
2. Add sugar, salt, mustard, dill, pepper, and pepper flakes. Bring mixture to a boil. Stir until sugar and salt dissolve.
3. Remove pan from heat and cool for 15 minutes.
4. Evenly distribute habanero peppers and garlic cloves between 2 jars
5. Pour hot liquid into the jars, leaving ¼" of space at the top
6. Place in the refrigerator for 24-48 hours before using.

Nutrition values:

Calories: 188
Total Fat: 8.5 g
Saturated Fat: 3 g
Cholesterol: 102 mg
Sodium: 115 mg
Total Carbs: 20.2 g
Fiber: 2.1 g
Sugar: 14.9 g
Protein: 32.7 g

65. Tangy Pickled Onions

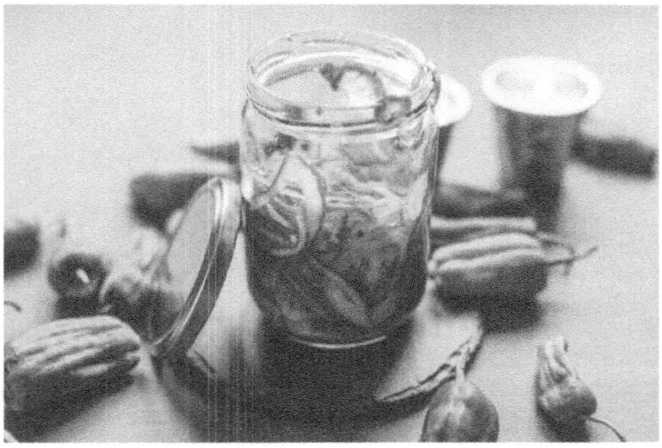

Preparation time: 15 minutes
Fermentation time: 3 days
Servings: 4 quarts

Ingredients:

- 4 canning jars with lids and rings, 1 pint
- 1 tsp. celery seed
- 1 tsp. yellow mustard seed
- 4 whole allspice berries
- 1 tsp. black peppercorns
- 40 oz. trimmed green onions, trimmed, sliced into 3" pieces
- 24 oz. water
- 24 oz. white vinegar
- ¾ oz. kosher salt

Directions:

1. Combine celery, mustard seeds, peppercorns, and allspice in a bowl and stir well.
2. Evenly distribute spice mixture among the sterilized canning jars.
3. Pack onions in the jars vertically.
4. Combine vinegar, water, and salt in a saucepan and bring to a boil. Pour hot brine into the jars, leaving ½" of space at the top. Seal and process jars.
5. Store jars in a cool dark place for one month before consuming.

Nutrition values:

Calories: 188
Total Fat: 8.5 g
Saturated Fat: 3 g
Cholesterol: 102 mg
Sodium: 115 mg
Total Carbs: 20.2 g
Fiber: 2.1 g
Sugar: 14.9 g
Protein: 32.7 g

66. White Kimchi

Preparation time: 15 minutes
Fermentation time: 3 days
Servings: 4 quarts

Ingredients:

- 1 head napa cabbage
- 1 ½ oz. salt
- 8 oz. water and more to cover
- 8 oz. white radish, thinly grated
- 2 sliced green onions, cut into thin strips diagonally
- 2 minced garlic cloves
- 2 slices of fresh ginger
- 1 tsp. granulated sugar
- 1 tsp. white vinegar
- 1 tsp. salt
- 3 pinches of dried Korean red pepper threads

Directions:

1. Keeping the leaves attached, slice cabbage along the length and then into quarters.
2. Rinse cold water and sprinkle 1 ½ ounce of salt between the cabbage leaves.
3. Put cabbage in a bowl and pour in enough water to cover. Let the cabbage stand for 5 hours until the leaves are tender.
4. Place salted cabbage in a colander and rinse with cold water 4-5 times. Drain in the colander for 20 minutes.
5. Mix 8 ounces of water, onions, radish, ginger, garlic, and sugar. Also, add one teaspoon of salt, vinegar, and pepper threads to a large bowl.
6. Distribute radish mixture between the cabbage leaves except for the large outer leaves.
7. Reserve juice from the radish mix.
8. Peel each large outer leaf, but leave it attached to the core.
9. Fold the inner leaves of the cabbage in half.
10. Wrap the outer leaf around the inner leaves and pack them into the sterilized canning jars.
11. Pour the juice into the jars, leaving ¼" of space at the top.
12. Seal jars and store them at room temperature for 24 hours.
13. Slice cabbage into 2" pieces.

Nutrition values:

Carbs: 250.86 g
Fat: 1.9 g
Protein: 7.09 g
Calories: 971

CHAPTER 4: MEAT AND FISH RECIPES

98. Cured Fermented Beef

Preparation time: 15 minutes
Fermentation time: 3 days
Servings: 4 quarts

Ingredients:

- 1 lb. ground beef
- 3.5 lb. cooked, sliced pork skin
- ½ tsp. salt or to taste
- 2 – 3 cloves garlic, peeled
- A handful of Vietnamese cilantro leaves
- 1 package of Nam powder seasoning mix
- 3 tbsp. sugar
- Crushed black pepper to taste
- Thai chili to taste

Equipment:

- Pan
- Large bowl

Directions:

1. Add pork skin and ⅛ teaspoon of salt into a pan. Place the pan over medium flame and cook for a couple of minutes. Turn off the heat and rinse the skin in cold water. Shake the skin to remove extra water.
2. Add the skin into a bowl. Add beef, sugar, pepper, and seasoning mix and mix well.
3. Cover and set aside for 24 hours. The color of the meat will change to brown in 24 hours.
4. Line a baking pan with cling wrap. Spread the meat mixture in the pan and spread it well. Wrap the meat with cling wrap. Spread it evenly with your hands.
5. Place something heavy on the wrapped meat and set it aside for 24 hours.
6. Unwrap the meat. Chop into bite-size pieces.
7. Slice the garlic and chili into thin slices. Chop the cilantro into small pieces.
8. Combine garlic, cilantro, and chili in a bowl and mix well.
9. Add the chopped meat to the bowl and toss until the meat is well coated with the mixture.
10. You can make the same recipe using ground pork instead of ground beef.

Nutritional values:

Calories: 18
Carbohydrates: 2.9 g
Sodium: 839.3 mg
Potassium: 4.9 mg
Fiber: 0.1 g
Sugar: 2.8 g

99. Meat Garum

Preparation time: 15 minutes
Fermentation time: 3 days
Servings: 4 quarts

Ingredients:

- 1.1 lb. lean meat, cut into pieces such that it fits in the meat grinder
- 1 ¾ c. of water
- 4.2 oz. kosher salt
- 3.5 oz. koji rice

Equipment:

- Meat grinder
- Fermentation container with lid
- Dehydrator
- Storage jar
- Cheesecloth

Directions:

1. Combine meat and koji rice and add to the meat grinder. Grind the meat and add to a bowl. Add salt and mix well.
2. Add water and mix until well combined. Transfer the mixture into the fermentation container. Press the mixture onto the bottom of the container.
3. Close the lid and place the container in the dehydrator. Adjust the temperature to 140° F. Check every few hours and remove any fat that floats. Do this for the initial seven days and every week after that until you will not find any fat floating. You may need to skim off the fat for about three weeks.
4. Once there is no fat floating, after about 1 – 2 days, tiny bubbles will be visible in the meat. This means that fermentation has started. Strain the garum after 70 days using a wire mesh strainer and place the liquid in the refrigerator. Skim off any fat that is floating.
5. Line the strainer with cheesecloth. Strain the mixture once again. Transfer into the storage jar. Make sure to label the jar with the name and date of preparation.

1. Refrigerate until use.

Nutrition values:

Calories: 188
Total Fat: 8.5 g
Saturated Fat: 3 g
Cholesterol: 102 mg
Sodium: 115 mg

Total Carbs: 20.2 g
Fiber: 2.1 g
Sugar: 14.9 g
Protein: 32.7 g

100. Fermented Thai Pork Sausage

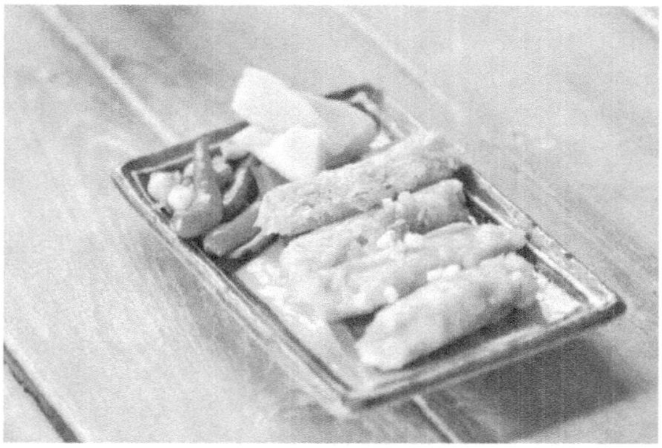

Preparation time: 15 minutes
Fermentation time: 3 days
Servings: 4 quarts

Ingredients:

- 1.1 lb. lean, minced pork meat, trimmed of fat
- 12 – 15 cloves of garlic
- 1 tsp. sugar
- ½ c. cooked, sticky rice
- 6.2 oz. pork skin
- 1 ¼ tbsp. sea salt
- ½ tsp. monosodium glutamate
- 20 bird's eye chilies
- White vinegar to clean
- Rough sea salt to clean

Equipment:

- Meat grinder
- Banana leaves of plastic wrap to wrap the sausages
- Saucepan

Directions:

1. Mince the meat in a meat grinder.
2. Using salt and vinegar, clean the pork skin. Rub the skin very well and rinse under running water.
3. Repeat the previous step a few times until the skin turns smooth.
4. Boil some water in a saucepan and add pork skin to it. Boil until the skin turns clear, and when you pinch it, it should break. This stage should reach in about 30 – 40 minutes.
5. Remove the skin and place it on your cutting board. Cut into thin strips of about 1 ½ inch in length.
6. Add minced pork, garlic, salt, monosodium glutamate, sugar, rice, and pork skin into a bowl and mix until well incorporated.
7. Place the banana leaves (7 – 8 leaves) on your countertop. Divide the sausage mixture into 7 – 8 equal portions and shape into sausages (like a log). Place one sausage on each leaf at the corner, parallel to the tip of the corner. Place a bird's eye chili on each and roll it a couple of rounds. Fold the sides inwards and continue rolling till the end. Place it with the seam side facing down.
8. Ferment it at 85° F for 3 – 5 days and humidity at 50%.

Nutrition values:

Calories: 138
Total Fat: 0.5 g
Saturated Fat: 0.1 g
Cholesterol: 0 mg
Sodium: 681 mg
Total: 27.1 g
Fiber: 5.9 g
Sugar: 6.3 g
Protein: 8.3 g

101. Salmon Gravlax

Preparation time: 15 minutes
Fermentation time: 3 days
Servings: 4 quarts

Ingredients:

- 1 ½ lb. salmon fillet, rinsed
- 1 tsp. coriander seeds
- 1 tbsp. fennel seeds
- 3 tbsp. kosher salt
- ¾ oz. vodka
- ½ bunch dill, chopped
- ½ tbsp. freshly ground pepper or to taste
- 1 tbsp. sugar
- 1 tsp. grated lemon zest
- 1 tbsp. chopped cilantro

Directions:

1. Dry the salmon by patting with paper towels.
2. Combine salt, spices, cilantro, dill, vodka, and lemon zest in a bowl.
3. Place two cling wrap sheets stacked on your cutting board. Place the salmon on the center of the sheet with the skin side facing down.
4. Spread the spice mixture over the salmon and wrap the salmon. Wrap more cling wrap over the salmon and place it on a plate. Place something heavy over it.
5. Place the salmon and the weight in the refrigerator for 12 – 16 hours.
6. It is now ready to use. It can last a week but ensure it remains wrapped in the refrigerator.

Nutrition values:

Calories: 138
Total Fat: 0.5 g
Saturated Fat: 0.1 g
Cholesterol: 0 mg
Sodium: 681 mg
Total: 27.1 g
Fiber: 5.9 g

Sugar: 6.3 g
Protein: 8.3 g

102. Fermented Beef Jerky

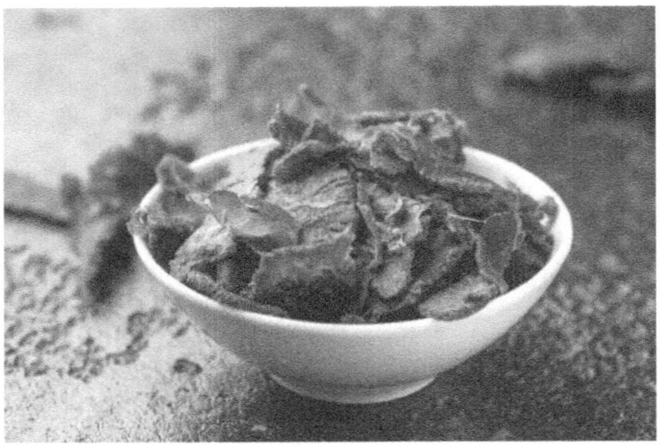

Preparation time: 15 minutes
Fermentation time: 3 days
Servings: 4 quarts

Ingredients:

- 2 lb. lean beef meat (or turkey or lamb or goat meat), trimmed of fat

For Kombucha Marinade:

- 1 c. wine
- 4 tsp. sea salt or fine salt
- ½ c. organic sugar
- ½ tsp. freshly ground pepper
- 2 tbsp. liquid smoke
- 3 c. kombucha vinegar
- 2 heads of garlic, minced
- ½ c. Worcestershire sauce
- 2 tsp. mustard seeds, slightly cracked
- 2 tsp. oregano
- 2 tsp. basil

Equipment:

- Glass container
- Dehydrator

Directions:

1. If the meat is fresh, place it in the freezer for about an hour. If the meat is frozen, remove it from the freezer and let it sit on your countertop to defrost for 3 hours.
2. To make the marinade: Add wine, sugar, and kombucha vinegar into the glass bowl and stir until sugar has dissolved. Kombucha vinegar is over-processed kombucha tea, i.e., it is fermented for longer than necessary.
3. Add the rest of the ingredients for the marinade and mix well.
4. Trim off the fat from the meat. Cut into ¼-inch slices along the grain.
5. Add the meat into the bowl of marinade and stir well. Cover the bowl and chill for 12 – 15 hours.
6. Transfer the meat into the dehydrator trays, set the temperature to 155° F, and dehydrate until crispy. It should take 14 – 16 hours, depending on the thickness of the slices.
7. Turn the meat slices over for four hours.
8. Alternately, you can place the slices on a baking sheet and bake in the oven at the lowest available setting. If your oven does not have an option of less than 155° F, keep the door slightly ajar while baking.
9. Let the jerky cool completely.
10. Transfer into a glass jar. Make sure to label the jar with the name and date of preparation.

Nutrition values:

Calories: 188
Total Fat: 8.5 g
Saturated Fat: 3 g
Cholesterol: 102 mg
Sodium: 115 mg
Total Carbs: 20.2 g
Fiber: 2.1 g
Sugar: 14.9 g
Protein: 32.7 g

103. Fermented Liver

Preparation time: 15 minutes
Fermentation time: 3 days
Servings: 4 quarts

Ingredients:

- 1 c. chopped chicken liver
- Fermenting liquid from kimchi or sauerkraut or whey liquid or kombucha

Directions:

1. Place the liver in the jar. Pour enough fermenting liquid into the jar to cover the liver.
2. Fasten the lid and place it on your countertop for 24 hours.
3. Refrigerate until use. Make sure to label the jar with the name and date of preparation.

Nutrition values:

Calories: 138
Total Fat: 0.5 g
Saturated Fat: 0.1 g
Cholesterol: 0 mg
Sodium: 681 mg
Total: 27.1 g
Fiber: 5.9 g
Sugar: 6.3 g
Protein: 8.3 g

104. Fermented Beef Liver Pate

Preparation time: 15 minutes
Fermentation time: 3 days
Servings: 4 quarts

Ingredients:

- 2 lb. raw beef liver
- Rosemary
- Cloves of garlic, peeled
- 2 tsp. Himalayan salt
- 4 tbsp. whey liquid
- 2 egg yolks
- 1 large sweet onion, chopped
- 2 tsp. peppercorns

Equipment:

- Food processor
- Mason's jar

Directions:

1. Add meat, spices, rosemary, yolks, onion, and whey into the food processor and process until smooth.
2. Transfer into the jar. Cover with a plastic lid and place it on your countertop at room temperature for 24 hours.
3. Shift the jar into the refrigerator. Make sure to label the jar with the name and date of preparation.

Nutrition values:

Calories: 22
Fat: 18 g
Carb: 0 g

Proteins: 22 g

105. Basic Salami

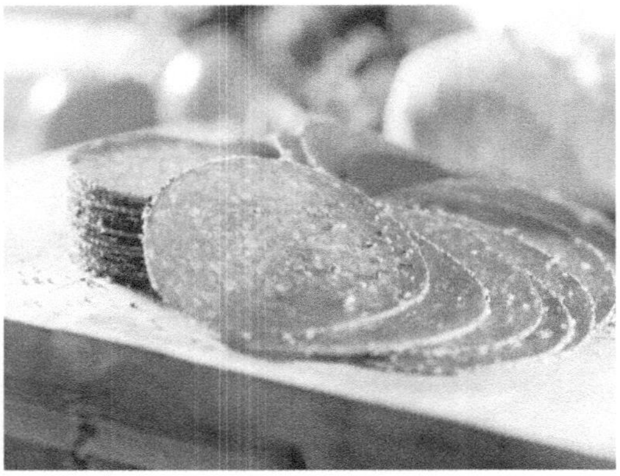

Preparation time: 15 minutes
Fermentation time: 3 days
Servings: 4 quarts

Ingredients:

- 2 lb. pork shoulder or wild boar meat
- 0.8 oz. salt
- 1 tsp. sugar
- 1 tbsp. minced garlic
- 2 tbsp. distilled water
- ½ lb. pork fatback
- 0.1 oz. Instacure No.2
- ½ tbsp. coarsely ground pepper
- Red wine
- ½ tsp. FRM=52 starter culture or T-SPX culture

Equipment:

- Hot casings (about 1 ½ inches diameter)
- Bowls
- Meat grinder
- Airtight containers
- Fermentation plastic container
- Sausage stuffer

Directions:

1. Take out about ⅓ pound of pork and finely dice it. The rest of the fat, pork fatback, and meat should be cut into bigger pieces (chop them so they can go into the grinder) and place the fat and meat chunks in different airtight containers (separate containers for the finely diced meat).
2. Sprinkle salt over the meat chunks and toss well. Place the containers in the refrigerator. The sinew and silver skin should be trimmed as well.
3. The following day, place the fat and the grinder parts in the freezer. Add garlic, Instacure, sugar, and ¼ tbsp. into the meat container and toss well. Place this container in the freezer as well. Take out the containers after 1 ½ hours.
4. Now, set up your grinder with the coarse die and add the finely chopped meat into the grinder. Grind the meat and place the meat in a bowl.
5. Fix the fine die and grind the chopped meat. Add it back into the container. Next, grind the chopped fat and add it back into its container. Place the containers in the freezer once again. Let the fat and meat chill until it is 35°F.
6. In the meantime, add starter culture and distilled water to a bowl. Stir until it dissolves completely.
7. Add the meat, fat, wine, starter mixture, and ¼ tbsp. of pepper into the fermentation container.
8. Mix using your hands for a couple of minutes. Place the container in the refrigerator. Now run the sausage casing under warm water for a couple of minutes.
9. Insert one end of the casing into the sausage stuffer. Stuff the casing with the meat mixture, ensuring you do not like stuff until the end. (You need about 6 inches on the other end of the casing to tie it up).
10. Press the casing gently to remove any air bubbles. Sterilize a needle and prick the casing at a few places for the air to escape.
11. Tie the bottom end into a knot. Remove the sausage from the sausage stuffer and knot this end as well. Fasten it once again with kitchen twine.
12. Now hang the sausage on some hook or nail in a warm and moist area of 35°F -85°F.

13. Spray some water over the sausage 1 – 2 times a day. Do this for 2 – 3 days.
14. Now hang the sausages in an area where the temperature is 50°F to 60°F and humidity of 80% to 90%. You may need a humidifier to maintain the humidity.
15. Let it remain like this for one week. Spray the sausage with water once daily.
16. Next, let the humidity be reduced to 70% to 80% and let it remain for one week.
17. Next, let the humidity be reduced to 65% - 70% and let it remain like this for 2 – 3 more weeks.
18. The salami is ready to eat now. If you want to store it for longer, vacuum seals the sausage and refrigerate it until use. Make sure to label the jar with the name and date of preparation.

Nutrition values:

Calories: 188
Total Fat: 8.5 g
Saturated Fat: 3 g
Cholesterol: 102 mg
Sodium: 115 mg
Total Carbs: 20.2 g
Fiber: 2.1 g
Sugar: 14.9 g
Protein: 32.7 g

106. Finocchiona

Preparation time: 15 minutes
Fermentation time: 3 days
Servings: 4 quarts

Ingredients:

- 2 ½ lb. fatty pork or wild boar shoulder
- 0.8 oz. salt
- 1 tsp. sugar
- ½ tbsp. minced garlic
- ½ tbsp. ground fennel seeds or fennel pollen
- 2 tbsp. distilled water
- 0.1 oz. Instacure No.2
- ½ tbsp. coarsely ground pepper
- ½ tbsp. fennel seeds
- 3 tbsp. ouzo or any anise-flavored liqueur
- ½ tsp. FRM=52 starter culture or T-SPX culture

Equipment:

- Hot casings (about 1 ½ inches diameter), 7.5 feet
- Bowls
- Meat grinder
- Airtight containers
- Fermentation plastic container
- Sausage stuffer

Directions:

1. Take out about ⅓ pound of pork and finely dice it. The rest of the fat and meat should be cut into bigger pieces (chop them so they can go into the grinder) and place the fat and meat chunks in different airtight containers (separate containers for the finely diced meat).
2. Sprinkle salt over the meat chunks and toss well. Place the containers in the refrigerator. The sinew and silver skin should be trimmed as well.
3. The following day, place the fat and the grinder parts in the freezer.
4. Add garlic, sugar, spices, Instacure, and ¼ tbsp. Pepper into the meat container and toss well. Place this container in the freezer as well. Take out the containers after 1 ½ hours.
5. Now, set up your grinder with the coarse die and add the finely chopped meat into the grinder. Grind the meat and place the meat in a bowl. Fix the fine dice and grind the chopped meat. Add it back into the container.
6. Next, grind the chopped fat and add it back into its container. Place the containers in the freezer once again. Let the fat and meat chill until it is 35°F.
7. In the meantime, add starter culture and distilled water to a bowl. Stir until it dissolves completely.
8. Add the meat, fat, liqueur, starter mixture, ouzo, and ¼ tbsp. of pepper into the fermentation container. Mix using your hands for a couple of minutes. Place the container in the refrigerator.
9. Run the sausage casings under warm water. Insert one end of the casing into the sausage stuffer. Stuff the casing with the meat mixture, ensuring you do not stuff up to the end. (You need about 6 inches on the other end of the casing to tie it up).
10. Press the casing gently to remove any air bubbles. Sterilize a needle and prick the casing at a few places for the air to escape.
11. Tie the bottom end into a knot. Remove the sausage from the sausage stuffer and knot this end as well. Fasten it once again with kitchen twine.
12. Hang the sausage on some hook or nail in a warm and moist area of 67°F -80°F. Spray some water over the sausage every 6 – 7 hours a day. Do this for three days.
13. Now hang the sausages in an area where the temperature is 50°F to 60°F and humidity 70% to 80%. You may need a humidifier to maintain the moisture.
14. Let it remain like this for three weeks. Spray the sausage with water once daily.
15. You can hang it for a couple of weeks more if desired.
16. The salami is ready to eat now. If you want to store it for longer, vacuum seal the sausage and refrigerate it until use. Otherwise, freeze until ready to use. Make sure to label the jar with the name and date of preparation.

Nutrition values:

Calories: 22
Fat: 18 g
Carb: 0 g

Proteins: 22 g

107. Authentic Roman Garum Fish Sauce

Preparation time: 15 minutes
Fermentation time: 3 days
Servings: 4 quarts

Ingredients:

- 1 lb. small, raw fish, rinsed and drained
- ½ tbsp. dried oregano
- Sea salt or pickling salt as required (mentioned in the directions)

Equipment:

- Fermenting container
- Bowl
- Strainer
- Storage container
- Cotton cloth or cheesecloth

Directions:

1. After you drain the fish, check the weight of the fish. Weigh out salt, 20% of the importance of the drained fish.
2. Combine salt, oregano, and fish in a bowl. Cover and set aside for 30 minutes.
3. Mix well and transfer into the fermenting container. Stir once daily.
4. Slowly, with the passing of days, only bones will be visible in the container, as the fish would have fully dissolved.
5. Strain the mixture into a bowl using a coarse strainer. Discard the bones and any solids.
6. Now line the strainer with a cotton cloth and strain the mixture a few times.
7. Pour into the storage container. Refrigerate until use. It can last for a couple of years or until it turns cloudy. Discard it once it turns cloudy. Make sure to label the jar with the name and date of preparation.

Nutrition values:

Calories: 118
Total Fats: 9.1 g
Carbs: 4 g
Protein: 7.3 g
Fiber: 0.6 g

108. Roasted Chicken Wing Garum

Preparation time: 15 minutes
Fermentation time: 3 days
Servings: 4 quarts

Ingredients:

- 3.3 oz. chicken wings
- 2.2 oz. chicken bones
- 8 oz. salt
- 8.5 oz. pearl barley koji

Directions:

1. Fill a pot with water (about 6 – 8 cups) and add bones into it. Place the pot over medium flame and let it boil.
2. Skim off any scum that rises on top. Lower the heat and cook for about 1 ½ - 2 hours. Strain the stock and let it cool.
3. Meanwhile, prepare a baking sheet by lining it with parchment paper. Spread the chicken wings on the baking sheet.
4. Bake the chicken wings in an oven that has been preheated to 355° F for about 40 – 45 minutes. Turn the wings every 12 – 15 minutes, roasting them evenly. Take out the baking sheet and let it cool completely.
5. Now weigh the roasted chicken wings and use only 1.1 pounds (chop them into smaller pieces). Use the rest of the wings in another recipe or as a snack with a dip of your choice.
6. Place koji in the food processor bowl and process until it is broken down into smaller pieces. Transfer into the fermentation container.
7. Add chicken wings, salt, and 28 ounces of chicken stock into the fermentation container and mix well.
8. Place a sheet of cling wrap on top of the liquid. Place the lid of the container and fix it less than fully tight. Place the container for fermentation at 140°F or place it in a rice cooker on the "Keep warm" mode for four weeks.
9. Remove any fat visible on top daily. Stir it well after discarding the fat. Do this for the first seven days.
10. Next, remove the fat and stir the mixture only once a week for the next three weeks. Strain the mixture into a bowl using a fine wire mesh strainer. Discard any solids.
11. Now line the strainer with a cotton cloth and strain the mixture a few times. Pour into the storage container. Refrigerate until use. Make sure to label the jar with the name and date of preparation.

Nutrition values:

Calories: 118
Total Fats: 9.1 g
Carbs: 4 g
Protein: 7.3 g
Fiber: 0.6 g

109. Vegan Mincemeat

Preparation time: 15 minutes
Fermentation time: 3 days
Servings: 4 quarts

Ingredients:

- 1 lb. dates, pitted, chopped
- 20 oz. raisins
- Juice of ½ orange
- Zest of ½ orange, grated
- Juice of ½ lemon
- Zest of ½ lemon, grated
- 1 apple, cored, grated along with the peel
- 1 oz. walnuts, chopped
- 2.5 oz. currants

- ½ tsp. ground cinnamon
- ⅛ tsp. ground nutmeg
- ½ tsp. ground ginger
- ⅛ tsp. ground cloves
- 2 tbsp. cider vinegar
- 1 tbsp. brandy (optional)
- 1 tbsp. cultured apple cider vinegar with mother

Equipment:

- Bowl
- Mason's jar

Directions:

1. Combine apple, dates, raisins, walnuts, currants, spices, lemon, orange juice, and zest in a bowl and mix well.
2. Add one tablespoon of cider vinegar and mix well.
3. Add brandy and cultured apple cider vinegar and mix well.
4. Transfer into the jar. Drizzle remaining cider vinegar on top. Fasten the lid and set it aside on your countertop for 24 hours in a cool and dark area.
5. Shift the jar into the refrigerator. Let it remain in the refrigerator for two weeks.
6. The mincemeat is now ready to use.
7. Add brandy just before serving.

Nutrition values:

Calories: 290
Fat: 36 g
Carb: 43 g

Proteins: 50 g

110. Beef Meatballs

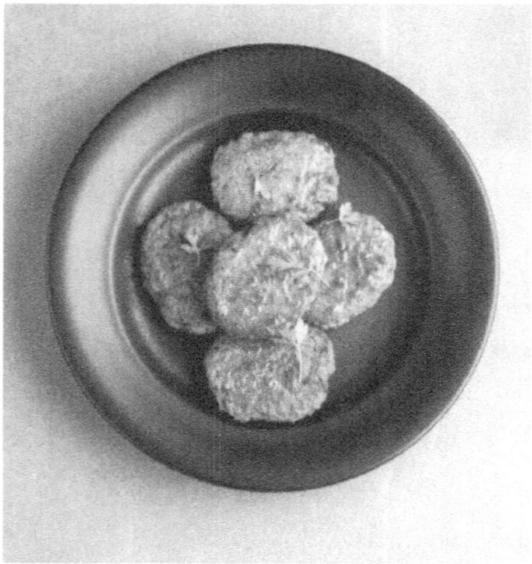

Preparation time: 15 minutes
Fermentation time: 3 days
Servings: 4 quarts

Ingredients:

- 6 lb. ground beef
- 6 c. soft breadcrumbs
- 6 large eggs
- 1½ c. water
- 1 c. onion, chopped finely
- 1 tbsp. salt
- ¼ tsp. ground black pepper
- 8 c. hot chicken broth

Directions:

1. In a glass bowl, add all ingredients (except for broth) and mix until just combined. Set aside for about 15–30 minutes.
2. Preheat your oven to 425°F. Lightly grease two shallow baking dishes.
3. Make 1-inch balls from the mixture. Arrange the meatballs onto the prepared baking dishes in a single layer.
4. Bake for approximately 15 minutes. In 8 (1-pint) hot sterilized jars, divide the meatballs.
5. Pack each jar with hot broth, leaving a 1-inch space from the top. Run a knife around the inside of each jar to remove any air bubbles.
6. Wipe any trace of food off the rims of jars with a clean, moist kitchen towel.
7. Close each jar with a lid and screw on the ring. Carefully place the jars in the pressure canner and process at 10 pounds pressure for about 75 minutes.
8. Remove the jars from the pressure canner and place them onto a wood surface several inches apart to cool completely.
9. After cooling with your finger, press the top of each jar's lid to ensure the seal is tight. Store these canning jars in a cool, dark place.

Nutrition values:

Calories: 525
Total Fat: 15.3 g
Saturated Fat: 5.3 g
Cholesterol: 222 mg
Sodium: 1,169 mg
Total Carbs: 30.4 g
Fiber: 2 g
Sugar: 3.3 g
Protein: 61.9 g

111. Beef in Wine Sauce

Preparation time: 15 minutes
Fermentation time: 3 days
Servings: 4 quarts

Ingredients:

- 1 tbsp. vegetable oil
- 2 lb. beef stew meat, cut into 1-inch cubes
- 1 c. carrot, peeled and shredded
- ¾ c. onion, sliced
- 1 large apple; peeled, cored, and shredded
- 2 garlic cloves, minced
- ¾ c. water
- ½ c. red wine
- 2 beef bouillon cubes

- 2 bay leaves
- 1 tsp. salt

Directions:

1. In a cast-iron wok, heat vegetable oil over medium-high heat and sear beef cubes in 2 batches for about 4–5 minutes.
2. Add in the remaining ingredients and stir to combine well. Adjust the heat to high and bring to a full rolling boil.
3. Set the heat to low and cook, covered for about 1 hour, stirring occasionally. Remove the wok of meat mixture from heat and discard the bay leaves.
4. In 3 (1-pint) hot sterilized jars, divide the beef mixture, leaving about 1-inch space from the top.
5. Run a knife around the inside of each jar to remove any air bubbles. Wipe any trace of food off the rims of jars with a clean, moist kitchen towel.
6. Close each jar with a lid and screw on the ring. Carefully place the jars in the pressure canner and process at 10 pounds pressure for about 75 minutes.
7. Remove the jars from the pressure canner and place them onto a wood surface several inches apart to cool completely.
8. After cooling with your finger, press the top of each jar's lid to ensure the seal is tight. Store these canning jars in a cool, dark place.

Nutrition values:

Calories: 354
Total Fat: 11.9 g
Saturated Fat: 4.1 g
Cholesterol: 135 mg
Sodium: 706 mg
Total Carbs: 9.4 g
Fiber: 1.7 g
Sugar: 5.8 g
Protein: 46.5 g

112. Chicken Marsala

Preparation time: 15 minutes
Fermentation time: 3 days
Servings: 4 quarts

Ingredients:

- 6 lb. boneless, skinless chicken, cut into bite-sized pieces
- Salt and ground black pepper, as needed
- 2-3 tbsp. olive oil
- 1 medium onion chopped
- 1 tsp. garlic, chopped
- 1 tsp. dried oregano
- 2 c. dry Marsala wine
- 8 c. chicken broth
- 5 c. mushrooms, sliced

Directions:

1. Rub the chicken pieces with salt and black pepper generously. In a cast-iron wok, heat olive oil over medium-high heat and sear the chicken pieces in 4 batches for about 3–5 minutes.
2. Transfer each cooked chicken batch to a colander to drain excess grease. Add the onion and sauté for about 3–4 minutes in the same wok.
3. Add in the garlic and oregano and sauté for about 1 minute. Stir in the wine and boil for about 1 minute.
4. Stir in the broth and cook until boiling. Set the heat to low and cook for about 3–5 minutes.
5. In 10 (1-pint) hot sterilized jars, divide the chicken pieces and mushrooms.
6. Pack each jar with a hot cooking mixture, leaving a 1-inch space from the top.
7. Run a knife around the inside of each jar to remove any air bubbles. Wipe any trace of food off the rims of jars with a clean, moist kitchen towel.
8. Close each jar with a lid and screw on the ring. Carefully place the jars in the pressure canner and process at 11 pounds pressure for about 75 minutes.
9. Remove the jars from the pressure canner and place them onto a wood surface several inches apart to cool completely.
10. After cooling with your finger, press the top of each jar's lid to ensure the seal is tight. Store these canning jars in a cool, dark place.

Nutrition values:

Calories: 259
Total Fat: 6.1 g
Saturated Fat: 1.5 g
Cholesterol: 105 mg
Sodium: 401 mg
Total Carbs: 2.2 g
Fiber: 0.3 g
Sugar: 1 g
Protein: 42 g

CONCLUSION

Thank you for reading this book! These recipes are sure to have something that will fit your needs. When you are craving a dill pickle or a savory pickled vegetable, give one of these simple dishes a try to fill your jars with tasty treats for the family.

This is an ideal book for people who are already fermenting and want to learn more, individuals who are just beginning and want to understand more about the process, and those who may not be extremely interested in health but simply want to experiment with making great food. You can discover something in this book that interests you no matter who you are or your background. The book itself includes many delectable recipes that use products that have undergone fermentation. It also demonstrates how to use fermentation techniques to enhance the flavor and appeal of food. The manual includes basic fermentation information, step-by-step recipes, and useful hints. Not everyone knows what to do when starting on the fermentation adventure.

While fermented foods contribute to a healthy diet, most people have started eating them because of their taste. The flavors of these foods are induced by the microbes that break the sugar in the food. Some common fermented foods include Asian miso, sauerkraut, kimchi, kvass, Russian kefir, and wine. People across the globe are embracing these foods and welcoming them to their diet.

It's simple to incorporate fermented foods into your diet. Replace your ordinary bread with a fresh slice of sourdough bread. Kefir is good to drink, and yogurt is preferable to milk. Smoothie recipes benefit from both. Why not even attempt some naturally fermented foods like pickled cucumbers, beets, onions, salsa, sauerkraut, and even kimchi?

Enjoy your fermented recipes!

CANNING MEAT
GUIDEBOOK FOR PREPPERS

The Safest Method to Preserve Meat for

3 Years While Retaining 97% of Nutrients

Tyler Gordon

CHAPTER 1: INTRODUCTION TO THE ART OF PRESERVING MEAT

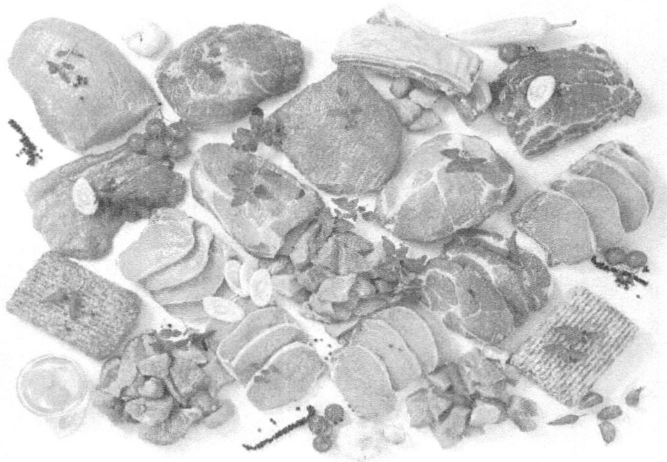

Canning Different Types of Meat

Canning is an excellent way to preserve tender cuts of meat, such as steaks and roasts. Trimmings with connective tissue, stew meat, and ground meat are also included, all of which are frequently made from less tender portions of beef. Bony bits are fantastic in soups. Organ meats such as hearts and tongues can be canned, but hog shoulders and hams are typically cured for smoking rather than canning. The canning process works especially well with pork loins and sparerib meat.

Because fat is undesirable in canned meats, it should be removed as much as possible, and cuts with high-fat content should be avoided.

Most types of meat can be canned at home. This includes both farm-raised and wild-caught meat. Examples are beef, veal, pork, lamb, mutton, moose, and bear. Canning meat from chicken, turkey, duck, goose, and rabbit, among other things, is possible.

Most (but not all) types of fish and shellfish can also be canned, but I'll cover that in a separate book because home canning them is a bit more difficult. Meat can only be safely canned in a pressure canner that reaches temperatures of more than 240F.

Boiling water bath canners cannot be used to can meat because they only reach 212F. That's fine for jams, pickles, and relishes, but it doesn't get hot enough to keep low-acid foods like meat safe.

Preparing the Meat for Canning

Depending on the type of meat you're working with, there are various processes for preparing it for canning. In this section, we will go over the basic steps for some of the more popular meats. Always follow the instructions provided with your pressure canner or the specific recipe you're working with when working with a particular type of meat.

Meat should be thoroughly cooked or heated before being packed into jars. This kills any bacteria in the meat. There are several methods for doing this, and certain methods are recommended depending on the type of meat you are preserving.

Meat Preparation

Cut your meat into cubes, strips, or chunks before canning.

Trim away any excess fat. If you are canning wild game, soak it in brine water, which is made up of 1 tablespoon of salt to every quart of water.

Allow at least an hour to soak to remove any strong game flavor. Large bones should be removed after soaking.

Meat Stew

Stew meat is one of the simplest meats to can. This can be beef, moose, elk, venison, or a combination of the three. This versatile cut of meat can be used in casseroles, chili, stews, barbecue, and Mexican dishes. Meat stew can be canned with or without a pressure cooker.

Red Meat Preparation

Thoroughly clean the meat. Cutting slightly frozen meat will go much faster because the ice crystals help firm it up.

Unless you have a specific recipe, cut the meat cross-grain into large chunks about one-inch thick. This is to provide you with meat cuts that can be used in various recipes.

As much fat and bone as possible should be removed. If you intend to use the bone in stews, keep in mind that it will take up space in your jars. If you choose this option, remove as much fat as possible. You want to preserve the highest quality portion of the meat, and if you leave too much fat on it, it may get stuck between the jar and lid during the sealing process, causing the seal to fail.

This is the time to "raw pack" or "hot pack" your meat. Poultry Deboning is recommended after thoroughly cleaning the poultry. Remove the skin, the fat beneath the skin, and the thin film that covers the chicken or turkey meat.

Seafood and Fish

Always remove the scales and, if possible, skin the fish before canning. Clean the fish thoroughly, just as you would if it were for a meal.

It is preferable to fillet the fish before canning it.

Keep oysters, crabs, lobsters, and other seafood alive until canning. This eliminates the possibility of spoilage before canning.

Before canning seafood, it is advisable to cook it for 5-10 minutes, depending on the type of seafood used.

CHAPTER 2: CANNING AND CURING PROCESS

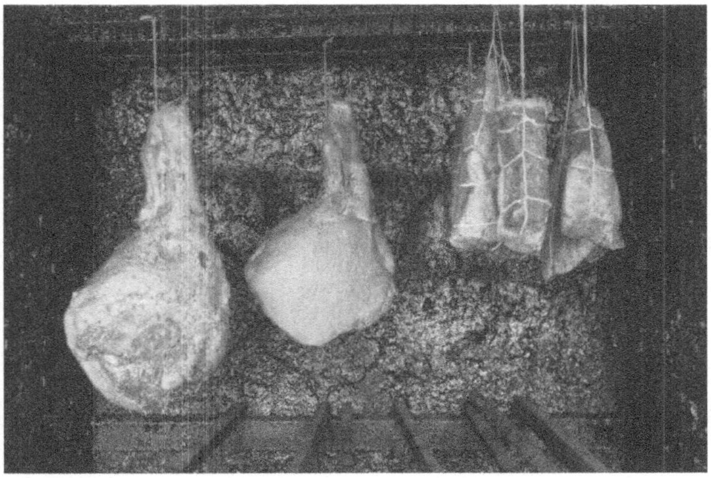

Preparing the Jars

Sterilize Your Jars and Lids

Preparing your jars and lids before canning is a fundamental process. You'll want to sterilize them to retard any bacteria growth. This is a very simple process and takes only about twenty-five minutes.

Materials:

- Large pot
- Water
- Canning jars

Directions:

1. Place jars and metal rings (not lids with adhesive strips) into a large pot, completely covering the jars with water.
2. Bring the water to a boil over high heat until at a rolling boil.
3. Boil the jars for fifteen minutes.
4. Turn off the heat and leave the jars in hot water while you prep the meat you're going to can. The jars can be left in hot water for up to an hour; however, if it goes over that, you'll need to repeat the sterilization process before filling them with the food.

Note: Do not boil the canning lids with the rubber seal, as this can harm the adhesive ring. After you've turned off the heat, these can be sterilized by adding them to the hot water.

Filling Jars

Once you have prepared the meat for canning and filled the jars with food (this is where the canning funnel is handy but not completely necessary), the air bubbles need to be released to remove as much oxygen as possible. This can be done by using a plastic or wooden spatula between the inside surface of the jar and the food. Making minor turns with the jar, slowly move the spatula up-and-down motion, causing air bubbles to escape the jar.

When canning meat and seafood, salt may be added for seasoning, but it is not a necessary step in preserving the food.

Be sure you leave a one-inch space between the food and the top of the jar. Clean the rim of the jar thoroughly with a dampened towel. Place the lid and adhesive strip down and fit the metal ring over the flat lid.

At this point, it is imperative to follow the manufacturer's instructions for tightening the lids to ensure the jars seal properly.

Canning Red Meat

First, use the "hot packing method" to prepare the meat for canning. Place the meat in a deep kettle or saucepan, fill it with water up to the point where the meat is covered, and cook it for 2-5 minutes. This will remove "air" from the meat and make it shrink.

Remember when canning ground or minced meat; always brown the meat before canning it.

Beforehand, you can create your meat broth, which you will use in canning the meat. Broths can be done by placing beef or pork bone into a saucepan, adding celery and onion, and bringing it to a boil. Add broth cubes to taste and set them aside.

After hot packing, the meat is drained and placed inside the "warm" containers. Make sure to limit the use of hands when doing this process, as bacteria can be easily transferred. Use tongs instead.

After placing the meat, pour in the broth. Remember to fill the jar only up to the lower part of the rim. This is called "head space." For meat products, the headspace must be from 1 to 1 ¼ inches. This is required as filling it to the brim may damage the seal when pressure canning.

After pouring the meat and broth, use a (plastic) spatula to release air bubbles. Insert the plastic spatula into the jar and move it up and down while turning the jar. This will release any trapped air bubbles. Clean the rim of the jar and place the cover.

Place the metallic lid on the top of the jar (remember that the metallic band and lid must be sterilized and heated before placing it on the container). After placing the metallic lid, make sure that the lid is perfectly placed on top of the jar to avoid sealing failures. Afterward, place the metallic band and screw it tight.

Place the sealed jars inside the prepared pressure canner and cook the meat until done. After cooking, remove the containers from the canner and allow them to cool. After cooling, inspect for any sealing failures. This can be done in three different ways:

The first is tapping the middle of the metallic lid with a spoon. A vacuum-tight seal will produce a sharp ringing sound, but a loose seal will create a dull sound.

You can press the middle of the metallic lid. If the lid pops back out after pressing, the seal is loose.

Lastly, you can inspect if the metallic lid is concave. Inspect the lid to see if its middle is depressed inwards. If the lid is bulging outwards, then the seal is loose.

If the seal is loose, never attempt to retighten it. Instead, remove the seal and repeat the process. If you cannot repeat the process, place the containers inside the freezer and consume them within 2 to 5 days.

Canning Poultry

When preparing poultry for canning, use the "hot packing" method as you would red meat. Remember to remove the skin, the fat under the skin, and the thin film that covers the meat before deboning the meat.

Place the meat in the container after it has been hot packed; however, unlike red meat, no broth is required. Poultry meat will cook entirely in its juices.

Before canning minced brown chicken or turkey meat, just remember that adding broth or any other liquid will cause the meat to disintegrate after cooking in a pressure canner.

After cooking in the pressure canner, remove the jars and let them cool. Inspect for sealing failures. If the seals are broken, repeat the process or store them in a freezer.

Canning Fish

As fish is a low-acid food, it is best to add any acidic liquid when in hot packing. Typically, the most popular thing added is either lemon juice or vinegar.

Placing it in jars after hot packing is acceptable for fish like salmon, trout, and other small types. However, baking it first is much preferred for tuna and similar types of fish.

When placing into the container, remember to add at least one teaspoon of oil and two teaspoons of salt per half a pint of water. In other cases, you can use oil instead of water when canning fish.

Canning Clams and Oysters

1. When preparing seafood for canning, keep oysters, clams, crabs, and other seafood alive until ready. Place the seafood in cold water at all times.
2. Open the shells of oysters and clams and steam until cooked.

3. Pour the weak brine solution over the cooked clams and oysters in canning jars. One teaspoon of salt per quart of water
4. Follow the same sealing and inspection procedures as described above.
5. Examine for seal failures.

Canning Crabs

There are two methods for canning crabs. It is possible to can them whole or in sections.

1. Break off the crab's shell, remove its back, and rinse it in running water, allowing it to bleed.
2. Cook the crab in boiling water and set aside to cool. Add flavor and keep the natural colors of the meat. Add lemon or any citrus juice.
3. Place it in cold water after cooking to speed up cooling and make removing the meat from the shell easier.
4. Before placing the meat in the container, gently squeeze it to remove any excess water.
5. Fill the jars with crab meat and 1 ½ teaspoon of vinegar for every pint of water to enhance the flavor. You can also flavor it with lemon juice.
6. Remove the jars after cooking and inspect them for sealing failures.

Packing

One of two methods can be used to accomplish this goal: the raw-pack method, which is not typically suggested, or the hot-pack method.

- **Raw-Pack Method.** This indicates that the meat is packed in glass jars before it is cooked; as a result, the meat is raw because it has not been subjected to any heat treatment.
- **Hot-Pack Method.** This requires the meat to be precooked before it is placed in the jars. Always ensure that the precooked meat is kept at a warm temperature.

To help you put food into jars, here are some helpful hints:

- If you pack too tightly, some liquid can leak out; leaving space between the items is better.
- If the directions for the hot pack say to add liquid, make sure the liquid is piping hot before adding it. Adding water is typically required before packaging raw foods.
- If you want to add broth as a liquid, put some meat in a pan, cover it with cold water, and cook it until the meat is tender. After that, separate the broth, let it cool, and remove the fat. After that, it is prepared to be rewarmed and put into the meat that has already been precooked.
- If you use glass jars with sides that are either straight or tapered outward toward the top, it will be much simpler to pack the jars' contents.
- You could use salt to add taste, but other flavors, like herbs and spices, are likely to lose their value or turn bitter if you do so. About one teaspoon of salt should be used for every quart of meat.
- Make sure you leave the required amount of headspace, as specified in the recipe or the directions.
- Use an implement made of plastic or wood to pop any air bubbles that have formed.
- To ensure that a proper seal is created, thoroughly clean the upper rim of the jar with a fresh towel.

Important Steps in the Jar Packing Process

Note: Make sure you have plenty of headspace, also known as the space above the food or liquid in jars. It provides for the expansion of the food when the jars are heated and allows for the formation of vacuums when the jars are cooled.

Put a spatula made of flat plastic or wood between the food and the jar, then slowly turn the jar while moving the spatula up and down to release any trapped air bubbles.

Using a paper towel or a wet dish towel, clean the rim of the jar. Seal failures can be caused by jar-sealing surfaces that have not been cleaned.

After cleaning the area that the lid will rest on, position it so that the gasket is facing down, and then place the metal screw band over the flat lid.

Jars should be loaded onto the canner rack.

Put a cover on the canner and secure it.

Put the filled jars on the rack at the bottom of the canner when there are 2 to 3 inches of boiling water in the canner. It is essential to position them so they do not come into contact with the walls of the canner or one another. Cold spots can form inside each jar if the steam is not allowed to circulate uniformly and fully around each jar. This can lead to food going bad as a result of insufficient processing.

After ensuring that the lid is secure, place it over the heat source and, for the next ten minutes, let steam escape from the canner through the petcock or any other opening that has been recommended. Why for the next ten minutes? Because the steam must expel all of the air from the canner, it cannot contain any. Again, cold spots may form if the air is not forced out of the container, leading to food deterioration. Even if not specified in the manufacturer's instructions, self-venting canners should have an additional 10 minutes of venting time.

Start timing the processing after the temperature has reached 240F (115C) and the dial or weighted gauge registers the correct pressure. The instructions with the canner, those with the jars, or those in your canning book will tell how long the temperature has to be held and at what pressure. During the processing phase, you must ensure that the temperature does not fluctuate, as temperature fluctuations can cause liquid to leak out of glass jars and prevent a seal from forming. If this happens, your efforts will have been in vain.

Remove the canner from the heat as soon as the allotted time has passed to stop any further cooking of the contents in the jars, which would otherwise cause them to turn into a mushy consistency. After the pressure is reduced to zero, remove the petcock or another mechanism for cautiously releasing steam. Next, hold the cover facing you while you open the canner to shield you from the steam coming at you. Finally, remove the glass jars, preferably using tongs explicitly developed for that purpose.

Do not use cold water in an attempt to bring the temperature of the canner down to zero! This has the potential to result in bodily harm as well as damage to both the property and the jars.

Steps in Using a Pressure Canner

1. Place the jars on the rack when two to three inches of boiling water are in the canner.
2. Open the vent port on the cooker and leave it open for ten minutes to allow all of the air in the cooker to escape.
3. Placing a weight on the vent port raises the pressure in the canner.
4. Start time when the weight begins to rock or jiggle or when the pressure gauge reads the correct pressure.
5. Adjust the temperature so the rocking or jiggling action is consistent or the dial gauge pressure is correct.
6. Take the object away from the heat and place it on a heat-resistant surface.
7. Open the vent port once the temperature has cooled. Please wait two minutes before opening the cooker and removing the lid.
8. Take the jars out of the oven and set them on a rack or a kitchen towel to cool down slowly.

How To Cool, Label, and Store

The canning process ends with several crucial procedures, the most significant being chilling, labeling, and storing jars.

Cooling

It is essential to perform a second inspection of the seals about twenty-four hours after removing the jars from the canner.

If you discover a can or jar that is leaking, or if inspecting the seal reveals that the seal has failed, you have two options: either store the contents in the refrigerator and consume them within a few days or within 24 hours, heat the contents, repack and reprocess for the whole period.

Labeling

Date, contents, and processing information should all be included on the labels of your containers. If you have to reprocess a meat container, put that on the label and mark it as one that needs to be used as soon as possible. It is a good idea to store your canned foods in such a way that the jars that have been in storage for the longest amount of time are the ones that are used first. Consider the phrase "First in, first out."

Storing

Keep the jars in a clean, cool, and dry spot. The optimal temperature range for storing them is between 38F and 45F (3.3C and 7.2C), but you should never keep them at a temperature higher than 95F (35C). Jars mustn't be exposed to light because this can cause the food's color to change, which can be an unpleasant experience. Do not allow the containers to freeze because this could cause the jars or seals to shatter.

Checking Jar Seals

After allowing the jars to cool for 12 to 24 hours, the screwbands can be removed. Perform one of the following three types of tests on the seals.

- **Option A**: You can use your thumb or one of your other fingers to press the middle of the lid. When you lift your finger off the lid, if it immediately returns to its original position, the lid is not properly sealed.
- **Option B**: Tap the top of the container with the spoon's bottom. Suppose the lid has not been properly sealed if it makes a droning sound. There will be a droning sound emanating from the container if food makes contact with the underside of the lid. A ringing, high-pitched sound should come from the jar if it has been properly sealed.
- **Option C:** Keep the jar at the same height as your eyes and peek over the top of the lid. It needs to have a concave shape curved down slightly in the center. It is possible that the lid will not seal properly if the middle of it is either flat or bulging.

Storing Tips

All canned meat must be stored in dry, humid-free environments. Remember that moist, damp, and humid storage areas are the perfect environment for bacteria and mold to thrive. Regularly checking your cupboards is vital to see whether they are still suitable for storing.

Checking for Food Spoilage

It is imperative never to taste food directly when checking for signs of food spoilage.

You can inspect the jar to see if many air bubbles are inside. If there are, it most likely means that the food inside is spoiled.

After opening the jar, check for any unnatural or foul odor. Also, check for mold growth in and around the jar's lid.

CHAPTER 3: CANNING INTRODUCTION

What is Canning?

You can consider canning as a form of cooking. You're preparing food that can be saved and kept for several months instead of one meal for immediate consumption. So, what's the point? Preserving food in cans allows you to save the best flavors at the season's peak to enjoy throughout the year. Consider how delicious it would be to eat tomato sauce straight from the garden in the dead of winter.

Canning is the process of preserving fresh food in jars by heating it to high temperatures to kill microorganisms and deactivate enzymes that could cause the food to spoil. When the jars are heated, the air inside them escapes, resulting in a vacuum seal once the jars have cooled. Mold, yeast, and bacteria cannot thrive without air, and food will not spoil.

Canning is a great way to keep fresh fruits and vegetables from the garden or farmer's market while they're still in season. It extends the bounty into the winter when locally and seasonally available items are scarce.

Canning can be done in two ways: in a boiling water bath or under pressure in a pressure canner. To safely store food in sealed jars at room temperature, you must understand the differences between the two methods. The simpler of the two methods is boiling water bath canning. It necessitates using a large, deep pot and canning jars with lids. The most important thing to remember about boiling water bath canning is that it is only suitable for high-acid foods.

What exactly do you mean by "high-acid foods"? High-acid foods include fruits, vinegar-based pickles (including chutneys), fruit-based sweet preserves such as jams and gellies, and tomatoes with extra acidity. The pH of the food contained in the jars must be 4.6 or lower for it to be adequately conserved in a boiling water bath.

Jars containing those items can be safely processed in a boiling water bath. Aside from pickled vegetables and soup stock, all other foods, including non-pickled meats and vegetables, should always be canned in a pressure canner.

Heat processing in a boiling water bath can extend the shelf life of food, but this does not guarantee that the contents are safe to consume. This leads to the conclusion that the acidity of the contents of each jar, rather than the heat of the processing, is what safely preserves the food when it is placed in a bath of boiling water. When combined with canning jars and lids, a boiling water bath creates a vacuum seal that prevents mold from growing within the jars. When the jars are opened, they must be refrigerated, just like store-bought canned goods.

You may come across old-fashioned methods for sealing your canning jars, such as turning them upside down while the food inside is still hot or baking them. It's not a good plan! Even if the jars seal, there is no guarantee that a true vacuum was formed.

Furthermore, the food within may not have reached the core temperature of boiling water using those methods. Canning times are determined by the density of the food and the jar's size, which influence how long it takes for all of the food to reach the hot water temperature in the surrounding area.

Canning significantly extends products' shelf life, and food remains edible for much longer than it would otherwise.

According to studies, canned foods have the same nutritional value as fresh foods and can serve as healthier alternatives.

Canning, when done correctly, is a significant and secure method of food preservation. During the canning process, foods are placed in jars and heated to a temperature that kills bacteria that could spoil the food or pose a health risk. Enzymes that could contaminate the food are also rendered inactive by canning. The jar's air is expelled during heating, and a vacuum seal is formed when it cools. The vacuum seal prevents air from returning to the product and contaminating the food.

Clostridium botulinum bacterium is the critical factor that makes pressure canning necessary for preserving low-acid food. Although boiling temperatures kill bacterial cells, they can still produce spores that can withstand these conditions. The spores thrive in low-acid foods like canned vegetables and meats without oxygen. Once the spores begin to develop, the lethal botulinum toxin is produced.

These spores can be eliminated by canning the food at a temperature of 240F or above for the appropriate time. This temperature can only be attained in a pressure canner because it is higher than the boiling point of water (212F).

History of Food Canning

People have been looking for ways to preserve food for longer since ancient times. Smoking, drying, and pickling are a few of these methods. Even in the 1800s, researchers could not develop an effective and successful method of preserving food.

In 1795, the French government decided to try to salvage the situation. During that year, the country was at war with the Germans, Italians, Dutch, and the Caribbean. These conflicts highlighted the importance of a consistent food supply for troops and sailors stationed in remote locations. The French government has decided to award a 12,000-franc prize through the Society for the Encouragement of Industry to a new idea that makes food preservation easier.

Nicolas Appert, a young chef from the Champagne region, was unwavering in his pursuit of victory. Appert, who previously worked as a chef for members of the French aristocracy, became interested in food preservation science. Finally, he devised a revolutionary idea: store food in champagne bottles and seal them with a combination of cheese and lime to ensure the bottles were airtight. Appert's invention was based on earlier, less-than-ideal methods that either eliminated air or preserved food by heating it, but not simultaneously. Appert's method was the first to achieve this dual objective.

Appert, who oversaw a busy lab and factory, quickly transitioned from using champagne bottles to wide-necked glass containers. In 1803 he delivered some of his preserved food to the country's military, which included meat, vegetables, fish, dairy, and fruit. The following year, he began putting meat in tin cans soldered shut and watched for any signs or symptoms of swelling for an extended period. Those that did not swell were then declared safe for sale and stored for an extended time.

Grimod de la Reynière praised Appert in 1806, stating that his canned, fresh peas were fresher, softer, and tastier than those consumed during peak season. Appert was officially awarded the government prize in 1809, but only with the condition that his method was made public. In 1810, he did so in his first publication.

Canners from all over the world adopted Appert's method, which was especially remarkable in England because it existed for more than fifty years before Louis Pasteur discovered germ proliferation and sterilization. Appert's method of canning food was also 30 years older than the can opener itself. The heavy lids of the early metal canisters had to be chipped open. They were made from tin-plated steel or even cast iron.

Appert worked on his methodology for many years after winning the award. While his factories remained innovative, they were unprofitable, and he died in 1841. Variations of his method were being used to can everything from Pennsylvania tomatoes and Italian produce to New York oysters and Nantes sardines by that time.

The accessibility of canned food was an essential factor in the nineteenth century. It was instrumental in feeding the massive armies that fought in the Crimean War and the American Civil War. It also gave explorers and colonists a taste of home in foreign lands. After the global depression that struck the world in 1873, the United States saw a surge in the exportation of canned foods led by different corporations. In 1904, the Max Ams Machine Company of New York received a patent for the double-seam procedure utilized in most modern food cans. Appert's pea-packed bottles have come a long way since the invention of the double-seam machine.

Things to Know Before You Start Canning

Always make sure you follow recipes and instructions accurately. There is no room for improvisation because the safety of your loved ones is dependent on you following this procedure accurately.

Put the jars in a pot of boiling water to keep them hot until you're ready to fill them. You can also use the dishwasher instead of a pot of boiling water to complete the task.

Use real canning jars with screw bands and new lids whenever possible. The Ball brand is recommended. Today's lids don't need to be heated to make the sealant work before they can be put on the top of a jar.

Don't fill the jars to the top. This is termed "head space," which can be ¼ inch or ½ inch, depending on the cuisine. If you put too much food in the jars, the food may get in the way of the sealant on the lid, and the jars won't seal perfectly.

Before placing on the lid and screw band, ensure you rinse the rim and threads of the jar to keep it tidy. The band should be finger-tight.

Put each jar on the rack in boiling water with the help of the jar lifter. Ensure at least 1 to 2 inches of water covering the jars. Put the lid on the pot and bring it to a boil. Once the water returns to a boil, you can start counting the time it takes to cook.

When the time is up, switch off the heat and take the lid off so the steam can escape from you. Using the jar lifter, take each jar out and set it straight up on a cloth towel about 1 to 2 inches apart. Give the jars twelve to twenty-four hours to cool.

To know that the jar has been sealed very well, you will hear a popping sound as it cools. You can't store jars that won't seal. Instead, put them in the fridge and use them within a few days.

If you store your canned foods in a cool, dry place, they should last all year. When the seal is broken, air can get in. The food has gone bad when the lid bulges or looks corroded or discolored.

If you open a can and see mold, bubbles, or cloudiness, the seal has been broken, and the food is bad.

CHAPTER 4: BENEFITS OF CANNING MEAT

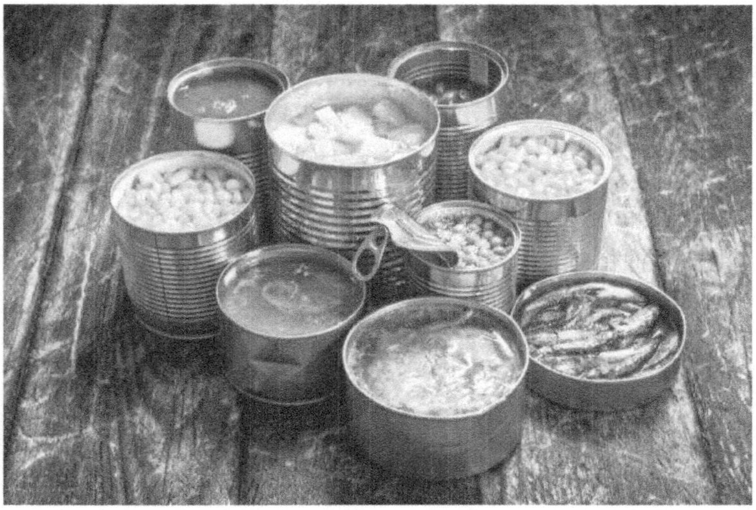

Why Can Meats, Poultry, and Fish?

Many of the millions of households in North America that preserve their food by canning it do so annually with beef. They do this for a variety of reasons, including the following:

- Canning is simple to do as long as specific procedures and protocols are adhered to and unauthorized shortcuts are avoided. Because of this, there is now access to meats that are exceptionally high in nutrients.
- Canning food is a cost-effective method. The initial financial commitment for the containers and the accompanying utensils is not too high. In addition, most of the equipment may be recycled and used multiple times, which means the investment cost can be spread out over a longer time.
- Canning enables one to purchase and store a large quantity of meat at a time when it is both the most readily accessible and most affordably priced. Canning food in this manner saves money in many ways.
- Canned food is simple to maintain because the containers are more or less the same size, which makes it possible to store the food conveniently.
- Because it is stored in transparent jars made of glass, food that has been canned is simple to locate and recognize. However, accurate labeling is still essential.
- Because of the variety of sizes available, the contents of the jars give manageable amounts that can be used without resulting in significant amounts of waste. In addition, a sudden increase in the number of guests can be easily met by simply opening several jars to satisfy hungry appetites at a moment's notice.
- Canning meat is an alternate method to freezing that is available to those who do not have access to freezers. Some individuals choose to freeze their meat, but others do not have this option.
- Preserving food in cans makes it more secure. If done correctly, the canning process will eliminate molds, yeasts, and bacteria that may otherwise be present in food and cause it to become contaminated.

Most people have limited freezer space, and frozen meat often takes up most of the space. If we can get the meat out of that precious space and into a canning jar on our own, that space can be much better used for things like ice cream and oatmeal. The important stuff, you know. Canning is also handy for avoiding the cost of ruined meals during a power outage. Once the freezer temperature reaches the unsafe level of 41F, meat is no longer safe to eat. If you've stocked your freezer with chicken, pork chops, bratwurst, and ground beef, it'll all have to be toed. So, can some of that meat now, store it at room temperature, and you won't have to worry much about power outages.

CHAPTER 5: WHICH NON-FOOD CHEMICAL PRESERVATIVES AND ADDITIVES TO USE

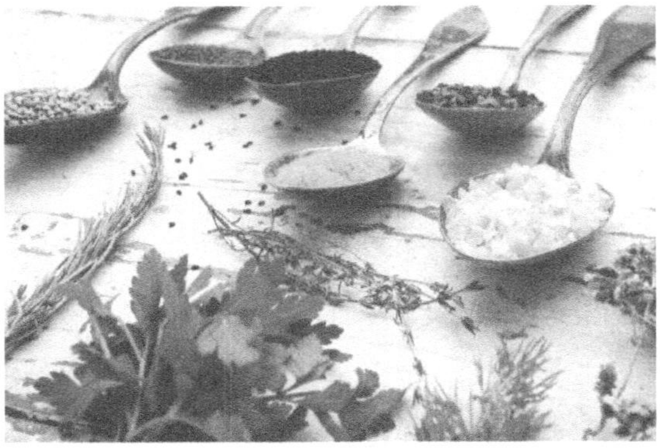

Sweetener

Sweetener has several uses in canning and is an essential component in preserving fruit, regardless of the sort of canned item you're producing. Sweeteners such as sugar, honey, maple syrup, and agave syrup can all be utilized. It improves the flavor of canned fruits and pickles, and soft spreads. It can, however, operate as a preservative by preventing germ formation in jars during storage. Sweetener also enhances the flavor of the fruit, aids in the gel formation required for a spread to set, and improves the shape and texture of the fruit.

Salt

Many canning recipes call for salt, and while standard table salt can be used, pickling salt without additives is preferred. Most table salt contains chemicals that keep it flowing smoothly. These same additives can cloud home-canned goods and reduce their flavor. Flake salt is also not recommended because its weight varies according to flake size, so one tablespoon of one size flake may be "saltier" than one tablespoon of another size flake. Kosher salt may also be used because it is additive-free.

Pectin

Pectin, a water-soluble carbohydrate that is a natural thickening and gelling agent, is found in all fruits. Some fruits, such as apples, grapes, gooseberries, and cranberries, have naturally high pectin levels, whereas others, such as strawberries, cherries, pears, and pineapple, have low levels. Fruit produces pectin as it ripens, with slightly underripe fruit containing the most pectin. Fruit with significantly underripe or overripe pectin does not form a solid gel. Commercial pectin is made from sour apples or citrus peels with high natural pectin content. Packaged pectin is available in powdered and liquid forms. However, they are not interchangeable in recipes due to manufacturing differences. Powdered and liquid pectin require different amounts of fruit, sugar, and acid to set. Use the pectin kind and package size called for in the recipe.

Using commercial pectin for preparing soft spreads such as jams, jellies, and marmalades are numerous benefits. Rather than using a significant amount of underripe fruit in feeds, commercial pectin allows you to use only the best-tasting, fully ripe fruit. The amount of time the fruit is cooked is also reduced, which results in a deeper flavor. Spreads can be made from any fruit combination with varying pectin levels.

Furthermore, commercial pectin yields a higher yield of finished spread because the fruit does not need to be boiled down as much to set.

Acid

The acid plays several critical roles in the canning process. For starters, it aids in the prevention of bacterial growth in canned foods during storage, which can occur if the acid level is too low. Acidic canned items, such as jams, jellies, fruits, and pickles, require the maximum acidity to be processed and preserved safely in a water bath. Low-acid foods, such as vegetables, must be pressure canned before they may be stored on a shelf. The lowered acid may render the preserve unsuitable for shelf preservation after processing. The two most popular acids in canning recipes are lemon juice and vinegar.

Lemon juice, freshly squeezed, is occasionally used to add acid to meals that lack natural acid, such as ripe peaches. Some recipes ask for a tiny amount of freshly squeezed lemon juice to improve the flavor of the fruit while also preventing the color of lighter fruits from fading during storage.

Some recipes that call for low-acid fruits, such as tomatoes and figs, require a consistent acidity, which can be found in bottled lemon and lime juice.

Canning is only appropriate for carefully prepared items. A vinegar with at least 5% acidity should be used. Check the acidity level on a bottle's ingredient list label. You can use white vinegar, cider vinegar, or wine vinegar.

Herbs

Preserves come in various flavors, from soft savory spreads to sauces. Fresh herbs give meals like pickles a delightful taste. Fresh herbs are more flavorful than dried herbs. Choose young, delicate, fresh herbs with dark green, unbruised leaves. Prepare the herbs as soon as possible. Wait until you're ready to utilize them for the best flavor.

Clear Gel

Clear gel is a modified maize starch used in the canning of pie fillings. Unlike conventional corn starch, clear gel is engineered to keep thickness during the canning process.

Salt, Sugar, and Dietary Restrictions

A frequently asked question is how to reduce salt and sugar in home-canned items. It is safe to do so if the following recommendations are followed:

- The salt in fresh-packed pickles (such as in this book) is simply for taste. Because salt is not needed to preserve the pickles, it is okay to leave it out.
- Jam includes a lot of sugar, yet it serves as a preservative. Sugar cannot be reduced while creating jams and other soft spreads unless the recipe calls for it and special low-sugar pectin is used.
- Fruit can be canned in water with no extra sugar. However, the result will not be as flavorful or hard as sugared fruit.

CHAPTER 6: CHEMISTRY BEHIND MEAT PRESERVATION

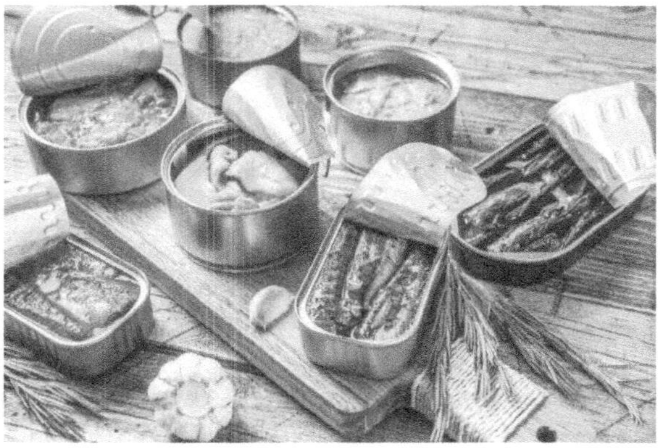

Canning takes oxygen from the cells, kills the bacteria, decimates the enzymes, and creates conditions where bacteria can't grow (high acid, low oxygen canning).

By putting your canned food through a water or pressure canner, you also create a powerful, tight seal that keeps the food inside the jar and keeps bacteria out. A stronger seal implies that the food can be stored for longer, and there is a much lower chance of contamination.

Understanding Food Acid Levels

Food with a pH above 4.6 needs to be pressure canned, or it can become the breeding ground for Botulinum spores. This rule was made specifically because of this bacterium. Fruits can usually kill these spores, but meat and vegetables can't. It's usually a safe bet to only pressure-can foods with high pH and only water-bath food with low pH. With any rule comes the exception, so make sure to research your product before you start to can it. However, this rule doesn't always consider food viscosity, taste, or heat transfer properties.

Not all acidic foods should be canned in a water bath canner alone. Tomato, the most indecisive of produce, requires the addition of lemon juice. This is because their pH levels are near 4.6. Other borderline foods, such as papaya and figs, have a similar pH level and need a supplement to increase their acidic levels. Cantaloupe and watermelon have pH levels that match some kinds of meat. Pressure canning these isn't recommended, though, because it will ruin the flavor. They can only be water-bath canned once they've been pickled.

Understanding Temperature and Time

A safe water bath product must consider both temperature and time. Although boiling water aids in the elimination of dangerous microorganisms, there are some points to consider. Throughout the processing time, the water must be boiling continuously. If the temperature of the water drops after the jars are placed in the canner, the processing is affected. This means the processing time must be restarted once the water returns to a boil.

Products must be maintained in boiling water for the period specified. The period specifies how long it takes for the heat from boiling water to penetrate the product and eliminate any hazardous microorganisms. You must retain a pot of boiling water on the stove when canning because it usually has the propensity to boil dry over a long processing time. By keeping a pot of boiling water, you may refill the water bath canner with boiling water without lowering the water temperature and having to start all over.

Understanding Acidity

The food's pH level is the most crucial factor in securely determining how to preserve foods for pantry storage—the more acidic the solution, the lower the pH. In a boiling water canner, foods with naturally high acid levels or those with enough acid added to reduce the pH level to 4.6 or lower can be prepared. While most jams, fruits, and jellies contain a high level of acid, some fruits, such as melons, figs, papaya, rhubarb, and tomatoes, necessitate the addition of additional acid, most commonly citric acid from lime or lemon juice. This ensures that the pH remains safe both during and after processing.

When combining high-acid and low-acid ingredients in a recipe, acidulation is required. Low-acid foods, such as chutneys and salsas, can raise the pH level and cause dangerous situations when canned, which is why thoroughly tested recipes and safe processing times are required. As you progress through this book, you will come across several recipes that call for fresh lime or lemon juice. This is done solely to maintain fresh flavor. Do not be concerned; every recipe for fresh lemon or lime juice has been thoroughly tested and proven safe.

Understanding Other Factors Related to Canning

Mold

Mold is a type of fungus that releases dry spores. These spores thrive in poorly sealed jars of highly acidic or pickled foods. They begin to grow when the spores fall through the air and land on one of their favorite foods. Initially, you will notice silken strands, color streaks, and fuzz that covers the meal. When high-acid and pickled foods are processed, mold spores are destroyed in a water-bath canner. Consume no food that has had the fuzz removed from it. This was once thought to be safe, but it is no longer. Carcinogens found in mold contaminate the remaining food. Although the food appears to be uncontaminated, eating it can induce disease.

Yeast

Yeast spores, like mold spores, thrive on food. They're incredibly fond of high-acid foods with a lot of sugar, such as jelly or jam. They form on the surface of your meal as a dry coating. By eliminating yeast spores in a water-bath canner, you can prevent them from fermenting in your food.

Enzymes

Enzymes are proteins found in all living things. If not deactivated, they induce rotting. Fortunately, enzymes can be easily inactivated by temperatures as low as 140F (60C). As a result, they are quickly neutralized by boiling water.

Bacteria

Certain bacteria flourish at temperatures that kill molds and yeasts and may survive without oxygen in a moist environment. Clostridium botulinum and staph bacteria toxin-producing spores must be eliminated by heating food in a sealed jar to 240F (116C). This high temperature is only possible with a pressure canner because the steam it produces can reach temperatures hotter than boiling water in a water bath canner.

Botulism

Botulism spores despise high-acid and pickled foods but adore low-acid ones. When these spores are placed in an airless container with low-acid food, such as a jar of green beans, the spores develop a poison in the food that can kill anyone who consumes it. Pressure canning is the only way to eliminate these spores in low-acid foods. To be safe, boil any home-canned, low-acid food for 15 minutes from the point of boiling at elevations of 1,000 feet or lower before eating. Add one minute for every 1,000 feet of elevation above 1,000 feet.

Food Spoilage

If you find that the lid of a jar you have stored has become unsealed or if there is any reason to suspect that food that has been canned has gone bad, throw it away. It should not be consumed and should not be given to animals. The USDA recommends storing jars without screw bands because it makes it simpler to identify some types of food spoilage. The proliferation of bacteria and yeast that cause food to spoil produces gas that causes the food to get pressurized, lids to bloat, and jar seals to fail. When you choose a jar from your stock, check the lid's seal to ensure that it is vacuum-sealed. Keep in mind that lids that have concave centers make for better seals.

Hold the jar upright at eye level and spin it before you open it. Check the jar's outside surface for dried food streaks that start at the top of the jar. Hold the jar for at least five seconds before opening it. Examine the contents to check for rising air bubbles and colors that are not natural.

When you first open the jar, sniff it to check for any strange odors. You should also check the bottom of the lid and the top surface of the food for mold growth that looks like cotton or is spurting fluids. The mold could be white, blue, black, or green.

Low-acid items that have gone bad, such as meat, fish, poultry, and game, might show a few signs of decomposition or various signs, depending on the circumstances. As a result, you ought to treat all containers that raise suspicion as having produced botulinum toxin. Take care when handling such containers in one of the following ways:

If the suspect glass jars still have lids, you should put them inside a strong trash bag. Put a lid on the bag, throw it away in a standard trash can or bury it in a landfill.

Before throwing away the potentially dangerous jars, check them to see if they are unsealed, open, or leaking. The method of detoxification recommended by the USDA can be found in the box.

Regarding properly canning meat, poultry, fish, and game, several issues we have been going over are of the utmost significance. Each one is relatively straightforward on its own, but collectively they are essential if we want to ensure that the food we buy in cans is safe to eat, well-sealed, aesthetically pleasing, delicious, and healthy.

Foods in cans that exhibit any signs of rotting shouldn't be tasted or used! Before opening any jars, give them a close inspection. A jar with a bulging lid or one that leaks indicate deterioration. When you open the jar, check for further symptoms like spurting liquid, an unpleasant odor, or mold. Canned foods that have gone bad should be thrown away wherever neither people nor animals will eat them.

All questionable containers of low-acid, damaged items, including fruits, vegetables, meat, fish, and tomatoes, must be handled with caution in one of two ways:

Put the jars or cans in a thick rubbish bag if they are still sealed. Close the bag and bury it in a local landfill or an ordinary garbage can.

Before being thrown away, the jars or cans should be detoxified if they are open, leaking, or not properly sealed.

Low-acid foods that are improperly canned can contain the toxin that causes botulism without showing any deterioration. Even if there are no signs of deterioration, jars of food that have not been adequately processed must also be thrown away. Likewise, if they are unsealed, open, or leaking, they must be detoxified and thrown away as instructed above. If any of the following are done, low-acid foods are deemed incorrectly canned:

- The food was not canned under pressure.
- The canner's gauge was incorrect.
- The size of the jar, type of pack, or type of food processed did not employ current researched processing periods or pressures.
- The components' proportions were altered from the recipe's approved original.
- The food was canned incorrectly for the processing duration and pressure.

CHAPTER 7: SANITATION RULES

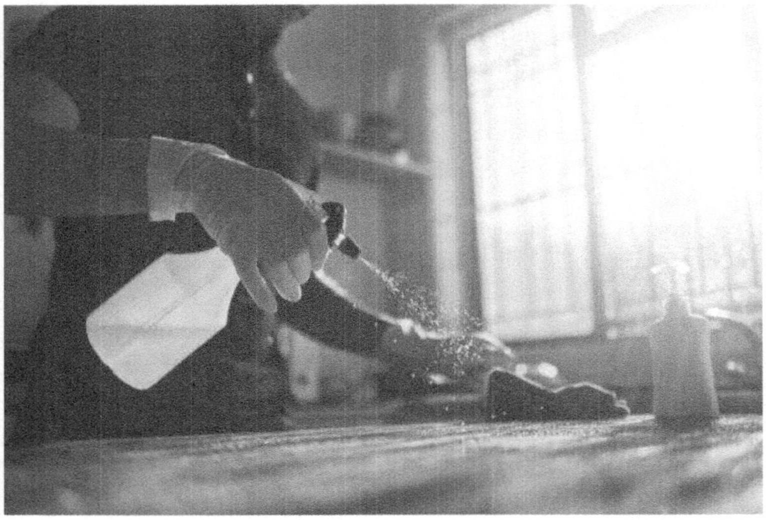

With the renewed interest in preservation comes a surge of popularity in seasonal and local consumption. Environmentally conscious individuals and those who enjoy seasonal food are now looking to canning and other preservation techniques to keep their seasonal goodies fresh at a low cost. However, food quality across the globe is not uniform. Not to mention, home-canned foods need to be prepared and bottled properly, or else they can lead to various health complications.

One of the most common issues associated with improper canning is botulism. It is an illness, sometimes even fatal, when you eat improperly prepared canned or bottled food. This disease is caused by a toxin, a bacteria called Clostridium botulinum, or CUP Botulinum for short.

This bacterium thrives in a moist and oxygen-free environment, which is exactly the conditions you might create if you do not preserve your food properly. In such a condition, the bacteria can multiply rapidly and produce the toxin, not to mention the readily available energy source from the food.

Funny enough, the bacteria itself is very common in nature. You can find it in soil and dust in the form of spores. You might wonder why everyone isn't sick from inhaling dust or getting a bit of dirt in their mouth. This is because they are exposed to oxygen, so they cannot grow.

Symptoms of botulism appear within 12 to 36 hours after consuming the contaminated food. These symptoms include:

- Fatigue
- Vomiting
- Nausea
- Dizziness
- Double vision
- Dryness in the nose and throat
- Headaches

More serious symptoms include paralysis, respiratory failure, and death. These symptoms will last between two hours to two weeks, though there have been cases where they lasted much longer. Pregnant women, children under the age of 5, adults over 60, and people with weakened immune systems are especially vulnerable to botulism.

Even worse, botulism does not change the food's color, odor, or even taste of the food. You cannot just eyeball it and tell whether it is safe to eat. When in doubt, just chuck it out. If you think you have food poisoning or botulism, seek a healthcare professional, or contact the local public health unit as soon as possible. Better be safe than sorry!

Cleaning Utensils and the Work Area

Everything that comes into contact with meat needs to be clean, and by clean, we mean spotless clean since bacteria will thrive, leading to the deterioration and contamination of food. Before and after handling meat, practice the following food safety procedures.

- Be sure to carefully follow the directions provided by the maker of your pressure canner and your canning jars.
- You are not allowed to take any shortcuts.
- Be sure to follow the directions on the cans on how to chill and store the food properly.
- Make sure you only use high-quality products and equipment.
- Canning under pressure is the only method recommended by the USDA.
- Keep in mind the enchanted number: 240F.
- Keep a sharp eye out for a flawless seal.
- Before you crack open the jars, check them for signs of deterioration.
- Before you eat the food, give it another heating.
- It is crucial to thoroughly clean any metal items that will be used, including knives, pans, saucepans, enamelware, and porcelain utensils, by washing them in hot, soapy water and then rinsing them in boiling water.
- Use a scraper to remove any traces of dirt and foreign material from wooden surfaces and equipment, such as work boards, butcher blocks, and wooden spoons. After that, disinfect them using a chlorine-based disinfectant such as bleach that has been diluted following the instructions on the packaging. It is recommended that the disinfectant containing chlorine be left on the surfaces and allowed to air dry. Do not attempt to wash it off. Take the appropriate precautions with food grinders.
- You should wash the cloths you use in water that has been soapy and then rinse them in very hot water.
- Wash your hands. Use soap and warm water. Clean between your fingers and under your nails. Take 20 seconds, at least, to do this. One way to count is to sing Happy Birthday. Alternatively, pretend that you have chili on your hands and need to rub your eyes; how would you wash your hands then?
- Use different boards when cutting up food. One for produce, one for raw meat, seafood, poultry, and fish.
- Wipe down kitchen surfaces with paper towels and change dishcloths daily to prevent contamination and the spread of bacteria. Never use sponges since they are difficult to keep clean of bacteria.
- Sanitize your countertops, cutting boards, and utensils before and after you prepare food. Ideally, you want to use a kitchen sanitizer or use a bleach solution for the job. Follow the manufacturer's directions if you use a kitchen sanitizer, use 5ml of bleach to 750ml of water if you use a bleach solution, and rinse the surface with water once you are done.
- At all stages of the cleaning process, clean your surfaces to minimize the risk of contamination.

Decontamination Process

If the inspection of unopened, open, or leaking jars leads you to believe that the food may be contaminated, you need to detoxify everything before you throw it away.

To decontaminate, lay the potentially contaminated containers and lids on their sides in a stockpot, pan, or canner that has a capacity of 8 quarts or more and fill it with boiling water. You should properly wash your hands. Add water to the saucepan in a careful manner. It is vital to ensure that the water covers the containers and that there is at least one inch of water above them. Try not to make any splashes in the water. Put the lid on the pot, then bring the water to a boil over high heat. The meal and all the container components should be boiled for half an hour to guarantee that any toxins are removed. After the containers have cooled, you may either throw them away with their lids and contents or bury them in the ground.

Cleanse all surfaces meticulously, including but not limited to countertops, containers, equipment, clothing, and hands that may have come into touch with food or containers. Put any washcloths or sponges that you think might have been used in the cleanup in a plastic bag, then throw them away. Finally, disinfect your workspace using a mix of dilute chlorine bleach and water.

Safety Precautions

The following safety precautions are not difficult to implement; they are based on good old-fashioned common sense. They are the result of tried-and-true procedures and years of experience gained by people in industry and government whose job is to determine what levels of food safety are acceptable. Remember that these safety precautions help you preserve food safely and nutritiously, so treat them with the respect they deserve.

- Pay close attention to the instructions for the size of the jar. Follow the instructions printed on the packaging. Similarly, treat your pressure canner with extreme caution and strictly adhere to the manufacturer's recommended use and maintenance.
- Make sure to carefully follow the instructions for rapid cooling and proper storage of canned meat.
- Make certain that you are only using high-quality products and equipment. It is critical to remember that spoiled and contaminated food can be produced using less-than-perfect equipment.
- Use only procedures that the USDA has approved. Do not be persuaded to employ methods that have not been tried and tested. According to the United States Department of Agriculture, there is only one safe way to preserve meat: to use a pressure canner. All other methods, such as an oven or microwave canning, processing in a boiling-water bath, using a steamer without pressure, or the open-kettle method, are potentially dangerous and should be avoided.
- Remember the magic temperature when canning meat or other items with low acid content. Botulism spores must be killed at 240F (115.6C). To preserve food in this manner, you will need a pressure canner because reaching this temperature under pressure is the only safe way to do so.
- Look for a flawless seal, just like it says on the page, and reheat the food before serving. Botulinum toxin can be deactivated by heat. You should bring the food to a rolling boil in an open kettle before tasting it, then boil it for 15 or 20 minutes while constantly stirring it.

This should be done even if you are certain that you have processed a low-acid food (such as meat) exactly according to the directions and have taken all precautions. The food must be thrown away immediately if it begins to foam or if it begins to smell rotten. Do not put it in your mouth, and do not offer it to your animals.

Cooking

Bacteria in your food should already be killed off when you cook your food at a high temperature. However, home canning is different since you want to create a vacuum seal, which presents the perfect environment for botulism bacteria to fester. So, what can you do to keep your food safe at this stage?

- Proper use of tools is crucial in the home canning process. You want to use a pressure cooker or a boiling water canner according to the acidity of the food.
- A bit of acid solution such as lemon juice or vinegar is recommended for certain food such as tomatoes to make them more acidic.
- Never substitute, especially for the processing time and pressure level. Cutting corners means giving the botulism bacteria a chance to fester.
- Check the cooking temperature now and again to ensure that your food is cooking at the right temperature.
- When using stream pressure, make sure that the pressure is maintained.
- Remember the preparation process for each batch.

Safe Equipment and Recipes

Similarly, the equipment you use and the recipe you choose to preserve your food should also be clean and safe.

- Use jars for bottling and home canning – not all vessels fit the job.
- Only use new self-sealing lids and ensure that the sealing compound is not damaged, as it can compromise the seal and spoil your food.
- Never reuse old lids, even if they look in good condition.
- When choosing recipes, it is best to stick to the ones that are popular/well-known since they are proven safe.
- Do not substitute the jar size or the number of ingredients recommended in the recipe.
- Most recipes will tell you how much space you want to leave in the jar. Always follow the instruction.

Safe Handling of Processed Jars

- Check the lid for a proper seal. Two-piece lids typically seal with a "pop" sound as they cool. Once the lid has wholly cooled, test it. When touched with a finger, it should have a downward curvature and be immobile.
- If a jar is not tightly closed, refrigerate it and use any undamaged food within two to three days, reprocess it within twenty-four hours, or freeze it.
- Instead of opening sealed jars, make plans to use them first. Even if the food is discolored, it is safe if it is sealed and the liquid is just below the food.
- Always label and date all jars before storing them.
- Always store your jars in a dark, cool, and dry location. The ideal temperature range is 50-70F.
- Keep canned goods away from hot appliances like a range or furnace, as well as direct sunlight. Depending on the temperature, they lose quality and may even spoil after a few weeks or months.
- Dry out any canned goods. If dampness corrodes metal covers and causes leaks, food may spoil. For the best quality, use canned foods within a year.
- Refrigerate leftovers once you've opened a jar for consumption.
- If you canned seafood and decide to open it, refrigerate it immediately and discard it three days after opening it.
- Consume all canned or bottled foods within a year for the best quality.

Food Reprocessing from Unsealed Jars

Food from jars that did not seal should be processed only if done within 24 hours. Remove the lid and inspect the sealing surface of the jar for any small nicks. Replace the jar if necessary, add a new, treated lid, and repeat the procedure using the same processing time. Use the re-canned goods first and label the jars with this information. They will be less nutritious than food that has only been processed once, and their texture will be softer.

When storing products for future use, food safety should always come first. Make sure everything is as fresh as possible and prepared in manageable proportions and small quantities as early as practicable. The greatest quality preserved foods are processed on the same day as they are collected and handled hygienically.

CHAPTER 8: EQUIPMENT

Pressure Canner

If you plan on canning meat, you simply cannot do so without this one piece of equipment. It is an absolute requirement. It is necessary to heat the cans and the food being canned to 240F(115.6C) to kill any potentially dangerous bacteria that may be present. However, this cannot be done safely without first building up 10 to 15 pounds of steam pressure, and the amount required varies depending on the altitude. Only with the use of a pressure canner is it possible to reach this temperature without risk. Canning canned meat without one is never a good idea.

One just cannot emphasize the significance of a pressure canner. Forget preserving meat in cans if you cannot locate one in good shape; consider other preparation methods.

Having a pressure canner around the kitchen is convenient for creating stews, baking beans, brown bread, cooking vegetables, and countless other purposes. A pressure canner can be used for many purposes other than for canning, and it is very beneficial to have one around.

A pressure canner must have a cover that can be sealed tightly, a petcock to let out steam for approximately ten minutes at the beginning of processing to ensure that all excess air is removed from the inside of the canner, a dial or pressure gauge to indicate the inside pressure when steam is built up, and a safety valve to let off excess steam if pressure is inadvertently allowed to approach the danger psi. A pressure canner that meets these requirements is in good working

Jar Lifter

You run the danger of scalding your fingers and breaking the jars if you take them from the pressure canner at the end of the processing period without first securing them with a clamp or similar suitable mechanism. You can access several solutions available today that fulfill your requirements while remaining within your budgetary constraints.

Bimetallic-Coil Thermometer

This kind of thermometer is required to guarantee that meat, poultry, and fish are cooked to the appropriate temperatures, which is necessary to prevent foodborne illness. Within the tip of the probe is a coil constructed out of two different metals that have been welded together. When the coil is heated, which causes it to be attached to the temperature indicator, the coil expands. The temperature may be read from the tip of this food thermometer up the stem, measuring between two and a half inches. The determined temperature is the same as the average of all the temperatures measured along the sensing region. This thermometer features a dial display and can be purchased with "oven-safe" and "instant-read" designations. Because of the disparities in the skills that each sort possesses, you might want to ensure that you have at least one of each kind.

Jars

This purchase is hard to go without, but quality canning jars are easy to find via garage sales, auction sites, and generous grandparents! Because they can be reused for many years, canning jars are an excellent investment for any beginning canner.

The best canning jars to use are mason jars, specifically those manufactured by Ball. These jars are purposefully designed for home canning. You may feel tempted to reuse a glass pickle or baby food jar; however, the mouths of these jars are not adequate for sealing lids, nor are they made out of heat-treated glass.

It is recommended that you purchase a variety of sizes so that you are prepared for a wide breadth of canning needs, from jelly jars to pints up to half-gallon jars. Canning jars are available in regular and wide-mouth tops.

Regular jars have shoulders and a smaller opening. Wide-mouth jars have straight sides and a larger opening. Ball recommends regular jars for pourable items like tomato sauce but wide-mouth jars for vegetables like pickles or green beans. I prefer wide-mouth jars because I can get my hand inside to clean the jar more easily than a regular-sized jar.

Lids and Bands

Canning lids are a purchase you will have to make every year, as they cannot be reused. The bands, however, can be used yearly so long as they have not formed rust.

Utensils

Whereas the latter two items were essentially mandatory items for the canning process, the rest of the items in this section can be fashioned out of other items around the house.

Jar lifters help remove hot jars from the canner. You could also use a set of tongs.

A jar funnel helps pour and pack liquid into canning jars without spilling. Any kind of funnel could be used for this, provided it is sterilized.

A lid wand is a magnetized bar that can remove lids from hot water. This is useful if you plan to sterilize your lids before canning (always recommended to ensure food safety).

Other useful tools include a stick or jar prod to remove trapped air bubbles, a timer, hot pads, plenty of dry, clean cloths, and a cutting board. Those who can make a large amount of food may also find it beneficial to invest in specialty items such as core removers and fruit skinners.

Many people opt to purchase a home canning kit when just starting. These are wise investments for the beginning canner because they include the canner itself and most of the tools listed above, including jars and lids.

Canning Funnel

A canning funnel is a wide-mouth instrument for canning food that keeps jar rims spotless. It can also be used to fill zip-top bags neatly.

Sealing Lid

Making sure that the can or jar is airtight is the main job of a sealing lid. It comes equipped with a rubber ring, so when the jar is in the pressure canner, it adheres to the mouth of the jar. It prevents oxidation by ensuring that pressure inside the jar does not escape. These should never be reused, as the rubber ring deteriorates.

Screw Bands

The metal rings are used to screw on after the sealing lid is securely in place. These can be used more than once.

Large Stock Pot

This is used for cooking and preparing your food for canning. You'll also need a large pot to keep your jars hot until ready to use.

Other equipment used is the following:

- Dishtowels (for cleaning the outside of the jars for storage)
- Potholders
- Cutting boards (non-porous)
- Permanent markers (for labeling)
- Canning funnel (helps reduce messes when transferring foods)
- Magnetic canning lid lifter (another cool tool)

CHAPTER 9: METHODS AND INSTRUCTIONS

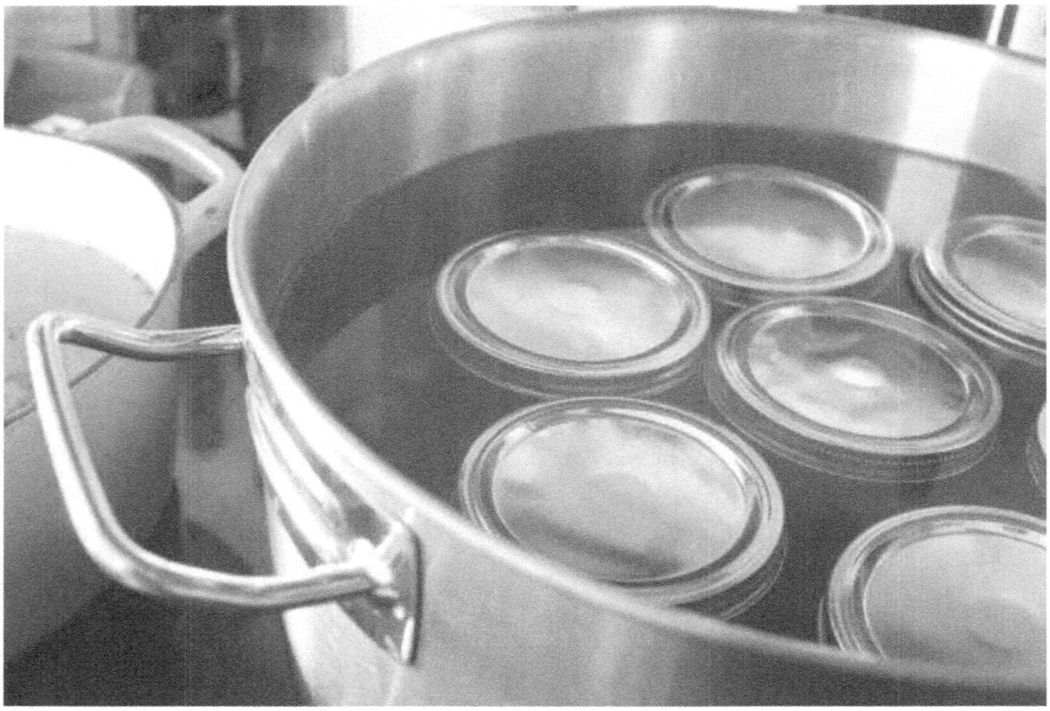

When it comes to canning meat, there are not several different approaches from which to pick. The steam pressure method is the only one that may be used, and using it is required. It is not recommended to use any other. Even if alternative methods are mentioned in certain texts written before the pressure canner was introduced, you should not attempt to use those methods. Canning meat, poultry, or fish using anything other than steam pressure is a dangerous and irresponsible notion that no responsible person would ever attempt to recommend.

Dry-Canning Meat

Dry-canning means no canning liquid added to the jar. The USDA Complete Guide (2015) allows for the dry-canning of raw-packed strips or cubes or large pieces of meat.

Note that dry-canning of ground meat is specifically and explicitly recommended against, whatever you see on the Internet. Many people feel that the quality of meat packed with a liquid in the jar is higher than dry packing it.

Hot Pack Canning Method

Hot packing is bringing freshly prepped food to a boil, letting it simmer for two to five minutes, and then loosely putting it in jars immediately. Regardless of whether the food has been hot-packed/raw-packed, the juice, syrup, or water that will be added to it should also be brought to a boil before being put in the jars. This helps get the air out of the food, shrinks the food, and keeps the food from bobbing in the jars. It also strengthens the vacuum in the sealed jars and makes the food last longer. When you preshrink food, it lets you put more food in each jar.

Hot-packing is the most effective method for eliminating air and is the packing technique recommended for foods prepped in a boiling-water canner. The color of hot-packed foods may not appear to be any different than raw-packed foods at first; however, after a short period of storage, the color and flavor of hot-packed meals will be improved.

The Hot Pack canning method is done by heating freshly prepared food to boiling, then simmering it for approximately 5 minutes (depending on the type of food you're canning). Once simmering is complete, the food is promptly placed into heated jars.

This method is the best way to remove air from your food. The more air/oxygen that is removed, the more food can fit into the jars, and more importantly, the more oxygen removed from the food before sealing, the longer shelf life will have. This is recommended for canning meats.

Raw/Cold Pack

The raw-packing method is used to tightly pack freshly prepped foods that have not yet been heated into jars. These foods, mainly fruits, will float inside the jars. Food discoloration caused by trapped air can occur as soon as two to three months after it is placed in storage. This method is ideal for vegetables that are prepped using a pressure canner.

The Raw Pack canning method is when jars are filled with prepared, unheated food and placed in a water-bath canner rather than a pressure canner. This method is generally used for fruits and vegetables or foods requiring little processing, and while it is not ideal for canning meat, we wanted to introduce the method to you.

Pressure Canning Method

At this point, you understand why you'd use a pressure canner and the differences between the most common types.

Once you've prepared your pressure-canning recipe, here's how to pressure can your food safely.

Before you start your first batch, there are a few things you need to do to make sure the canner is in good working order.

Check the seals and gaskets to make sure they look good. On a gasket-less canner, the metal-on-metal contact point is oiled with a tiny bit of olive oil periodically to ensure a good seal. Take a bit of olive oil on your finger and run it along the seal before you get started.

When you're ready, here's how to do the pressure canning method.

1. Gather materials. Ensure all canning jars are clean by washing in hot, soapy water and rinsing well and air drying. Make sure all jars, lids, and bands fit properly. There shouldn't be any nicks or cracks on the jar's rim.
2. Pre-heat jars. Place jars in a large pot with enough hot water to cover the jars with water. Add lid. Bring water to a simmer (180°F) for ten minutes.
3. Set up your pressure canner with the rack and 2-3 inches of water brought to a simmer and kept simmering until ready to fill with jars.
4. The lids sold today do not need to be placed in simmering hot water to activate the sealing compound before placing on the jars.
5. Follow one of our low-acid, pressure-canning recipes when preparing your produce. Fill each jar with the prepared food and liquid needed, using a ladle and funnel.
6. Release any trapped air bubbles using a rubber spatula or a plastic canning wand between the jar and food to release trapped air. Leave appropriate headspace (¼", ½", or 1" per recipe directions).
7. Wipe rims of jars with a clean, damp cloth and remove any food residue.

8. Put the lid on each jar, apply the screw band and tightened only finger tight. Using the jar lifter, put the jars on the rack in the pressure canner with 2 – 3 inches of simmering water. Don't allow the jars to touch each other.
9. Process the jars: Lock the canner lid in place, leaving the vent pipe open. Adjust heat to medium-high to get steam flowing through the vent pipe. Allow steam to escape through vent pipe for ten minutes or until steam forms a constant flow to ensure there is no air (only steam) left in the canner. Close vent using weight or method described for your canner. Monitor and adjust heat to achieve the recommended pressure.
10. Maintain the recommended pressure for the time indicated in the recipe, adjusting for altitude (see altitude chart). Turn off heat. Let canner stand undisturbed (do not remove the weighted gauge) until pressure returns to zero. Wait 10 minutes, remove weight and unlock the lid, tilting away from yourself. Allow jars to cool for an additional ten minutes.
11. Remove jars from the pressure canner using a jar lifter and set upright on a towel. Leave jars undisturbed for 12 to 24 hours.
12. Remove the screw bands and inspect lids for seals. There should be no flex when you gently press the center of each lid. If the lid flexes, gently try lifting the lid at the rim with your nail. Properly sealed lids will remain attached. If a lid fails to seal within 24 hours, immediately refrigerate the product.

CANNING MEAT
COOKBOOK FOR PREPPERS

The Safest Method to Preserve Meat for
3 Years While Retaining 97% of Nutrients

Tyler Gordon

CHAPTER 10: CANNED MEAT RECIPES

1. Beef Meatballs

Preparation Time: 20 minutes
Cooking Time: 15 minutes
Canning time: 1¼ hours
Servings: 16

Ingredients:

- 6 lbs. ground beef
- 6 c. soft breadcrumbs
- 6 large eggs
- 1½ c. water
- 1 c. onion, chopped finely
- 1 tbsp. salt
- ¼ tsp. ground black pepper
- 8 c. hot chicken broth

Directions:

1. Add all ingredients (except broth) to a glass bowl and mix until combined. Set aside for about 15–30 minutes.
2. Preheat your oven to 425°F. Lightly grease two shallow baking dishes. Make 1-inch balls from the mixture.
3. Arrange the meatballs onto the prepared baking dishes in a single layer—bake for approximately 15 minutes.
4. In 8 (1-pint) hot sterilized jars, divide the meatballs. Pack each jar with hot broth, leaving a 1-inch space from the top. Run a knife around the insides of each jar to remove any air bubbles.
5. Wipe any trace of food off the rims of jars with a clean, moist kitchen towel. Close each jar with a lid and screw on the ring. Carefully place the jars in the pressure canner and process at 10 pounds pressure for about 75 minutes.
6. Remove the jars from the pressure canner and place them onto a wood surface several inches apart to cool completely.
7. After cooling with your finger, press the top of each jar's lid to ensure the seal is tight. Store these canning jars in a cool, dark place.

Nutrition:

Calories: 525
Total fat: 15.3g
Saturated fat: 5.3g
Cholesterol: 222mg
Sodium: 1,169mg
Total carbs: 30.4g
Fiber: 2g
Sugar: 3.3g
Protein: 61.9g

2. Beef Paprika

Preparation Time: 10 min
Cooking Time: 1 hour
Servings: 6

Ingredients:

- 1 sliced onion
- 2 tbsps. Flour
- ¼ tsp. Black pepper
- ¼ tsp. salt
- 2 minced cloves of garlic
- 2 chopped red bell peppers
- 2 tbsps. sweet paprika
- ½ c. beef broth
- 2 tbsps. tomato paste
- ½ c. sour cream
- 1 tsp. caraway seeds
- ¼ c. chopped fresh dill
- 2 lbs. canned beef

Directions:

1. Place onions in a slow cooker. Toss the beef in flour with salt and pepper in a small bowl.
2. Top onions with seasoned beef. Spread over garlic and bell peppers in the slow cooker. Mix paprika, broth, caraway, and tomato paste in a separate small bowl.
3. Pour sauce over beef—cover to cook. Put on high for 4 hours or low for 8 hours.
4. Uncover and turn off the heat; let stand for 10 minutes. Stir in dill and sour cream.

Nutrition:

Calories: 768

3. Mexican Beef and Sweet Potato Soup

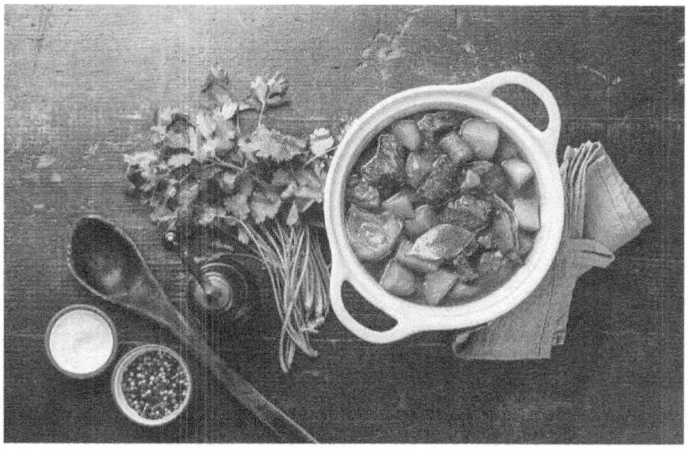

Preparation Time: 90 minutes
Cooking Time: 80 minutes
Servings: 8

Ingredients:

- 1 tbsp. vegetable oil
- 2 ½ qt. beef broth
- 2 ½ pounds Beef chuck roast, trimmed of fat and sliced into one-inch dice
- 4 Roma tomatoes, seeded and sliced
- 1 medium sweet potato, peeled and sliced
- 8 1-inch diameter carrots, peeled and cut into ¼-inch rounds
- 1 c. frozen or fresh whole-kernel corn
- 1 large onion, sliced
- 2 jalapeño peppers stemmed, seeded, and thinly sliced
- 2 poblano peppers stemmed, seeded, and sliced
- 1 tbsp. salt
- 6 cloves garlic, minced
- ½ tbsp. ground black pepper
- ½ tbsp. chili powder

Directions:

1. Pour ½ tablespoon veggie oil into a 6-quart pot and place over low-medium heat. Add half of the beef cubes. Fry and stir to turn brown. Move beef into a small bowl.
2. Do the same with the remaining ½ tablespoon of oil and beef. Transfer all the meat to the pot and add broth. Reduce heat and allow it to boil. Simmer covered until beef is soft.
3. Ladle vegetables and beef into the canning jars by filling each halfway. Pour hot broth into every jar and leave one-inch headspace. Remove air bubbles, wipe jar rims, adjust lids, and screw band.
4. Set the filled jars in a pressure canner at 11 pounds pressure for dial-gauge or 10 pounds for the weighted-gauge canner. Process heat jars for seventy-five minutes, adjusting for altitude.
5. Switch off the heat and let pressure drop naturally. Remove the lid and cool the jars in the canner for five minutes. Take out the jars and cool. Inspect the lid seal after twenty-four hours.

Nutrition:

Calories: 377
Fat: 6g
Carbs: 6.2g
Protein: 3g

4. Pot Roast in a Jar

Preparation Time: 20 minutes
Cooking Time: 50 minutes
Servings: 6

Ingredients:

- 2 lbs. stewing beef, cut into chunks
- 1 c. chopped onions
- 2 tsps. dried thyme
- 2 cloves of garlic, minced
- 2 bay leaves
- 1 c. beef broth
- 1 c. dry red wine
- 2 tsps. salt
- 1 tsp. ground black pepper
- 1 c. chopped carrots
- 1 c. diced potatoes
- ½ c. chopped celery

Directions:

1. Sterilize the jars in a pressure canner as indicated in the general guidelines of this book. Allow the jars to cool.
2. Place the beef in a pot and add the onions, thyme, garlic, bay leaves, broth, and wine. Season with salt and black pepper. Close the lid and turn on the heat. Bring to a boil for 10 minutes and allow to simmer for 10 minutes.
3. Add in the vegetables and simmer for another 5 minutes. Turn off the heat. Transfer the mixture to sterilized jars.
4. Remove the air bubbles and close the lid. Place the jars in the pressure canner. Place it in a pressure canner and process for 25 minutes.

Nutrition:

Calories: 234
Protein: 34.2g
Sugar: 2g
Fat: 6.2g
Carbs: 9.3g

5. Crumb Meatballs with Sauce

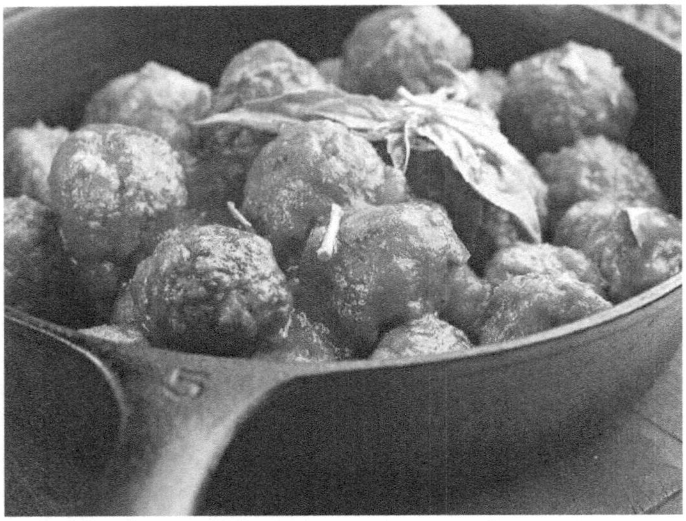

Preparation Time: 15 minutes
Cooking Time: 1 hour and 40 minutes
Servings: 1 quart

Ingredients:

- 5 lbs. ground meat
- 2 c. very fine crumbs
- 2 tbsps. salt
- 2 tbsps. dried parsley
- 1 tbsp. garlic powder
- 1 tbsp. onion powder
- ½ batch marinara spaghetti sauce

Directions:

1. Combine the meat, breadcrumbs, salt, parsley flakes, garlic powder, and onion powder in a large bowl, using your hands to mix well. Form very firm meatballs.
2. Place 8 to 10 meatballs into each sanitized quart jar. Don't overfill the jars with meatballs because you want to leave room for the sauce.
3. Heat marinara sauce until it is simmering, about 10 minutes. Cover the meatballs with hot marinara sauce.
4. Use a rubber spatula to remove air pockets, so the sauce occupies the jar, leaving some headspace. Can for 90 minutes in a pressure canner at 10 PSI, adjusting for altitude.

Nutrition:

Calories: 219.1
Fat: 8.5g
Carbs: 15.6g
Protein: 20.3g

6. Pressure Canned Fish

Preparation Time: 15 minutes
Cooking Time: 1 hour and 40 minutes
Servings: 10 pints

Ingredients:

- 20 11-inch blue backs
- Onions
- 2 tbsps. pickling salt
- 9 tbsps. white vinegar
- 9 tbsps. ketchup

Directions:

1. In a sizable bowl, mix salt, vinegar, and ketchup. Now layer the ingredients in the sterilized jars so that you start with fish, onions, and a tablespoon of the vinegar mixture.
2. Repeat with all the jars, leaving a headspace of ¼ inch. Arrange the sealed jars in the pressure canner and process them at 11 pounds for 100 minutes.
3. Wait for the pressure canner to depressurize to zero before removing the jars. Arrange the jars on a cooling rack for 24 hours, then store them in a cool, dry place.

Nutrition:

Calories: 137.7
Fat: 3.6g
Carbs: 0g
Protein: 25.3g

7. Beef, Lamb, and Venison

Preparation Time: 15 minutes
Cooking Time: 1 hour and 25 minutes
Servings: 8 pints

Ingredients:

- 8 lbs. ground beef, lamb, or venison
- 4 tsps. salt, divided
- White vinegar

Directions:

1. Prepare the jars by cleaning them well. Set a rack in a pressure canner, then put 3 to 4 inches of water. Fill your jars with a couple of inches of water, so they do not float, then place them in the canner. Simmer until ready to fill the jars. Do not boil the water. Add water to a large pot and boil.
2. Cook the meat within 10 minutes or until lightly browned in a large skillet set over medium-high heat. Drain off any fat.
3. Remove it from the canner, empty it into the sink, and place it on a cutting board on a nearby countertop.
4. Pack the meat into the prepared jars, leaving 1 inch of headspace. Add ½ teaspoon of salt per pint. Ladle in the boiling water, leaving 1 inch of headspace. Release any air bubbles using a nonmetallic utensil.
5. Rinse the rim of the jar with a solution of diluted vinegar and water to remove any greasy films. Seal with the lid and ring. Repeat with the remaining jars, meat, and salt.
6. Arrange the jars on a rack in your pressure canner. Lock the lid, boil, and let the canner vent for 10 minutes. Place a weighted gauge or pressure regulator on the vent.

7. Process for 1 hour and 15 minutes at 11 pounds (454 g) on a dial gauge or at 10 pounds (4.5 kg) on a weighted gauge. Adjust your temperature to maintain an even pressure. Turn off the heat. Let the pressure drop to zero before opening the lid.
8. Remove the jars from your canner. Set aside to cool, undisturbed, for 12 hours.
9. Check the lids for proper seals. Remove the rings, wipe the jars, label and date them, and transfer them to a cupboard or pantry.
10. Refrigerate any jars that don't seal properly, and use them within three days. Properly sealed jars will last in the cupboard for 12 months.

Nutrition:

Calories: 29.8
Fat: 18.8g
Carbs: 0g
Protein: 19.2g

8. Buttered Chicken Breast

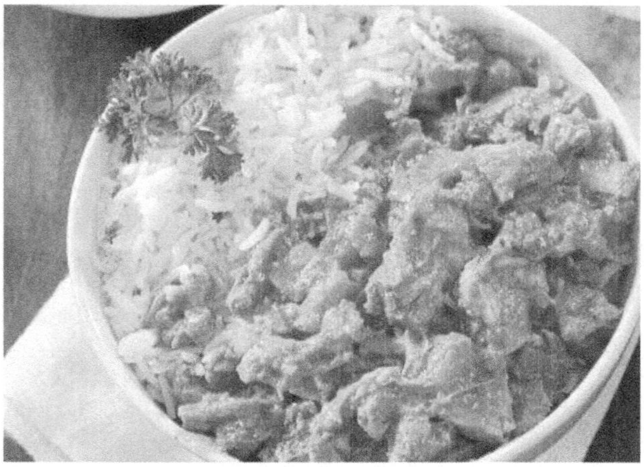

Preparation Time: 15 minutes
Cooking Time: 1 hour and 30 minutes
Servings: 8 pints

Ingredients:

- 18 medium boneless and skinless chicken breasts
- 1 ½ tbsps. salt
- 4 ½ c. water
- Butter or olive oil for frying in a skillet

Directions:

1. Cook each side of the chicken in a skillet with butter or olive oil for about 8-10 minutes. Remove from the heat when the chicken is white and cooked through. If you poke it with a fork, the juices should run clear.
2. Place ½ teaspoon of salt and two chicken breasts in each pint jar. Fill the jar with water.
3. Can for 70 minutes at 10 pounds of pressure for the weighted gauge of the pressure canner or 11 pounds if the pressure canner has a dial gauge.
4. Remove the jars and let them cool until it is at room temperature, which may take about a day.

Nutrition:

Calories: 44.8
Fat: 0.9g
Carbs: 0g
Protein: 9.2g

9. Beef Stew

Preparation Time: 10 min
Cooking Time: 30 min
Servings: 4

Ingredients:

- 3 tbsps. flour
- 2 lbs. canned beef
- 1 package of beef stew seasoning mix powder
- 2 tbsps. vegetable oil
- 5 c. frozen bagged vegetables
- 3 c. water

Directions:

1. Toss beef in flour, then browns in oil in a skillet over medium-high heat.
2. Stir in water and seasoning.
3. Add frozen vegetables and bring to a boil.
4. Turn to low.
5. Cover and simmer for 15 minutes.

Nutrition:

Calories: 443
Fat: 8g
Fiber: 1g
Carbs: 8g
Protein: 3g

10. Canning Boston Pork And Beans

Preparation Time: 10 min
Cooking Time: 1 hour
Servings: 6

Ingredients:

- 1½ pounds bacon, diced
- 1 c. brown sugar
- 3 bay leaves
- 1 tsp. black pepper
- ½ c. ketchup
- 3 tbsps. kosher salt
- ¾ c. molasses
- ¼ c. apple cider vinegar
- 3 large yellow onions, sliced
- ½ tsp. ground cloves
- 3 pounds dried white/navy beans
- 2 tbsps. ground dry mustard
- 5 cloves garlic, cut
- 2 tbsps. Worcestershire sauce

Directions:

1. Wash the beans and quickly boil them in water for two minutes, don't add salt. Switch off the heat, then put the lid on and allow it to soak for one hour. Take out and throw away the liquid.
2. Bring the beans back to the pot with 6 liters of water and get it to a boil. After that, drain instantly again, but reserve the liquid this time. Keep the beans and liquid aside.
3. Bring out a big stockpot, fry the bacon until golden, and then get rid of the fat. Add onions and then cook until it's tender and caramelized. Follow up by adding the garlic and cook for further minutes.
4. Go ahead and add the rest of the ingredients, together with the beans and liquid. Bake for three to four hours, stirring once or twice, at 350°F. You can add a small amount of water if desired.
5. Add it to hot and purified canning jars, allowing for 1-inch headspace, then cover each jar with seals and rims.
6. Process at 10 pounds for 1,000 ft (weighted gauge) or 11 pounds at 1,000 ft (dial gauge). Then adjust for pressure above the altitude.
7. Take away your pressure canner from the heat and let the pressure naturally go away. Take out the jars, put them on a dishtowel, and allow them to sit for twenty hours.

Nutrition:

Calories: 226
Total Fat: 8.8g
Carbs: 3.62g
Protein: 33.11g

11. Canning Venison Spaghetti Sauce

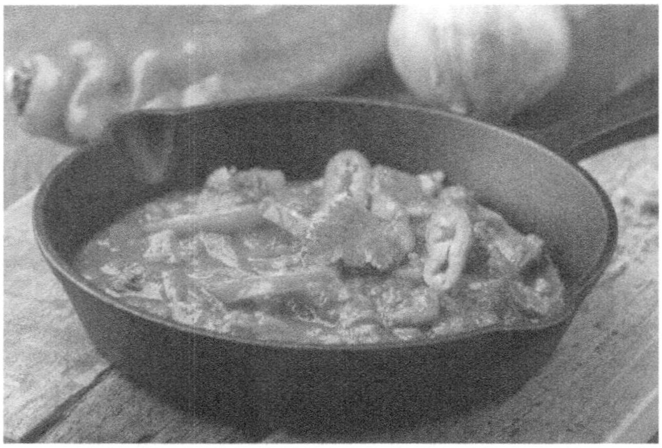

Preparation Time: 10 min
Cooking Time: 3 hours
Servings: 6

Ingredients:

- ¼ c. olive oil
- ½ tsp. red pepper flakes
- 2 28 oz. cans of crumpled tomatoes
- 1 c. red wine
- 1 6 oz. can of tomato paste
- 1 large yellow onion, sliced
- 2 tbsps. dried oregano
- 2 ½ lbs. ground venison
- Salt, black pepper, and sugar to taste
- 6 cloves garlic, sliced
- ¼ c. chopped fresh parsley
- 1 qt. venison/beef stock

Directions:

1. Bring out a big Dutch oven and brown the venison on medium-high heat.
2. When the meat turns golden, go ahead and add the onion; keep stirring and cooking for eight minutes. Continue stirring and cooking for a minute or two. Add the tomato paste and stir to mix properly. Allow cooking for a few minutes until it turns brown.
3. Add the wine and stir it, then add the herbs and red pepper flakes. Allow the wine to boil down to half. After that, add the crumpled tomatoes as well as the stock. Allow it to thicken to a thick simmer, and keep cooking for thirty minutes. Season with salt, pepper, and sugar.
4. Set out your pressure canner while the sauce is simmering down. Bring out a neat quart jar. Moisten your dishtowel with vinegar and use it to clean the rims of the jar.
5. Then, pour the hot sauce into the jars, leaving 1-inch headspace. Turn and seal the lids, then keep the jars in the canner.
6. Follow the canner's instructions on sealing, venting, and setting the gauge. Increase the heat until it reaches your required pressure. Ensure you switch the heat to medium and set the timer for 70 minutes.
7. Once the time expires, switch off the heat and let the canner sit for about an hour or two. Then gradually open the canner. Hold on for all the jar lids to tootle. Then drop the jars onto a chopping board and allow them to sit till the next day.
8. Make sure to label it and keep it in a cool and dry place. You can store it for up to 2 years.

To Make Bone Broth:

1. Make some homemade bone broth to get things started. Fill a 5-gallon stockpot about halfway with bones from the freezer. Because they come from a meal, the bones are usually already roasted. If you have already boned your raw meat, roast the bones in the oven before you start making your stock to give it a deeper flavor.
2. Add about five carrots or three onions in each batch.
3. Fill the pot with water and allow for 2 inches of headspace.
4. Get it to a low boil, and simmer on the cooktop for about 4 hours.
5. Remove any solids from the bone broth by straining it. Start by putting it over a colander and then through a filter with a fine mesh.
6. If your bone broth has too much fat, you can let it cool and then skim off the fat. This isn't necessary, but it will make the result look better.

To Can Bone Broth:

1. Add about 2 inches of water to the bottom of the canner to get it ready. Put the bottom rack in and let the water boil.
2. On a different stove, let your bone broth boil. After that, pour the hot bone broth into the canning jars, allowing for 1 inch of headspace.
3. Put the canning jars on top of the bottom rack using a jar lifter. If you own a double-decker canner, attach the divider and fill up the second rack.
4. Closely tighten the bolts and seal the pressure canner lid. Before adding the canning weight at 10 lb of pressure for elevations below 1,000 feet, let the steam drain from the pressure valve for about ten minutes.
5. Keep the stove on high until the canner reaches the proper temperature and the canning weight begins to twirl to let the pressure out. Start timing after the canner has reached pressure. At 10 lbs of pressure, it takes twenty-five minutes to can filtered bone broth without meat.
6. Reduce the stove's heat. The canning weight should move at least once every minute to confirm that pressure has been managed. Reduce it so it isn't wobbling because that would leak too much water.
7. Turn off the heat and let the pressure canner return to room temperature gradually after 25 minutes of cooking time have passed. Do not take out the canning weight until the canner has returned to ambient temperature. Decreasing pressure too quickly can cause jars to break, which is a safety hazard for everyone involved.
8. The dial gauge will not read "0" pounds of pressure until the canner has cooled for at least an hour. Wait for any leftover steam to dissipate, then take off the weight, uncover the canner, and take out the jars.
9. Take out the jars. When it has fully cooled, take out the canning rings to store it. The moisture that is tucked inside can make them rusty.
10. Clean the jar and store it in a cool dark location. You can store your canned bone broth for a year and six months.

Nutrition:

Calories: 302
Total Fat: 10.4g
Carbs: 8.9g
Protein: 14.6g

12. Basic Canned Chicken, Rabbit, or Squirrel

Preparation Time: 10 min
Cooking Time: 20 minutes
Servings: 6

Ingredients:

- Poultry or small game meat
- Broth for seasoning, optional
- Salt

Directions:

1. Cook chicken (or other meat) until the meat no longer has a pink color. Pack the meat loosely into the jars, and add hot broth, if desired, leaving standard 1-inch headspace
2. Add salt, if desired. ½ teaspoon per pint jar or one teaspoon per quart jar.
3. Clean jar rims, then add sealing lids and rings.
4. It is now time to add jars to the pressure canner and follow the manufacturer's instructions. Typical processing recommends setting the canner at ten pounds pressure and cooking pint jars at one hour, 5 minutes, or quart jars at one hour and 15 minutes.

Nutrition:

Calories: 300
Total Fat: 9.6g
Carbs: 8.3g
Protein: 14.8g

13. Potato and Veal Meatballs

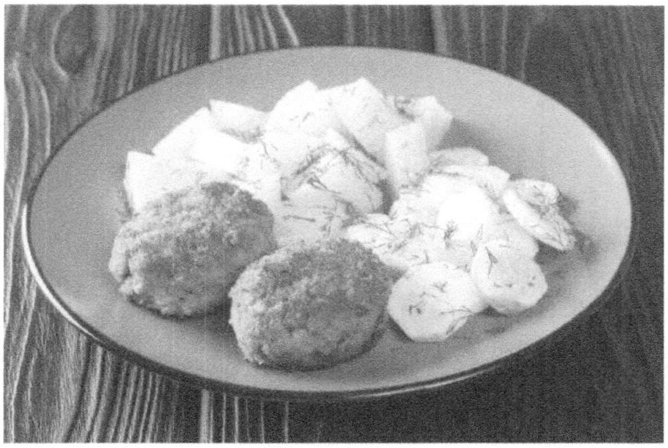

Preparation Time: 10 min
Cooking Time: 10 minutes
Servings: 6

Ingredients:

- 7 oz. (200 g) ground veal
- ½ pounds (250 g) of potatoes
- 1 large egg, beaten
- 3 ½ oz. (100 g) or about 1 cup Parmigiano-Reggiano cheese, grated
- Freshly grated nutmeg to taste
- Vegetable oil for frying
- Salt and pepper to taste

Directions:

1. Boil the potatoes in a large pot of salted water until tender when pierced with a fork, 15 to 20 minutes. Peel and rice the potatoes.
2. Mix the ground veal with the potatoes. Season with salt and pepper and a bit of nutmeg. Add the Parmigiano-reggiano and the egg.

3. Form the meatballs and flatten them lightly. Fry the meatballs in the oil over medium heat, turning them to cook evenly for about 5 to 10 minutes.
4. Transfer to paper towels to drain.

Nutrition:

Calories: 302
Total Fat: 9.6g
Carbs: 8.3g
Protein: 15.8g

14. Roast Veal Shank

Preparation Time: 10 min
Cooking Time: 30 minutes
Servings: 6

Ingredients:

- 2 ⅔ pounds (1.2 kg) veal shank
- 1 ¾ oz. (50 g) bacon, minced
- ⅓ oz. (10 g) fresh rosemary, minced
- Extra-virgin olive oil, as needed
- 3 oz. (80 g) onion, diced
- 2 oz. (60 g) carrots, diced
- 1 ½ oz. (40 g) celery, diced
- ¾ c. + 1 ½ tbsp. (200 ml) white wine
- ½ cup (100 g) crushed tomatoes
- Beef broth, as needed
- Minced garlic to taste
- Salt and pepper to taste

Directions:

1. Trim the excess fat off the veal shank, make deep slits all over the meat and season with salt and pepper.
2. Mix together the garlic, rosemary and bacon and insert it into the slits you have made in the meat.
3. Heat the oven to 350F (175C). Heat the oil in a pot over medium heat and brown the meat.
4. Add the onion, carrot and celery and cook until tender.
5. Add the white wine and cook until it evaporates. Add the crushed tomatoes and stir to combine.
6. Transfer to a baking pan and cook in the oven; add broth if necessary during cooking. When the meat is fork tender, in about one hour, remove from the pot to rest.
7. Let the sauce simmer; if necessary, thicken with a little cornstarch dissolved in a spoonful of water.

Nutrition:

Calories: 289
Total Fat: 9.2g
Carbs: 8.3g
Protein: 14.3g

15. Beef Tartar

Preparation Time: 10 min
Cooking Time: 45 minutes
Servings: 6

Ingredients:

- 14 oz. (400 g) beef tenderloin
- ¾ cups + 1 ½ tbsp. (200 ml) extra-virgin olive oil
- 2 salted anchovies, rinsed well and minced
- 15 capers in salt, rinsed well
- 1 tbsp. chopped fresh parsley
- 3 ½ oz. (100 g) red onion, or about one medium, finely chopped
- Juice of one lemon, as needed
- 4 large eggs
- Salt and pepper to taste

Directions:

1. Finely chops the beef tenderloin with a knife and divides it into four portions. Separate the eggs, putting each yolk in a small cup (the whites are not used), and season with salt, pepper and lemon juice to taste.
2. Arrange each serving of beef tartare on a plate together with the egg yolk in its cup. Arrange the anchovies, capers, parsley and red onion on the plates.
3. Each person will add these to the beef tartare according to to taste. Season to taste with salt, pepper, and extra-virgin olive oil.

Nutrition:

Calories: 304
Total Fat: 9.2g
Carbs: 8.2g
Protein: 16.2g

CONCLUSION

Thank you for reading this book. Canning and preserving food are long-established kitchen activities. Glass mason jars have been used to store, seal, and save all types of foods since before refrigeration, and they are still popular today. Some foods are easier to can than others, but they can all be enjoyed if you have the proper knowledge and can safely and easily preserve them.

Some cooks prefer to preserve whenever possible, while others only do so on rare occasions, such as when making batches of in-season fruit jellies. This book is here to help you no matter how you plan to incorporate canning into your life!

You've learned everything you need to know about safely canning and storing various types of meat on these pages. You have received health advice, equipment information, and other information.

To avoid Bisphenol A (BPA), many people have returned to home canning and preserving; store-bought canned foods frequently contain BPA. However, when you can for yourself, you can be sure you are not consuming harmful additives.

It is also much less expensive to buy canned foods than store-bought foods. Aside from the glass mason jars (which are very inexpensive to begin with), the only ingredients you'll need to buy are the ones you'll put in the cans. This can be a very cheap way to eat.

Canning is also highly eco-friendly. Instead of adding to the waste in landfills across the country, thoroughly wash your mason jars and lids, and they will be ready for another use!

It can also be very satisfying to do your canning; you can feel proud of yourself for completing such a large project! It may also be enjoyable to reconnect with your past. For example, if your grandmother canned frequently as a child, you would carry on the family tradition.

Whatever you want out of your cooking life, canning and preserving can help you get it!

Good luck.

SMOKING & SALT CURING

GUIDEBOOK FOR PREPPERS

1000 Days of Recipes to Preserve Meat and Fish for Survival

Tyler Gordon

INTRODUCTION

Prepping means being prepared for any disaster that may occur in the future. It is the process of actively preparing for any disaster or emergency. Natural disasters, such as earthquakes and floods, can occur as well as man-made disasters, such as terrorism. Our preparation gives us three major advantages when a disaster strikes.

When a disaster strikes, people rush to markets and hardware stores searching for provisions, fixtures, tools, medical supplies, etc. You may forget what you require due to your fragile state of mind during a disaster, and the items you need may have already been sold by the time you return to the stores. Thus, prepping gives us the advantage of having a head start on others.

If you already have a lot of supplies and the necessary medicines, items, and provisions, you probably don't need to worry about getting more supplies. Also, if disaster strikes, you will have a handy kit with all the necessary items, making it easier to flee during such events. As a result, having everything under control increases your chances of survival. Furthermore, you will only have to worry about minor details when you prepare rather than searching for supplies.

Another issue with disasters is that you may have to survive without technology or electricity. You can meet these unforeseen events by having a handy survival kit and being well prepared. It will also lessen your reliance on emergency services.

Another advantage of prepping is that you will have to live without modern conveniences on which we humans are inherently dependent. We have become overly reliant on technology and power in recent years. We also take them for granted, assuming that there will never be a time when we will need them. Thus, prepping will assist us in overcoming such dependency and difficulties when a disaster strikes.

You must understand the fundamentals of prepping and ask yourself why you must prepare for any situation. Modern-day preppers attempt to prepare for a specific time when life becomes difficult. They intend to be self-sufficient and independent enough to face any challenge, no matter how difficult. These challenges could take the form of almost anything or everything, and they all fall under the SHTF umbrella. It could be as simple as a harsh winter, an earthquake, or a pandemic. Everything that interferes with your usual way of life is a challenge for you. Every prepper takes the initiative to prepare for all risks unique to them or their location.

Prepping is the process by which preppers adapt to be capable of dealing with almost anything that violates the peace around them. The approach promotes anticipating and planning for potential risk factors and the necessary needs to overcome them. As a result, this is the best way to mitigate the adverse effects of a disaster or emergency that the SHTF situation may cause for your livelihood. Prepping promotes the idea that 'Change' is a constant in life. Everyone who considers caring for their families in a disaster without relying on government assistance is a prepper. All governments launch counter-measures to natural disasters and pandemics to keep people safe in the modern era. They are also preparing on a large scale rather than focusing on a single individual.

Prepping is the process of preparing for survival without the use of complex infrastructure. It is the action that promotes being ready to face life before, during, and after an apocalyptic event. You may have heard most of the time during natural disaster alerts when people raid grocery and essential stores right before storms, tsunamis, and other such events. However, preppers plan for such common problems far in advance. They have the idea and consideration to have water, food, first aid, and other supplies that one might require due to the inaccessibility of grocery stores for the next few days or weeks. Preppers risk stockpiling pantry items, bottled waters, battery lamps, candles, first-aid kits, antibiotics, generic medications, and other similar items. The most fundamental level of prepping is gathering all the items required for a camping or outdoor trip.

An important consideration is how you will obtain the items you require. Food, water, fuel, and shelter are all included. If you live in an area where growing your food will be difficult or impossible due to the climate, consider moving to a more suitable location if you are passionate about farming. Many people have gardens for growing food, but they do not live in climates that allow them to garden all year. This means that if you rely on your garden for everything, the same winter freeze that kills it could also kill you. Learning how to preserve food by canning or smoking will be critical if this is the case. If you live in an area where hunting is permitted, learning how to hunt and gut a deer will provide you with a backup plan if necessary.

Getting enough food and clean water can be difficult when you have to rely on yourself for everything. A first-aid kit, essential medicines, and a first-aid class will come in handy here. These should be addressed as soon as possible to ensure you understand how to treat injuries following an accident or other event. Many classes on first-aid are available through the Boy Scouts, churches, and other organizations. If having the supplies isn't enough to pique your interest in learning these skills, consider how much it will cost you to keep going to the doctor when there isn't anyone else for miles.

In this book, you will learn the fundamentals of smoking and salt curing for preppers. Our goal is to teach you the fundamentals of smoking. Once you've mastered the fundamentals, you can progress to more complex techniques and recipes. We've included tips on improving your smoking skills, whether cooking your first brisket, learning how to use an injection marinade, or creating the perfect candied salmon or smoked chicken. Let's get started!

CHAPTER 1: UNDERSTANDING SMOKING AND SALT CURING

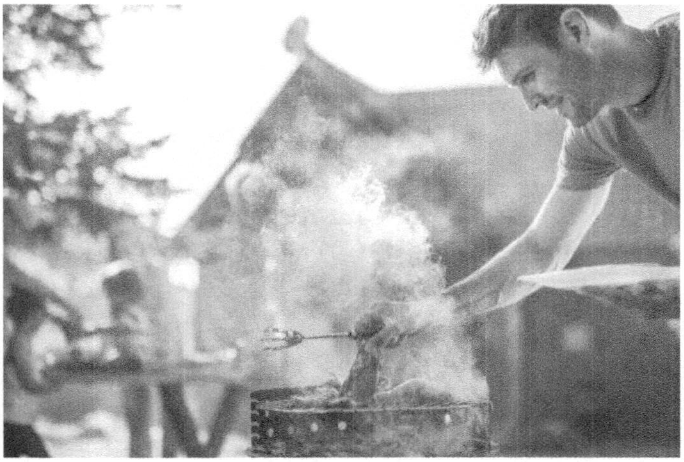

Smoking Meat

Smoking is the process of flavoring, cooking, or preserving food by exposing it to smoke produced by burning or smoldering plant materials such as wood, mainly hardwood wood. Food smoking is practiced both commercially and at home. The meats are hung or placed on racks in an enclosed area, preventing smoke from escaping and penetrating the foods. Steam pipes are sometimes used in commercial smoking to supplement the wood fire.

Because it is antimicrobial and antioxidant, smoke is used to preserve foods. Smoking is most likely the oldest method of food preservation, emerging shortly after the discovery of fire. Because of the use of chemical preservatives, smoking as a preservative has declined in popularity, but it is regaining popularity because it is considered natural. The most commonly smoked foods are meat and fish, but cheeses, nuts, vegetables, and beverages such as tea and whisky are also smoked. In Scandinavia, smoking fish is popular, whereas ham is famous in Europe and the United States.

Smoking evolved from ancient traditions, beginning as a method of preserving meats and fish for the long winters and eventually becoming a popular outdoor activity and a staple of our modern-day patio culture. Cooking with smoke has recently become something of a craze. Smokers and grills are more widely available than ever before, and many supermarkets stock wood pellets, chunks, planks, and almost anything else you might need to add smoke to your cooking.

Smoking is fundamentally similar to roasting or baking in many ways. You cook in an enclosed, heated chamber, either quickly at a high temperature or slowly at a low temperature. If you imagine this as a cooking process in your oven, all you need to learn is how to add smoke. That is the subject of this book.

To properly add smoke, you'll need the right kind of wood. There are numerous wood "flavors" to choose from, ranging from heavy and robust to light and sweet and everything in between. Consider the cooking equipment next. You can use strategies to produce a good dose of smoke, whether you own a large smoking rig or a small gas grill. Once you've mastered a few fundamentals, which we'll go over in this chapter, you'll be able to smoke the perfect barbecue brisket, holiday turkey, or weeknight salmon fillet, as well as delicious appetizers and side dishes to round out the meal.

Smoking is a preservation method that extends the shelf life of a product while also improving its flavor profile. It flavors, cooks, and preserves food by exposing it to a consistent smoke. Smoke is produced when plant material, such as wood or hardwood is burned. While it is primarily a commercial process, it can be done at home with the proper equipment.

The smoke required to cook food is extremely precise. Fortunately, achieving it is not difficult, but you must be prepared. Because smoke can be powerful, it must flow properly around the food. Even if you're cooking low and slow, it should be generated by hot, fast combustion. This is what produces the much-desired thin blue smoke.

Dark gray or black smoke will impart a bitter, tongue-numbing flavor to your food. Slowly billowing white smoke can cause a stale aroma from your cooker. Worse, both of these can indicate creosote buildup. This thick, tar-like substance is caused by smoke that lingers too long and is tainted with resins, lighter fluid, or charcoal additives.

The following is how smoking meat works: You cook at a much lower temperature than you would grill a steak, and the smoke slowly absorbs into the meat. This "low and slow" process infuses maximum flavor while gently breaking down and melting the intramuscular fat, collagen, and tough tissues to produce a uniquely tender, succulent, smoky, and savory bite. It's not something you can rush. Each roast or cut of meat has a different internal temperature at which it goes from tough to tender. Generally, this smoking temperature can be achieved by cooking with an external indirect heat source ranging from 225°F to 250°F, and occasionally even 275°F. An accurate thermometer is always helpful, but don't worry about the temporary temperature swings when adding wood chips or fuel.

When you go slowly, a few things happen. First, the tissues degrade into juiciness. Bark eventually forms on the outside of the meat. The combination of smoke, protein, and seasonings should produce a firm, deep, dark brown color. Not entirely black, but close. The color is caused by a chemical reaction on the meat's surface. In the following pages, we'll go over the smoke ring and the burning sugar.

Finally, with enough time and smoke, you'll be able to tenderize the meat fibers. With a bite and an easy chew, they should gently break apart. When you marinate meats or bite into filet mignon, you expect this level of tenderness. The difference is that cuts like filet mignon remain tender at lower (rare) internal temperatures of 125°F to 130°F. In contrast, traditional low-and slow-smoked meats achieve pull-apart tenderness only when topping internal temperatures over 190°F (considered an insult to prime steaks).

Smoking Methods

Hot and cold smoking are both popular. Hot smoking occurs when food is directly exposed to smoke in controlled environments. Smoked foods can be cooked or reheated as needed. These foods can also be eaten right away without further preparation. The temperature range for hot smoking is typically between 125 and 180°F. This temperature is considered normal for food. 180°F is the ideal temperature for most meats. If the ingredients are exposed to heat and smoke, they can be eaten immediately. Foods retain moisture and texture when heated to this temperature. When a smoky flavor is added to food, it can cause it to dry out. Foods can lose moisture if the temperature rises above this level and fats begin to dry. Smoking is frequently used with other preservation methods, such as drying or curing. Salt-cured foods can be smoked to extend their shelf life.

The next method of smoking is cold smoking. This smoking technique is more of a flavor enhancer than a cooking technique. It's frequently used to season chicken breasts, pork chops, scallops, steaks, and salmon. This is done at temperatures ranging from 68 to 90°F. This temperature is maintained to ensure moisture retention. It is not intended for food storage. It is simply used to give food a smoky flavor. Cold-smoked foods should not be consumed immediately. They must instead be dried before being cold-smoked. Curing removes moisture from meats, preventing bacteria from growing. Cold smoking meat after it has been cured in any other way is possible.

Benefits of Smoking Meat

Smoke is thought to have antimicrobial and antioxidant properties. This means that any pathogens on the surface of the meat are destroyed, as are their chances of resurfacing. Smoking, on the other hand, cannot be used as a stand-alone preservation technique. The issue is that the smoke compound only adheres to the outer surface of the food and does not penetrate the meat or food you are attempting to preserve. As a result, smoke's antioxidant and antimicrobial properties are limited to the meat's outer surfaces. This is why smoking must be used with other preservation methods such as salt curing or drying.

When wood is burned, the smoke contains phenol, and other phenolic compounds thought to be natural antioxidants. Oxidation is the process by which the structure of molecules changes as a result of oxygen exposure. Rancidity is a common example of food damage caused by oxidation. When food is exposed to the elements for an extended period, it spoils. As a result, the beneficial compounds in wood smoke slow the rancidification of fats found in meat, fish, and even poultry. This, in conjunction with antimicrobial agents such as formaldehyde, acetic acid, and a variety of other beneficial organic acids, lowers the pH of smoke. The pH of smoke is typically around 2.5. Pathogens struggle to survive in this environment due to the low pH.

Smoking not only extends the shelf life of food but also improves the flavor profile. Smoked meats are delectable! Once smoked and preserved, the meats can be stored at the proper temperature for up to a year! This allows you to access the necessary ingredients whenever you want to cook easily. This makes the meat more flavorful and appetizing. The color of the meat changes as well when it is smoked. The meats appear to be shinier and redder. This simply adds to their allure.

Meat Smoking Tips

Always Cook Meat Slowly

When you taste authentic barbecue for yourself, you will quickly realize that it is not made by smothering your meat in barbecue sauce. The secret to authentic barbecue is slow cooking your meat for several hours over low heat. This is how most authentic barbecued meat stays moist and tender, and it is something you should keep in mind when smoking your meat.

Always Begin Early

When it comes to smoking meat, one of the best ways to ensure that your meat has a ton of flavor is to start prepping early. It is best to begin preparing your meat while it is still raw if you want it to absorb all of the smoky flavors as soon as possible. This is the time to get your meat into the smoker as soon as possible. Remember that the longer your meat sits out, the more dried it will become.

Keep the Air Flowing At All Times

The most important thing you can do while your meat is smoking is to keep it well ventilated throughout the cooking process. You should keep the vents of your grill or smoker open while your meat is smoking. This will assist in drawing smoke from your charcoal or woodchips and causing it to swirl around your food while properly exiting the top.

Use a Pan of Water to Control the Temperature Inside Your Smoker

When the temperature inside your smoker fluctuates dramatically, it can cause your meat to become too tight or dry. The best way to prevent this is to place a pan filled with water inside your smoker. This pan of water will help to stabilize the temperature inside your smoker and even add some humidity, keeping your meat moist and tender.

Never Go Overboard

Overdoing it is one of the most common mistakes that new smokers make. They frequently add far too many woodchips to their smoker or overseason it. When it comes to smoking, the general rule is that you should only smoke your meat for half the time it takes to cook. If you follow these steps, your meat will taste delicious every time.

Keep in Mind that Black Smoke is a Bad Thing

You may notice a few puffs of white smoke escaping your smoker while smoking your meat. White smoke is a good sign because it means your meat is being layered with that addictive smoky flavor you crave. This is a bad sign if you start noticing black smoke coming out of your smoker. This can be caused by several factors, such as your smoker not receiving adequate ventilation or your food is cooked directly over the fire. The general rule of thumb is always to aim for your smoker's white smoke. Avoid inhaling black smoke.

Never Leave Your Smoker Unattended

While smoking meat requires many hours of your time, this does not mean you should ever leave your smoker unattended during this time. You want to ensure a safe cooking environment, so check the temperature of your smoker every hour or two to ensure that it isn't reaching dangerous levels.

Don't Look At Your Food While It's Cooking

One thing you might have to fight yourself against is peeking at your food while it cooks. You should remember that opening your grill or smoker loses heat and adds time to the cooking process. That said, never peek at your food to see how it's doing. Open your grill or smoker only when you need to add more woodchips, tend to the fire inside, add a water pan, or check the doneness of your meat as it approaches the end of its cooking time.

Check that Your "Bark" Darkens Evenly

The special glisten with a dark brown crust we all love and wish for is a sign of authentic barbecued and smoked meat. This is referred to as the "bark" of your meat and is the hallmark of good smoking. Before you remove your meat from the smoker at the end of its cooking time, make sure the "bark" on the surface is the perfect shade of mahogany brown to ensure it tastes like a little slice of heaven.

Always Season Your Meat to Perfection

Every flavor should play a role in the overall taste, which is one of the critical ingredients of any perfect smoked recipe. You want to avoid having one flavor that overpowers the others and instead strives for the ideal balance of all of your spices.

Salt Curing

Salt curing produces and preserves meats such as bacon, ham, sausage, chorizo, and even corned beef. Salt is the foundation for preventing bacteria and keeping meats fresher for longer without using a refrigerator.

Curing is essentially a salt-preserving technique for meat. Salt aids in their death and prevents this process. When pathogens consume and metabolize meat, the meat's texture, color, and flavor change. These are all indicators of food spoilage.

So, how exactly does salt aid in food preservation? Through a process known as osmosis, salt removes all of the moisture or water present within the meat cells. Osmosis has two positive effects. The first effect is that it dries the meat, and the second effect is that it kills all pathogens. It's important to remember that salt does not refer to regular table salt in this context. Instead, it refers to a mixture of salt, salt cures, and a small amount of sugar.

Bacon, ham, and corned beef are the most common salt-cured meats. Other salt-cured meats include pancetta, liverwurst, summer sausage, salami, and chorizo. Even if salt-curing meats take several weeks, the flavor it produces is worth the wait. During curing, various enzymes in the meat undergo chemical changes that contribute to the meat's flavor. Aside from that, the salt used in curing enhances the natural flavor. This, combined with sugar, herbs, and spices, further balances and elevates the flavors. When salted meat is smoked later, it develops a fantastic and well-rounded flavor profile. Salted meats have not been cooked. Some salted meats are further dried to ensure they are safe to eat.

It works because salt kills any bacteria already present in the meat. It also draws moisture from it, which inhibits the growth of bacteria. It's the perfect one-two punch for long-term meat preservation.

Salt curing, on the other hand, is not simply coating a steak in table salt and leaving it on the counter until dinnertime. It's not a creative or interesting way to use table salt. Instead, salt curing combines regular salt, salt cures, and sugar to keep everything together. Balance is crucial when it comes to salt curing!

Salt, like sugar, draws water out of food and inhibits bacterial growth. At a high level, it may destroy the cells of microscopic organisms, though the food is logically unappealing by this point.

Curing Methods

There are three methods for curing meat with salt. There are three methods for salt curing meats: dry curing, wet curing, and injecting. For at-home curing, wet curing is the best option. We will go over these options and how they work.

Dry Curing

Remember the different curing methods we discussed in the previous section? The most common is dry curing.

When dry curing, plenty of curing powder should be applied. Rub the meat in the curing mixture before placing it in a container. Place the meat in a refrigerator or other cold area that can keep a temperature of 36-40°F. The most important aspects of curing meat are temperature and humidity control, so pay close attention to them.

Wet Curing

Wet curing is the most effective method for curing meat in small quantities. This is especially useful if you intend to re-cook the cured meat. You'll need to make a brine solution and immerse the meat. The brine aids in the removal of excess moisture and the creation of an ideal balance that prevents pathogen growth.

This method makes it simple to adjust the amount of salt used. This ensures that the salt is evenly distributed throughout the meat and that there are no salt pockets.

Place the meat in the refrigerator or freezer once you've finished curing it. You must keep the meat submerged in the brine at all times and turn it every few days to ensure even exposure to the brine. The meat should not be left out in the open. Keeping the meat in a separate area is best to avoid cross-contamination.

Injecting

As the name implies, you will inject salty brine into your meat using a syringe. It can be difficult to distribute the salty brine evenly utilizing this method, especially if the equipment is not professional. This is not a recommended do-it-yourself solution. This technique may result in salt pockets in the meat.

A lot goes into salt curing meats; it isn't the easiest thing in the world. Measuring, judging weight, and being cautious is all essential. Curing powders are safe and effective in small amounts.

Salt-cured meats are still popular today, not only for their convenience but also for their distinct flavor. If you understand how curing works, you can make cured meats like bacon, sausage, ham, and corned beef at home.

The most apparent advantage of salt curing is that it extends the shelf life of ingredients. For example, if the meats are properly cured and then dried or smoked, their shelf life is extended by a few months. Cured meats can be kept at the proper temperature for nearly a year if stored properly. This is an excellent method for preserving meats, poultry, fish, and even game meats.

Another benefit of salt curing is that it kills any pathogens in the meat. The salt dries out the meat and absorbs any remaining moisture. Pathogens are automatically killed when this occurs. Pathogens that cause disease become unwelcome in the meat.

Salting can also improve the flavor and texture of certain meats. After the meats have been cured, they can be cooked in various ways. Bacon, for example, tastes different from a regular strip of pork belly, doesn't it? This is due to the curing process it goes through.

Types of Salts To Use

Numerous curing salt options are available, and the evidence is frequently contradictory. Previously, regular salt was used to cure meat, but saltpeter was added to the curing mixture in the 1600s. The common name for sodium nitrate or potassium nitrate is saltpeter. Salt is primarily used to preserve food. Saltpeter, on the other hand, does not directly preserve the food.

Certain bacteria cannot be killed by salt alone. As a result, saltpeter is added to guard against them. Bacteria in food consume the nitrates in saltpeter, producing nitrites in the process. Following this, another reaction occurs, converting the nitrites to nitric oxide. Nitric oxide begins to form bonds with various proteins found in meat. This turns the meat pink and reduces the possibility of oxidation. Nitric oxide preserves the meat while killing Botulism spores and other harmful bacteria. When using saltpeter, it is always used in conjunction with salt. Saltpeter is not a salt substitute.

This brings us to what is commonly referred to as pink salt or Prague powder. It is another name for saltpeter, which is used to cure meat. Pink salt is so named because it contains a food coloring that prevents consumers from mistaking it for regular salt. The pink color of the cured meat caused by salt-curing is unrelated to the red dye used in the cure. Remember that the activation of nitric oxide is what gives the meat its pink color. Pink salts come in two varieties: Prague powder #1 and Prague powder #2. Pink salt #1 and pink salt #2 are their other names. The former comprises 93% common table salt, and the remainder is sodium nitrite. When cooking meat, poultry, or fish after curing, use Prague powder #1. Pink salt #2, on the other hand, contains 4% sodium nitrate, 6.25% sodium nitrite, and the rest is table salt. This is a dry cure for meats, such as prosciutto, which will not be cooked further.

Aside from that, Morton Tender Quick is used in some recipes. It contains salt, sodium nitrite, sugar, and sodium nitrate. It is not pink as its counterparts are. If you use it at home, keep it separate from regular table salt. Most beginners make the mistake of believing that all curing salts are the same. Curing salts are not interchangeable, so please avoid this error. Follow the instructions if a curing recipe calls for a specific curing salt. Try not to change it. The salts are selected based on the preservation process.

Now that you've learned about the various types of curing salts used for food preservation, it's time to address some common concerns about curing salts. Curing salts are extremely toxic, contrary to popular belief. Curing salts are toxic only in large and excessive amounts. Curing salts should not be consumed directly. You should not inhale it or rub it in your eyes. It should be kept out of the reach of children. Don't be concerned because home curing recipes do not require such large amounts of salt. Furthermore, it does not endanger your health because you are not constantly exposed to it.

Another common concern about nitrites is their link to increased cancer risk. Natural foods contain nitrates. They are more common than you might think. For example, a single serving of spinach contains more nitrites than a serving of salami.

The only thing to be concerned about when curing meats is the risk of botulism. Aside from that, there's nothing else to be worried about. Botulism risk is reduced when the curing recipe is followed correctly, and the required salting and smoking temperatures are maintained.

Curing salts are not the only option. The only reason to use curing salts is to remove all Botulism spores from the meat. You can cure with regular salt, but there are a few things to remember. The presence of iodine in regular or table salt is a significant concern. Table salt is always iodized, and iodine can give the cured meat an odd flavor. Table salt's anti-clumping active ingredients make the dry cure lumpy. If you use it to make a brine, it may contain sediments. Stick to the recipe and use non-iodized salt when curing the meat with regular salt.

If you're using regular salt, consider the size of the salt granules. This can impact the amount of salt used in a recipe. For example, a cup of kosher salt weighs about 5-8 ounces, whereas one cup of table salt weighs about 10 ounces. So, one cup of table salt differs from one cup of kosher salt. When curing meats at home, a weighing scale is an efficient way to measure the ingredients.

Choose celery juice if you want a natural source of nitrate, as these can be found in celery juice. Celery juice causes a reaction similar to saltpeter during the curing process. This, however, is not a substitute for the results obtained with saltpeter.

CHAPTER 2: SMOKERS AND OTHER MUST-HAVE TOOLS

Cooking has been overlooked as a necessary survival skill in the age of convenience and technology. Fresh-grown produce and local meats are more readily available than ever, but the question remains about storing them without canning or smoking correctly. Will you know how to start a fire if you get lost in the wilderness?

To start a fire, you'll need three things:

- **Tinder:** A small, dry, flammable substance used to catch a spark and ignite a fire.
- **Kindling:** A slightly larger but flammable material that catches the tinder's flame and spreads it until it becomes a bonfire. Dead twigs and branches the size of your thumb make excellent kindling.
- **Fuel:** A larger material, usually hardwood or deadfall, is used to keep the fire going once it's started.

You'll need matches or another heat source, such as flint and steel, to start a fire. If you're using matches, keep them in a tight, waterproof container to ensure longevity. Tease apart a piece of cattail fibers until they are fine and fluffy to make a matchstick. Then, using your fingers, roll the fibers into a tight bundle, careful not to crush them. Roll a thin strand of dry grass around the center of the bundle and secure it with another piece of grass. When you have enough, strike your heat source along the side of the bundle, and it should light instantly.

Once you have a flame, carefully add kindling. Smaller pieces of wood will catch more easily than larger ones, so start by placing your kindling around the edges of the fire. When you have a nice medium-sized flame, add larger wood pieces.

We must control the fire when using charcoal. This entails closing the lid and adjusting the vents so that the grill maintains the desired temperature. When you open the lid, you let out heat and oxygen. As a result, the temperature drops, jumps, and then stabilizes. Don't freak out. This is normal; low and slow cooking has been practiced for decades.

Begin with a large fire when cooking with charcoal. You want a lot of charcoal burning, and once the coals are cleanly burning, close the vents and the grill lid to reach your desired temperature. If you plan to cook for more than 6 to 8 hours, you may need to add more fuel. In this case, light more charcoal with a charcoal chimney and add it to the grill when the first charcoal has burned to one-third of its original size. Adding more fuel early in the cooking process is always preferable rather than later.

When burning wood for smoke, you want clean and consistent combustion. You don't want a smoldering, steamy smoke with little aroma. As a result, do not soak your wood chips and chunks. That has been the advice for a generation, but it has resulted in poor smoke production.

Whatever wood you choose, it must be dry. It should be carefully stored to keep it dry. Even in moderately humid environments, dry wood will absorb moisture from the air, leading to mold growth and bad smoke. So, until you're ready to use it, keep your smoking wood in an airtight container.

The first thing you'll need to start smoking meat at home is the smokers themselves. Smokers come in various sizes and shapes; you can buy them commercially or make your own out of barrels, as Nonno did. Smoking is essentially the process of hanging or placing meat on a rack with a smoldering pile of slow-burning wood beneath it. An electric griddle or a small metal bucket filled with charcoal and terracotta pots can be used to make your smoker. You can even smoke meats on your grill if you know what you're doing.

Salt Curing Equipment

You will need basic equipment, regardless of whether you are dry curing or smoking meats. Here are a few things to get the most out of salt curing.

Grinder

A grinder is essential if you plan on making your own cured sausages. Consider the shape of most salt-cured meats... Isn't it ground meat that's been processed, seasoned, and then cured? You'll have difficulty producing cured sausages if you rely on your butcher to do all your grinding.

Instead, purchasing a meat grinder will save you time and trouble in the long run and provide a much better final product. Aside from your curing chamber, a meat grinder may be your most expensive purchase. These range from $50-60 to hundreds of dollars.

At the very least, your cutting blades should be stainless steel. These will last much longer and cut through frozen or semi-frozen meat the most easily. They are also the simplest to clean and sanitize, which is extremely useful when working with raw meat.

There are vital points to remember if you're looking for a separate stuffer.

One consideration is capacity; if you plan on making 10-20 pounds of sausage or processing most of a deer, boar, or elk, you'll need a larger stuffer. It will make your life much easier because you won't have to reload every 3-4 pounds until you've stuffed it all.

Thermometer

A good, easy-to-use thermometer is essential when smoking meats, in addition to everything else mentioned above! A long cord and a clear digital readout are essential for finding something you can easily read without opening the smoker. You don't need those fancy Bluetooth ones you can control with your phone, though they are convenient.

Curing and Smoking Ingredients

Aside from keeping Instacure in your kitchen, you can keep a few other items in your pantry or kitchen to help you produce the best final products.

In my opinion, high-quality spices are essential. Don't season your game meat with a generic branded spice blend, especially if you're curing it. Starting with a new, high-quality product will produce the best-finished product.

Like a quality spice, a quality herb is essential when using a recipe that calls for herbs. Fresh is always preferable to dry, and if you have a small area with adequate sunlight, such as a porch or windowsill, you can probably grow your own.

The most common spice is ground pepper, which comes in several varieties: black, white, and green. The fruits of the future spice grow on pepper vines and, when ripe, take on their distinctive color. Right before cooking, ground pepper is thought to be the most aromatic.

Smokers

Smokers made of wood or fire are the most basic and have been used for centuries. These will provide a richer, woodier flavor. However, because you are dealing with naked fire, it will require constant tending and attention - definitely not for beginners, as mastering temperature control with these smokers will take longer.

Making use of charcoal is another old way of smoking meat. It will give your meat a different flavor when compared to wood smokers. It's not inferior to wood smoke - it's simply different and ultimately depends on a person's preferences. And like fire, it will be hard to maintain the temperature with these smokers and need constant tending - and fanning for those old-school charcoal smokers. It's not recommended for beginners.

Refrigerator for Storage

A refrigerator or cool place is an essential thing when curing meats. The critical aspect of curing is temperature regulation. Incorrect temperature can lead to pathogens breeding in your meats if you aren't careful. The final product is not suitable for consumption. Curing and storing meats should be kept at 40°F. Anything higher than that, and you run the risk of getting pathogens. You will need a fridge, freezer, or other cold place to keep the meat at this temperature as long as it is cured.

What Kind of Smoker Should You Use?

You can choose between gas, electric, and charcoal smokers based on your needs and preferences.

Charcoal smokers produce the best smoky flavor, but they can be challenging to control at first.

Gas and electric smokers are simple to use and regulate the temperature; they also cook meat slightly faster. The smoky flavor may not be as authentic as if charcoal were used. If you go with gas, ensure your gas bottle is full enough to last the duration of your smoking session.

After some practice, move on to chicken or turkey, keeping in mind that the meat is leaner and can become tough, so choose a whole bird and smoke for a shorter time to avoid this. If you want to try seafood, go for a robust, oily fish like salmon.

Selecting the Wood

If you want good smoking results, pay special attention to the wood you use. Yes, the type of wood is important here. Different types of wood tend to pair with different meat flavors and would need to complement the meat flavor. Let's take a look at some of the most common smoking woods.

Apple wood has a fruity, sweet flavor. It's mild and goes great with poultry, ham, and fish. Alder is another commonly used smoking wood. Alder has a delicate flavor profile and natural sweetness that complements the flavor of pork, fish, poultry, and other light meats. Hickory is the best way to add some hearty smokiness to red meats and ribs. This is the most commonly used word in barbecues. The pungent and strong aroma of hickory perfectly complements the hardness of red meats. This brings us to another popular wood, oak. Oak is ideal for smoking large cuts of meat for extended periods. It has a pleasant smoky flavor that is not overpowering. This is an excellent choice of wood for short brisket or game meats. Mesquite is another popular material, but it can be overwhelming. Mesquite should be used in the same way that peppers are. When combined with other woods, it is ideal for short-term use.

Maple has a light and sweet flavor that complements ham and poultry. However, use caution when using maple because it can darken the color of meat. Maple, like mesquite, is combined with other woods such as oak and apple. Use pecan sparingly because it has a strong fruity flavor. It also burns cooler than other woods, making it ideal for smoking larger cuts of meat. Add some cherry wood to any meat to improve its color. It goes great with pork and beef.

If in doubt, go with oak or alder. These are the most secure options for smoking meats.

Different types of wood complement various types of meat. For example, lighter and sweeter woods like apple and cherry would pair better when smoking poultry and fish because they can absorb more flavor from the smoke. Whereas heavier, stronger-smelling woods like walnut and mesquite pair well with beef and pork, which require more time for the smoke to impart flavor.

You must now decide on the size and shape of the wood you will use. The largest is the wood chunks. Most commercial smokers use larger chunks of wood because they last longer and can smoke the meat for hours or days. Wood chips are smaller and have a shorter lifespan than wood chunks.

If you want, you can soak the wood as well. Although it is not required, dry wood burns much faster than wet wood. If you soak the wood, properly drain it before putting it in the smoker. This will increase the burn time as well as the smoldering time. Larger sizes, such as chunks, require an hour of soak time, whereas chips require only 30 minutes. Another option is to soak the wood in beer or juice. This will give the smoked meat an extra kick of flavor. Mix some dried herbs and spices with the wood to add even more complex flavors. To control the smoke, adjust the moisture and oxygen levels inside your smoker. Moisture in the wood causes it to burn longer and produce more smoke. More oxygen inside the smoker means larger flames consuming fuel and wood faster.

You need to choose your wood carefully because the wood you will use greatly affects the meat's flavor and taste. Here are a few options for you:

- **Maple:** Maple has a smoky and sweet taste and goes well with pork or poultry
- **Alder:** Alder is sweet and light. Perfect for poultry and fish.
- **Apple:** Apple has a mild and sweet flavor. Goes well with pork, fish, and poultry.
- **Oak:** Oak is great for slow cooking. Ideal for game, pork, beef, and lamb.
- **Mesquite:** Mesquite has a smoky flavor and is extremely strong. Goes well with pork or beef.
- **Hickory:** Has a smoky and strong flavor. Goes well with beef and lamb.
- **Cherry:** Has a mild and sweet flavor. Great for pork, beef, and turkey.

In general, there are essentially three different types of charcoal. All of them are porous residues of black color made of carbon and ashes. However, the following are a little distinguishable due to their specific features.

- **BBQ Briquettes:** These are the ones that are made from a fine blend of charcoal and char.
- **Charcoal Briquettes:** These are created by compressing charcoal and are made from sawdust or wood products.
- **Lump Charcoal:** These are made directly from hardwood and are the most premium quality charcoals. They are entirely natural and are free from any form of additive.

CHAPTER 3: SELECTING THE MEAT

We need to talk about the best meats for smoking. Essentially, any meat can benefit from the deeper flavor that smoking provides. However, larger cuts will perform better in the smoker, especially if they have an excellent marbling of fat on and in them. Slow smoking causes the fats to melt slowly, giving the meat that desired fall-off-the-bone texture.

Here are some cuts that will be good for smoking:

- Pork roast
- Pork shoulder
- Pork butt
- Whole poultry (chicken or turkey)
- Ribs
- Beef brisket Prime rib

Consider jerky, smoked salmon, or smoked potato casserole. Consider the s'mores you made over a campfire. We've got you covered for all of this and more. So many classic foods enjoyed for generations have had a touch of smoke, and we now have the equipment, wood, and know-how to do it properly.

Before even considering smoking, you should figure out what ingredients you want to use. Smoking can be used on various foods, including poultry and other types of meat. What is the significance of taking the cut of meat into account? The time it takes to smoke depends on how thick the cut is.

The most popular smoking cuts are all motion muscles. Spareribs from the loin, belly, beef brisket and ribs are among the most popular cuts of meat for smoking.

Fatty cuts are preferable for smoking. The meat has fat will absorb the delicious smoky flavors better. When smoking meat, choose cuts high in fat and connective tissue. Fattier cuts of meat keep it moist and tender. The fat melts and coats the meat in juices. This improves the flavor and makes it easier to incorporate the smokiness into the meat.

While reading the various chapters on food preservation in this book, remember that smoking is the final step in the preservation process. Before being smoked, the ingredients, whether fish, poultry, meat, or game, are salt-cured.

Everything from poultry and various types of meat to fish can be smoked. Why is the cut of meat significant in this case? The time required for smoking will vary depending on the thickness of the cut. The most common smoking cuts include all of the motion muscles. Spareribs from the belly, loin, beef brisket, and ribs, for example, are the most popular meat cuts for smoking.

It is always preferable to smoke fatty cuts. The fat aids in the absorption of the delicious smoky flavors of the meat. So, when selecting meat to smoke, look for cuts with a lot of fat and connective tissue. Choosing fattier cuts of meat keeps it tender and moist. When the fat begins to melt, it coats the meat in its juices. This enhances the flavor profile while easily incorporating smokiness into the selected meat.

SMOKING & SALT CURING
COOKBOOK FOR PREPPERS

1000 Days of Recipes to Preserve Meat and Fish for Survival

Tyler Gordon

CHAPTER 4: RECIPES

1. Smoked Trout with Orange & Basil

Preparation and Cooking Time: 4 hours and 30 minutes
Servings: 4

Ingredients:

- 1 Orange zest, grated
- 6 lbs. (2.7kg) ground trout
- ½ c. fresh oregano
- ½ c. Kosher salt
- Apple wood chips

Directions:

1. Butterfly the fish and remove the insides.
2. Mix oregano with orange zest in a dish.
3. Apply salt to the trout on both sides.
4. Sprinkle oregano on the inside of the fish and refrigerate overnight.
5. The next morning, wash off the salt on the trout and refrigerate for a day.
6. Place the trout on a preheated smoker for 3-4 hours and serve.

2. Kelp-Cured Blue Mackerel with Fennel Salad

Preparation and Cooking Time: 3-8 hours
Servings: 2

Ingredients:

- 2 whole blue mackerel, headless, remove pin bones, gutted, made into 2 fillets
- ½ c. rice wine vinegar
- ½ tsp. brine from a jar of preserved lemons
- ½ tbsp. finely chopped chives
- 3 tbsp. broken pomelo segments
- ½ tbsp. fine salt
- 2 sheets of dried kelp (kombu)
- Extra-virgin olive oil, to drizzle
- Microgreens like red garnets, shallots, etc.

For Dressing:

- 1 tbsp. Mirin
- ¼ tsp. finely chopped red Asian shallots
- 2 tbsp. Soy sauce
- ¼ tsp. Finely grated ginger
- ½ tsp. Finely grated lemon zest

For Salad:

- 1 young fennel bulb shaved
- 1 tbsp. fresh lemon juice
- Salt to taste
- Freshly ground black pepper to taste
- ¾ tbsp. Extra-virgin olive oil

Directions:

1. With the flesh side facing up, lay the fish fillets on a tray. Sprinkle it with salt. Keep in the refrigerator for 30 minutes.
2. Add rice wine vinegar into a bowl. Dip the fish fillets in the vinegar one at a time and keep them on a plate—brush the remaining vinegar over the kelp sheets.
3. Brush lemon juice on the flesh side of mackerel and keep each on a piece of kelp, with the flesh side touching the kelp.
4. Cover mackerel with the remaining two pieces of kelp and place them on a tray. Keep the tray covered with cling wrap in the refrigerator for 3 – 8 hours, depending on how much time you have on hand.
5. To make the dressing: Whisk together mirin, shallots, soy sauce, ginger, and lemon zest in a bowl. Cover and set aside a couple of hours for the flavors to fuse.
6. Sprinkle salt and pepper over the fennel. Drizzle lemon juice and olive oil over the fennel and toss well. Spread over a serving platter.
7. Discard the skin from the mackerel and cut it into thin slices across the grain.
8. Place mackerel slices over the fennel—drizzle dressing over the fennel and mackerel.
9. Sprinkle chives, pommel, and microgreens over the salad. Trickle some extra-virgin olive oil on top and serve.

3. Tasty and Easy Smoked Turkey

Preparation and Cooking Time: 3 hours and 30 minutes
Servings: 4

Ingredients:

- 1 (12 lbs.) entire turkey, defrosted if solidified, neck and giblets expelled
- ¾ c. salt
- ¾ glass unsalted spread softened

Directions:

1. Place turkey in a cooking dish. Rub salt all over and inside the turkey. Let sit for 60 minutes.
2. Preheat smoker to 250°F (120°C). If your smoker is outfitted with a water dish, fill it.

3. Wash salt off the turkey and pat dry with paper towels. Come back to the cooking dish and treat with liquefied better. Spread with aluminum foil and place in smoker.
4. Cook for around 3 hours; expel aluminum foil. Keep on cooking, revealed until a moment read thermometer embedded into the thickest part of the turkey thigh peruses 165°F (74°C), 3 to 3 ½ hours.
5. Expel turkey from the smoker and tent with aluminum foil. Allow it to rest in a warm region before cutting, 45 minutes to an hour.

4. Marinated and Smoked Venison Tenderloin

Preparation and Cooking Time: 8-12 hours
Servings: 4

Ingredients:

- 4 venison tenderloins (6 – 8 oz. each) remove silver skins
- ½ c. extra-virgin olive oil
- 2 tsp. brown or Dijon mustard
- 1 small onion, diced
- 2 tsp. dried rosemary
- 2 tsp. cracked black pepper
- ⅔ c. dry red wine
- 2 tbsp. soy sauce or tamari
- 2 tsp. honey or maple syrup
- 4 cloves of garlic, minced
- 2 tsp. sea salt

Directions:

1. In a bowl, combine olive oil, mustard, onion, rosemary, pepper, red wine, soy sauce, honey, garlic, and sea salt.
2. Take 2 – 3 large Ziploc bags and put the tenderloins in them. Drizzle the marinade over the tenderloins. Seal the bags after removing extra air from the bags.
3. With the bag sealed, massage the meat so that the meat is coated with the marinade. Keep the bags in a dish and chill for 8 – 12 hours.
4. About 20 minutes before starting the smoker, remove the meat from the refrigerator.
5. Take a grill rack from the smoker and place it over paper towels.
6. Set up your smoker and preheat it to 250°F. Keep the top vent open. Place the venison on the rack and discard the marinade. Place the rack in the smoker and smoke the venison until the internal temperature of the meat in the thickest part shows between 140°F - 150°F on an instant-read thermometer or meat thermometer, depending on how you like it cooked. Add wood chunks or wood chips as and when required. (Follow the manufacturer's instructions on how to use the wood chips). See that the temperature of the smoker is maintained between 240°F and 225°F. It should be cooked for 2 – 2 ½ hours.
7. Once cooked, place the venison on your cutting board. Cover loosely with foil.
8. After about 20 – 25 minutes, cut into thin slices and serve with a side dish of your choice.

5. Spicy Smoked Trout

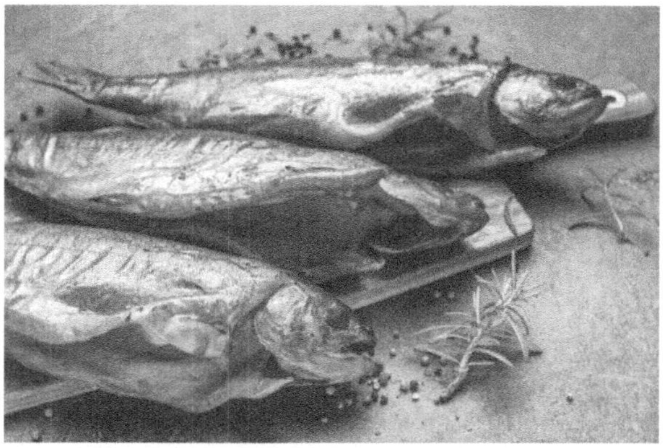

Preparation and Cooking Time: 3 hours and 30 minutes
Servings: About 10

Ingredients:

- 6 lbs. trout
- ½ c. white sugar
- ½ c. brown sugar
- 1 tbsp. kosher salt
- 1 tbsp. smoked paprika
- 1 tbsp. ground ginger powder
- 4 garlic cloves, minced
- 1 tbsp. chili powder
- 1 tbsp. onion powder
- 1 tsp. cumin
- 1 tsp. mustard powder
- 1 tbsp. Dried oregano, powdered
- ½ tsp. cayenne pepper
- 1 tbsp. dried basil
- 1 tsp. ground black pepper
- Wood chips or chunks

Directions:

1. Mix brown sugar with paprika, white sugar, kosher salt, smoked paprika, garlic powder, ginger powder, mustard powder, cumin, cayenne pepper, black pepper, and oregano in a large bowl.
2. Marinate the fish with the above mixture on the inside and outside.
3. Refrigerate the marinated fish for about 3-4 hours or overnight.
4. Soak the wood chips for about an hour and preheat the smoker.
5. Smoke the fish for 2-3 hours until flaky and serve.

6. Perfectly Smoked Salmon

Preparation and Cooking Time: 4 hours and 30 minutes
Servings: 8

Ingredients:

- 5 lbs. (2.2kgs) salmon
- ⅓ c. Diamond Crystal Kosher salt
- 1 qt. cool water

- ½ c. maple syrup
- 1 c. brown sugar
- Maple wood chips

Directions:

1. Prepare the brine by mixing water, Kosher salt, maple syrup, and brown sugar.
2. Cover the fish with the brine and put it in a zip lock bag. Refrigerate overnight.
3. Remove the salmon the next morning, pat it dry, and leave it in a cool and dry place to form the pellicle.
4. Put fish in the smoker and gradually increase the temperature (120°F, 50°C for about 2 hours, 140°F, 60°C for about one more hour, and finally 175°F, 80°C for the last hour).
5. Ensure basting the fish every hour with the maple syrup.
6. Serve as per individual preferences.

7. Smoked Pork Loin with Raspberry Chipotle Glaze

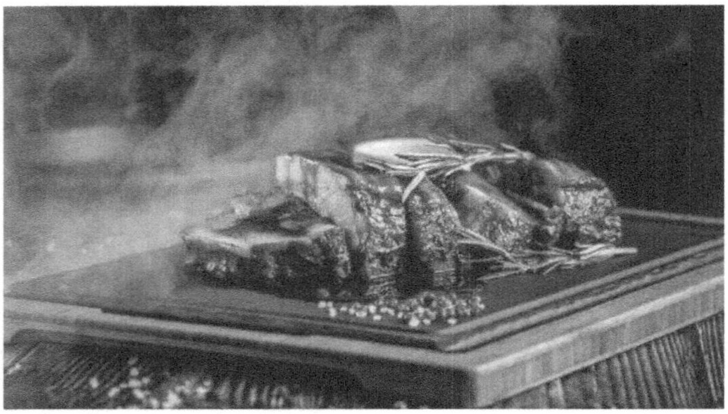

Preparation and Cooking Time: 2 hours and 10 minutes
Servings: 4

Ingredients:

- 1 jar raspberry jam, seedless (10 oz.)
- 1 pork loin (4 lbs.) white silver skin trimmed
- 3 tbsp. Spice rub, dry for pork
- 1 bottle (5 oz.) Tabasco chipotle hot pepper sauce
- Extra-virgin olive oil, as needed

Directions:

1. Preheat your outdoor smoker or stovetop to approximately 230°F in advance.
2. Coat the entire loin lightly with olive oil. Liberally sprinkle the rub on the loin, preferably on all sides.
3. Arrange the pork in a smoker & smoke for an hour or two until a meat thermometer reflects an internal temperature of pork as 150°F. Remove the pork from the smoker & lightly wrap them in aluminum foil.
4. In the meantime, preheat your broiler.
5. Place the jam in a bowl, preferably medium-sized & stir in approximately ⅓ of the chipotle sauce; mix well. Feel free to add more chipotle sauce until you get your desired level of heat & taste.
6. Unwrap the pork & cover them with the glaze. Place the pork on a preheated broiler pan & broil for three minutes until the glaze starts bubbling. Slice the pork against the grain. Serve & enjoy.

8. The Original Juice and Succulent Alabama Pulled Pig Pork

Preparation and Cooking Time: 12 Hours and 10 Minutes
Servings: 8

Ingredients:

- 2 c. soy sauce
- 1 c. Worcestershire sauce
- 1 c. cranberry grape juice
- 1 c. teriyaki sauce
- 1 tbsp. of hot pepper sauce
- 2 tbsp. of steak sauce
- 1 c. light brown sugar
- ½ tsp. of ground black pepper
- 2 lbs. flank steak cut up into ¼-inch slices
- 4 c. wood chips

Directions:

1. Take a non-reactive saucepan and add cider, salt, vinegar, brown sugar, cayenne pepper, black pepper, and butter
2. Bring the mix to a boil over medium-high heat
3. Add in water and return the mix to a boil
4. Keep saucing the pork with the mixture before smoking
5. Place your pork butt on a slow smoker using apple wood chips
6. Smoke it for about 6-10 hours. Make sure to keep basting it with the sauce every hour or so
7. After the first smoking is done, take an aluminum foil and wrap up the meat forming a watertight seal
8. Place the meat in the center of your foil and bring the edges to the top, cupping up the meat complete
9. Pour one cup of sauce over the meat and tight it up
10. Place the package back into your smoker and smoke for two hours until the meat easily pulls off from the bone
11. Once done, remove it from the smoker and pull off the pork, discarding the gristle and fat
12. Place the meat chunks in a pan and pour one cup of sauce for every four pounds of meat
13. Heat until simmering and serve immediately!

9. Oregano Pecan Rub Smoked Lamb Leg with Yogurt Marinade

Preparation and Cooking Time: 5 Hours and 10 Minutes
Servings: 10
Ingredients for 10 Servings:

- 5-lb. (2.3-kg.) Lamb leg

For the Marinade:

- 3 c. Greek yogurt
- 2 tbsp. Ground cumin

- 2 tsp. Ground coriander
- ½ tsp. Ground turmeric
- ¼ tsp. Allspice
- 2 tsp. Kosher salt
- 1 tsp. Black pepper

For the Rub:

- 1 c. Roasted pecans
- 1 c. Chopped fresh oregano
- 1 c. Chopped thyme leaves
- 3 tbsp. Minced garlic
- ½ c. Brown sugar
- 2 tbsp. Smoked paprika
- 1 tsp. Pepper
- 1 tsp. Grated lemon zest
- 1 tsp. Kosher salt
- ½ c. Vegetable oil

For the Water Pan:

- 2 c. Water

For the Heat:

- Oak wood chunks

Directions:

1. Season the yogurt with cumin, coriander, turmeric, allspice, kosher salt, and black pepper. Mix well.
2. Add the lamb leg to the yogurt mixture and marinate it for at least four hours. Store it in the fridge to keep the lamb leg fresh.
3. In the meantime, place the roasted pecans in a food processor and process until becoming crumble.
4. Mix the pecan crumbles with oregano, thyme, minced garlic, brown sugar, smoked paprika, pepper, grated lemon zest, and salt.
5. Pour vegetable oil into the dry spice mixture and stir until becoming a paste.
6. Take the marinated lamb leg out of the fridge and coat it with pecan paste. Set aside.
7. Prepare the smoked grill and fill it with fuel.
8. Add wood chunks to the smoker grill and start the fire. Set the smoked grill for indirect heat.
9. Place a disposable aluminum pan in the smoker grill and pour water into it.
10. Set the temperature of the smoker grill to 225°F (107°C) and wait until it reaches the desired temperature.
11. Place the seasoned lamb leg in the smoker grill and smoke it for five hours.
12. Check the smoked lamb leg and once the internal temperature reaches 135°F (57°C), remove it from the smoker grill.
13. Place the smoked lamb leg on a serving dish and serve.
14. Enjoy!

10. Aromatic Cloves Smoked Lamb Ribs Tender with Pineapple Marinade

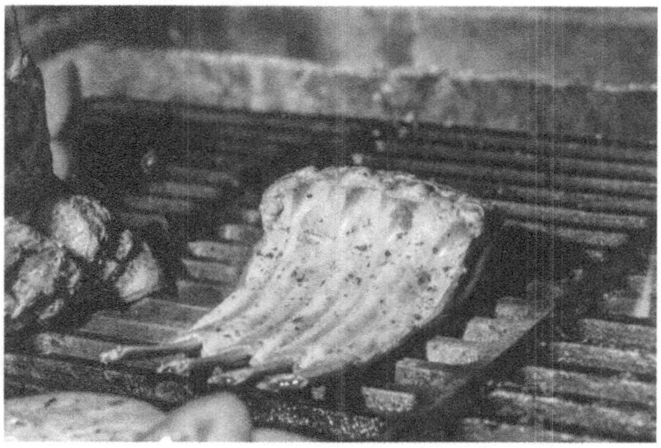

Preparation and Cooking Time: 5 hours and 10 minutes
Servings: 10
Ingredients for 10 Servings:

- 6-lb. (2.7-kg.) Lamb ribs

For the Marinade:

- 3 c. Pineapple juice
- ½ c. Pineapple preserves
- 1 c. Ginger beer
- 2 tbsp. Worcestershire sauce
- ½ c. Brown sugar
- 2 tbsp. Minced garlic
- 2 tbsp. Kosher salt

For the Glaze:

- ½ c. Maple syrup
- 2 tbsp. Olive oil
- 2 tbsp. Fish sauce
- 2 tbsp. Soy sauce
- ½ tsp. Chili powder
- ½ tsp. Grated lemon zest
- A pinch of Ground clove
- ½ tsp. Pepper

For the Water Pan:

- 2 c. Water

For the Heat:

- Oak wood chunks

Directions:

1. Combine pineapple juice with pineapple preserves and ginger beer. Stir until incorporated.
2. Season the pineapple mixture with Worcestershire sauce, brown sugar, minced garlic, and salt. Mix well.
3. Add the lamb ribs to the pineapple mixture and make sure that the lamb ribs are entirely coated with the pineapple mixture.
4. Marinate the lamb ribs for at least six hours or overnight and store the ribs in the fridge to keep the lamb ribs fresh.

5. The next day, remove the marinated lamb ribs from the fridge and thaw them at room temperature.
6. Prepare the smoked grill and fill it with fuel.
7. Add wood chunks to the smoker grill and start the fire. Set the smoked grill for indirect heat.
8. Place a disposable aluminum pan in the smoker grill and pour water into it.
9. Set the temperature of the smoker grill to 225°F (107°C) and wait until it reaches the desired temperature.
10. Once the smoke is ready, place the marinated lamb ribs in the smoker grill and smoke the ribs for approximately five hours.
11. In the meantime, combine maple syrup with olive oil, fish sauce, and soy sauce.
12. Add chili powder, grated lemon zest, ground cloves, and pepper. Stir until dissolved.
13. After 3 hours of smoking, baste the glaze mixture over the smoked lamb ribs and repeat it once every thirty minutes.
14. Regularly check the smoked lamb ribs and once the internal temperature reaches 135°F (57°C), remove the smoked ribs from the smoker grill.
15. Lightly baste the remaining glaze mixture over the smoked lamb ribs and wrap the ribs with aluminum foil. Let the ribs rest for approximately 25 to 30 minutes.
16. Unwrap the smoked lamb ribs and transfer them to a serving dish.
17. Serve and enjoy.

11. Gourmet Smokehouse Beef Jerky

Preparation and Cooking Time: 12 hours and 10 minutes
Servings: 6

Ingredients:

- 2 c. soy sauce
- 1 c. Worcestershire sauce
- 1 c. cranberry grape juice
- 1 c. teriyaki sauce
- 1 tbsp. of hot pepper sauce
- 2 tbsp. of steak sauce
- 1 c. light brown sugar
- ½ tsp. of ground black pepper
- 2 lbs. flank steak cut up into ¼-inch slices
- 4 c. wood chips

Directions:

1. Take a bowl and whisk in the soy sauce, cranberry grape juice, Worcestershire sauce, teriyaki sauce, steak sauce, hot sauce, brown sugar, and black pepper
2. Mix them well and pour the mix into a re-sealable bag
3. Add the flank steak to the bag and coat it well with the marinade
4. Squeeze out any excess air and seal it up
5. Let it refrigerate for about 8-10 hours
6. Remove the flank steak from the marinade and wipe off any excess
7. Place the steak onto the wire racks of your smoker, then place the racks into the smoker
8. Smoke for about 6-8 hours and keep adding pans of wood chips (1 pan every hour) until perfectly done!
9. Serve!

12. Tipsy Maple Glazed Smoked Bacon

Preparation and Cooking Time: 15 hours and 20 minutes
Servings: 8

Ingredients:

- 1 ½ gal. of water
- 2 tbsp. sodium nitrate
- 1 c. sugar-based curing mix
- 2 c. coarse salt
- 1 c. brown sugar
- 1 14 lb. whole pork belly
- Maple, apple, or cherry woods

Directions:

1. Take a large-sized kettle and add water, sodium nitrate, brown sugar, curing salt, and maple syrup
2. Bring the whole mix to a boil over high heat and cook it for about 15 minutes until everything dissolves perfectly
3. Pour the bring into a 5-gallon plastic bucket and let it cool to room temperature for about 8 hours
4. Cut the pork belly against the grain into about 4-6 slabs (keeping the skin on) so that you can fit them in your smoker
5. Place them into your brine bucket and weight them down so that they are fully submerged
6. Cove r them up and let them refrigerate for seven days
7. When you are ready to smoke, remove the pork from the brine and rinse them well under cold water
8. Allow the pieces to stand under the fan for about 1-3 hours until the skin is dry and glossy
9. Smoke the belly slabs at a temperature of 110°F for about 8-12 hours
10. Remove the rinds and slice up to serve!

13. Honey Drizzled Citrus Smoke Turkey

Preparation and Cooking Time: 12 hours and 10 minutes
Servings: 7

Ingredients:

- 1 gal. hot water
- 1 lb. kosher salt
- 2 qt. vegetable broth
- 8 oz. jars of honey
- 1 c. orange juice
- 7 lbs. bag of ice cubes
- 15 lbs. whole turkey with giblets and neck removed
- ¼ c. vegetable oil
- 1 tsp. poultry seasoning
- 1 granny smith apple, cored and cut up into large chunks
- 1 celery stalk, cut up into small chunks
- 1 small-sized onion, cut up into chunks

- 1 quartered orange

Directions:

1. Take a 54-quart cooler and add kosher salt and hot water. Mix them well until everything dissolves.
2. Add vegetable broth, orange juice, and honey. Pour ice cubes into the mix and add the turkey to your brine, keeping the breast side up.
3. Lock up your cooler's lid and let it marinate overnight for 12 hours. Make sure that the bring temperature stays under 40°F.
4. Remove the turkey from the brine and discard the brine. Dry the turkey using a kitchen towel.
5. Take a bowl and mix vegetable oil and poultry seasoning. Rub the turkey with the mixture. Place apple, onion, celery, and orange pieces inside the turkey cavity.
6. Preheat your smoker to a temperature of 400°F and add one cup of hickory wood chips. Set your turkey onto your smoker and insert a probe into the thickest part of your turkey breast.
7. Set the probe for 160°F. Smoke the turkey for 2 hours until the skin is golden brown.
8. Cover the breast, wings, and legs using aluminum foil and keep smoking it for 2-3 hours until the probe thermometer reads 160°F.
9. Make sure to keep adding some hickory chips to your heat box occasionally. Remove the vegetables and fruit from your Turkey's cavity and cover it with aluminum foil.
10. Let it rest for one hour and carve it up!

14. Smoked Salmon Fillets with Whiskey

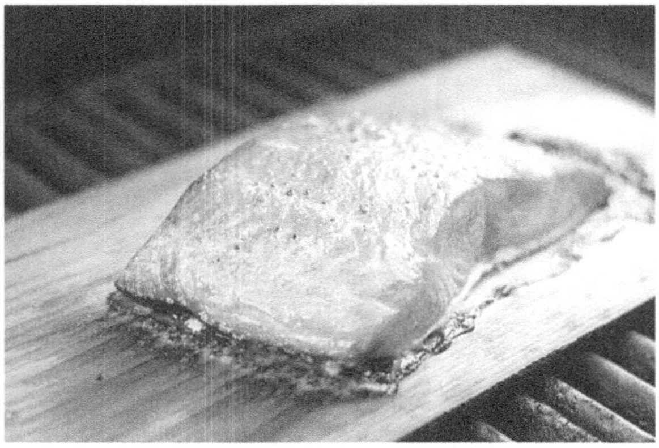

Preparation and Cooking Time: 12 hours
Servings: 3

Ingredients:

- 1 salmon fillet
- 1½ c. Bourbon whiskey
- 1 qt. distilled water
- 4 tsp. non-iodized salt
- ½ c. brown sugar
- 1 tsp. fresh ground black pepper
- 1 tsp. garlic powder
- Wood chips as per choice

Directions:

1. Prepare the brine with whiskey, brown sugar, salt, garlic powder, and black pepper.
2. Cover the fish with the brine and put it in a zip lock bag. Refrigerate overnight.
3. Remove the salmon the next morning, pat it dry, and leave it in a cool and dry place to form the pellicle.
4. Preheat the smoker and cook for 10 to 12 hours between 100°F (40°C) to 150°F (65°C).
5. Ensure to change the wood chips at least three times before the dish is finally prepared (i.e., every 4 hours).

15. Tasty Smoked Beef Filets

Preparation and Cooking Time: 1 hour and 30 minutes
Servings: 5

Ingredients:

- 4 lbs. hamburger filets
- 2 tbsp. olive oil
- 4 garlic cloves, squashed
- Fit salt
- Ground pepper

Directions:

1. Preheat smoker to 225°F.
2. Season meat with garlic cloves, salt, and pepper. Heat olive oil in an expansive griddle. Burn/cocoa meat on all sides. This will seal in juices before smoking.
3. Wrap every filet in aluminum foil, leaving the highest points of each revealed. Sprinkle somewhat olive oil on top of every filet.
4. Place foil-wrapped filets in the smoker and cook for roughly 1 to ½ hours for medium-uncommon. The cook's reality of the situation will eventually become obvious in the thickness of the filet. Consider a longer cooking time for medium and well-done. Deliberately screen the inner temperature of the meat.

CONCLUSION

Thank you for reading this book. Smoking meat, poultry, and fish is not a new concept. Our forefathers were able to preserve fish and other games to extend their shelf life. The most common methods of food preservation are salt curing and smoking. Almost any meat, from fresh fish and game to processed meats, can be smoked or cured. Once you're at ease with it, the sky's the limit. Learn how to salt cure and smoke meat, fish, and other foods!

Now that you have the necessary tools and knowledge, what are you waiting for? It's time to gather your supplies, gather your ingredients, and get started on something amazing. All you need right now is patience. You'll get the hang of it with practice and patience.

After you've mastered the theory, you can begin to explore the delectable recipes included in this book. These recipes are simple to understand and execute. All that remains after selecting a recipe is to gather the ingredients. You're done if you follow these simple steps!

Have a good time, good luck, and happy smoking!

ROOT CELLARING
FOR PREPPERS

Learn How to Build your Root Cellar to Preserve Food for the Next 10 Years of Crisis

Tyler Gordon

INTRODUCTION

Learning how to store or preserve food, in general, is critical for anyone attempting to become more self-sufficient, whether for financial, family, health, or disaster reasons. This book will teach you everything you need to know about the humble root cellar, from its origins to modern applications. By the end, you will clearly know what you want to do, how you intend to do it, and when you plan to do it.

You can now store and eat all the fantastic, organic, healthy food you can grow in your garden all year! Forget about grocery store vegetables wrapped in harmful plastic and food you know has been sprayed with chemicals or imported from a foreign country at great expense. Consider the rows of carrots and potatoes, the corn, onions, beets, and dozens of other things you can grow in your garden and store for the winter.

This book will teach you how to build a root cellar from scratch rather than digging one into the ground. After all, not everyone has a large garden and enough space to begin digging a cellar. You might be surprised at what you can use to store your vegetables, and this book includes some intriguing suggestions for you to try.

What Exactly is a Root Cellar?

Root cellars are technically underground rooms that use the earth's natural humidifying, cooling, and insulating properties. They are a traditional method of storing and preserving food to help people get through the winter. While cellars were once rooms beneath the house, they are now any type of storage that keeps food fresh for longer by controlling light, temperature, and humidity. Your refrigerator is the modern root cellar, but if you don't want to rely on electricity, learning how to make a root cellar is essential.

Every root cellar, regardless of design, performs the same basic function. It can keep your food up to 40°F cooler than ambient summertime temperatures if properly constructed. Low temperatures have significant benefits during the winter, as storing food at temperatures just above freezing point can slow rot and deterioration. Even in a basement, the temperatures inside your home are slightly higher, which means stored foods spoil much faster. Most vegetables will become tough, sprout, and spoil if the temperature rises above 45°F.

However, root cellar temperatures vary from one corner to the next. Because the temperature near the top is around 10 degrees warmer than the lower part of the cellar, it is critical to organize the root cellar efficiently. Place vegetables that can withstand higher temperatures on top.

What if your garden is too small or you don't want to grow vegetables? No problem—root cellars are intended to store produce that you did not grow yourself. If you can find great deals at your local farm or farmer's market, you can easily store them in your cellar.

A Brief History of the Root Cellar

The root cellar has a fascinating history that dates back at least 40,000 years. Indigenous Australians were the first to use the earth's natural insulation and cooling properties to store food. Records show that over 40,000 years ago, they were growing massive amounts of yams and devised a method of long-term storage, namely burying it in the ground. They discovered another process, fermentation, while developing their technique, which is why alcoholic beverages are commonly stored in cellars.

Iron Age storage rooms beneath the ground have also been discovered, which Etruscans still use to store immature wine. Although the first alleged use of a walk-in root cellar was in seventeenth-century England, the most notable uses came from English colonists in North America.

During ancient times, China and Egypt had already mastered food preservation methods such as salting, pickling, using spices, and drying. On the other hand, cold winters and widespread famines drove the British to invent the walk-in root cellar.

Across the eastern parts of Canada and America, the land is scattered with thousands of old root cellars. Elliston, a small town in Newfoundland, has even claimed the title of "Root Cellar Capital of the World," with over 135 root cellars, some around 200 years old.

Benefits of Having A Root Cellar

Root cellaring may sound like an exaggeration, but the effects it could have on your diet and lifestyle would be nothing short of life-changing. This simple, age-old idea of simply burying your food can serve as the foundation for a more sustainable diet and lifestyle, making healthy eating more convenient and affordable.

Let us take a step back for a moment. Before you can decide whether a root cellar is something you should incorporate into your own life, we need to discuss what it is and how it works. A root cellar is simply an underground chamber where food deteriorates much more slowly. The underground environment is ideal for food storage, allowing you to stockpile everything from potatoes to rhubarb wine without using chemicals or canned food.

For millennia, root cellar stockpiling was the only way many people could survive winters when no fruits, vegetables, or grains could grow. Modern refrigeration changed all of that, and since the end of WWII, most of us have had no trouble finding, say, strawberries in the middle of February at the grocery store.

Convenience

The beauty of a root cellar is that after you go through the effort of building it, you can have your produce section waiting for you at home, whether you grow your vegetables or buy them from a local farmers market. Yes, a lot of work is involved, but anyone reading this book is unlikely to turn back at the prospect of working up a sweat.

Delicious and Healthy Food

Having your stockpiles of locally grown produce makes it simple to eat healthily. It will then take you the same amount of effort to make something from the freezer that is unnaturally high in processed flour and fructose as it will to walk to your root cellar and grab a handful of fresh tomatoes and spinach. Then, once you've tasted a real tomato, grown naturally, and eaten in season, you'll never return.

Affordability

We've only touched on it so far, but it bears repeating. Every year, storing nutritious food in a root cellar will save you hundreds of dollars in grocery bills. If you grow everything and have a large enough storage capacity, you could save thousands of dollars.

Of course, there will be an initial investment in building your root cellar, but the return on this investment will be well worth it.

Growing populations and rising fuel prices will only make food more expensive in the future; this was evident when food prices abruptly spiked globally in 2007 and 2008. We have also seen that eating healthy food costs more money in the United States, Canada, the United Kingdom, and many other Western countries. Paying a premium for healthy living is opposed to the concept of self-sufficiency.

Dietary self-sufficiency begins with providing a space to collect and store all of the natural produce you require, and root cellars are explicitly designed for this purpose. Anyone can build a root cellar with limited construction experience in their spare time or throughout the weekend.

Natural Refrigeration

Despite what the modern world would like you to believe, it is currently possible to live without electric-powered refrigeration. In truth, the solution to long-term food storage and preservation was solved generations ago; it has just been pushed aside by a modern society primarily concerned with instant gratification and a population full of individuals unconcerned with ensuring they have what they need to survive when push comes to shove.

CHAPTER 1: CREATING A ROOT CELLAR

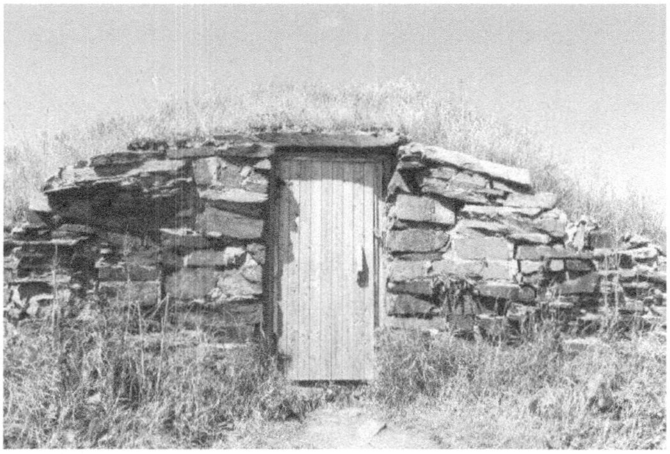

Planning Your Root Cellar

Now begins the most crucial step: making plans for your root cellar. It would be imprudent to run into your backyard and start digging a hole. You must first consider many things to ensure that your root cellar is successful, sustainable, and even scalable.

Your Needs

Why do you think about a root cellar? If you only have a small garden plot that produces a limited number of vegetables, consider the size or style best suits your storage needs.

Suppose you want it to serve as a storm shelter or another emergency shelter. In that case, you'll need to consider construction strength, occupancy capabilities, and storage space for necessities.

Before you even consider root cellar plans, you must first determine what you require from your root cellar. Will it simply be a large underground pantry for farmer's market purchases? Do you have a garden that is producing more and more each year? Do you want to make beer or cider as well? Do you have young sons who will be teenagers in a decade or so and thus capable of consuming roughly half of their body weights per meal? How you answer these questions will determine your capacity needs.

As a rule of thumb, consider an area of 10 feet x 10 feet more than sufficient for storing anything your family could consume. More space might be necessary if you have commercial aspirations or might try home brewing. If you have a small family, have a small garden, and supplement your food supply with weekend trips to the farmers market, 5 feet x 8 feet might be enough room for you.

Your Environment

Produce should be stored in cool, humid environments where air can circulate freely. Because the earth is a fantastic temperature regulator, root cellars are typically underground. An ideal climate has a long enough growing season (if you grow your produce) and a cold enough winter to keep the ground below the frost line, no warmer than 50°F (10°C). That encompasses the majority of the populated continent of North America.

For most vegetables, you'll want to create an environment inside your root cellar that approaches the low-40°Fs (5-6°C) because this temperature range prevents them from freezing or sprouting. The ability to maintain this temperature all year is the most important factor in the efficient operation of a root cellar. That means you can't guess the temperature; instead, get a thermometer.

After temperature, you should consider humidity. The ideal humidity range is 70-90%. Much more will spoil your food. It will shrivel if you use less. It is important to note that humidity will fluctuate at different levels within your cellar. A hygrometer is a device that measures humidity, and perfectly useful hygrometers can be purchased online for between $10 and $20.

Later, you'll be regulating the temperature and humidity of your root cellar through simple air circulation, so your climate should provide you with cooler and warmer days according to the season. If you live near Miami or Fairbanks, Alaska, your extreme weather does not preclude you from having a root cellar entirely, but it does make your job more difficult.

If excavating ground, you must consider what may be below the surface in terms of utility supplies; bursting a water main or an electricity supply can ruin your day. Contact your local utility providers if you have any concerns about previous installations.

Keep an eye out for your local water table or freshwater spring. This can mean that any hole dug into the ground will quickly (or slowly) fill with water. A little damp, however, is perfectly acceptable and essential for a root cellar.

Climatic Conditions

Depending on where you stay, water, cold, and heat will play a different part in your construction details. A cellar in Nevada, for instance, is more likely to be bothered with excess heat than it is to be troubled by water, so waterproofing is maybe not such a big deal – whereby insulation is. And a cellar in Wisconsin has to withstand bitter cold winters to stop the roots from freezing and withstand a fair amount of rainfall. This means more concentration of waterproofing and insulation.

Cost

This is usually a top consideration for most folks and has to be weighed against any advantage gained in the construction.

Consider whether or not a temporary structure would do, even one that you can renew on an annual basis.

Such temporary ‘cellars’ can be made from straw bales, lumber, or corrugated iron and covered with turf to form a simple yet effective shelter. These shelters are cheap to make and removable at short notice if necessary.

Local Authority Permissions

Something to bear in mind with a more permanent structure is that it may need a building permit or planning permission from your local authority.

This is not usually a problem, especially in rural areas – but better safe than sorry!

Finding the Right Location for Your Root Cellar

This is purely for practical reasons, as trudging through 3 feet of snow to get carrots for dinner is no laughing matter!

If possible, keep it close to the kitchen door, as that is where you will most likely be approaching it (along with the veggie plot).

Your options for location will certainly be limited, especially if you are attaching the root cellar to an existing structure. Here are a few key things to look for in a potential root cellar building site:

- Somewhere higher or elevated so that water runs away from it

- Somewhere away from trees, or specifically tree roots
- Somewhere with no traffic, even if it's just your lawnmower
- Somewhere away from prevailing winds or intense mid-summer sun, possibly on the north face of a hill (south face for anyone in the Southern Hemisphere)

Don't be concerned if your location does not meet these requirements. During the construction and maintenance of your root cellar, you can compensate for any geographical shortcomings.

Also, keep in mind the soil that will surround your cellar. If the terrain is too difficult, you will need professional equipment to locate your location. If the soil is sandy, it may require additional reinforcement or a modified root cellar design. Above all, ensure that the location is sufficiently deep in the earth to allow for proper temperature regulation.

Finally, consider the location's accessibility for yourself. This is a place you will visit daily, so putting it a 10-minute walk from your kitchen or garden would be inconvenient. No problem if your root cellar connects to your basement. However, if you intend to build your root cellar on a nearby hillside, be prepared for a hike in freezing temperatures and torrential downpours, not to mention that you will need to shovel a path to it during the winter. An inconvenient root cellar would miss the point entirely.

Plans for Drainage, Airflow, and Lighting

As mentioned before, drainage and airflow will play key roles in the maintenance of your root cellar. Later, we will discuss what materials you need to drain water from your root cellar properly; for now, know that you will have to consider this. The same goes for airflow and ventilation. You will need to create some way for outside air to get in while keeping pests and other creatures out.

The Basics of Root Cellaring

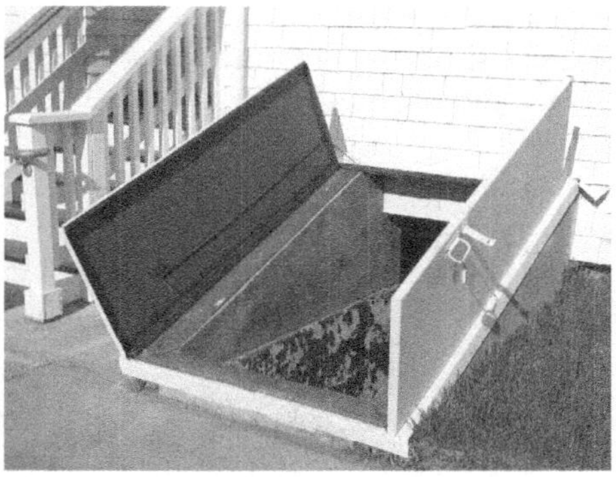

Humidity

Root cellars require high humidity levels of 85-95%. This prevents your stored produce from drying out and becoming shriveled. There are three ways to achieve the right levels of humidity in your root cellar:

- **A Dirt Floor:** Dirt floors retain moisture much more easily than concrete or stone floors. Assume you dug a root cellar into the ground. You already have an advantage in that case because the soil will provide some humidity. The earth should be packed in tightly, followed by a layer of gravel. This serves two purposes: it keeps your feet dry when things get wet and aids in moisture retention. If your cellar becomes dry, spray some water (carefully) over the gravel. Water evaporates quickly, adding moisture and humidity to the air.
- **Adding Water:** There are other options if you do not want to add gravel or if your floors are made of concrete. You can add water by lightly spraying the floor, spreading damp burlap bags over the vegetables (but not soaking them), or placing a few water pans on the floor. These measurements are usually required in the fall when you first put your produce into storage. Dug-in root cellars are less likely to require humidity assistance than basement root cellars. In areas where the air is very moist, keep root vegetables in uncovered bins to keep them firm and smooth.

If your humidity falls below optimal levels, there is a third option: sawdust, moss, or sand. You can pack your fruits and vegetables with damp sawdust, moss, or sand. This is especially effective for parsnips, beets, and carrots, as it reduces surface evaporation.

One of the most critical considerations is that warm air absorbs more moisture than cool air. The environment will be somewhat unstable if your root cellar is damp and cold. If your air temperature is 34°F, it has room to absorb a little more moisture. If the temperature falls a few degrees, the air will become saturated. The "dew point" is the temperature at which the air can no longer hold excess moisture. This water will condense on your ceiling, walls, and fruits and vegetables. The most secure way to ensure your humidity levels are correct is to purchase a hygrometer, which can be found at any hardware store or garden center.

Ventilation

Each root cellar is unique and will necessitate its methods of regulating ventilation and humidity. The most important thing to keep an eye on is the conditions inside your root cellar, and make sure you can change your design if necessary, preferably before you start building. Alternatively, make sure your design allows for changes to be made later.

The simplest way to vent your cellar is with two 3- to 4-inch-wide vents. To ensure proper air circulation, place the first near the ceiling and the second near the floor.

Proper ventilation is just as important as humidity. Air must be allowed to enter and circulate through the cellar to keep the temperature low. Adjusting the air intake is critical for reducing extra humidity and preventing condensation from ruining your hard work. When air moves efficiently, it eliminates the ethylene gas that some fruits emit and other vegetable odors that may alter the flavors of other vegetables and fruits.

Understanding how air circulates through your root cellar necessitates recalling basic physics—hot air rises (lighter) and cold air falls (heavier). A large or enclosed cellar requires an air intake system and an air outlet. The intake should be low in the room to bring cool air from outside. The outlet should be elevated to allow warmer air to escape. To allow for efficient air circulation, place the outlet and inlet on opposite sides of the room.

If your storage area is small or there are many cracks allowing air in (think old stone foundations), you may only need one high-up outlet to remove the warm air. Keep it a couple of inches above the ground when storing your produce to allow air to circulate beneath it.

Lighting

Finally, consider the lighting in your cellar. A root cellar should essentially be as dark as possible—too much light can cause rotting and sprouting. Have a single light bulb in your cellar, but don't leave it on for any longer than necessary. You can also use burlap to keep the light out while allowing for adequate air circulation and ventilation. Cover any windows that you use for ventilation with dark material.

Temperature

Temperature is the most critical variable to consider in a root cellar. A good root cellar does two things: it borrows cold and keeps it cold. How do you borrow when it's cold? It's simple: dig a hole in the ground. The earth will remain at a temperature of around 52 degrees below the frost line. This is because the deeper earth temperature is less affected by freezing temperatures above, providing your vegetables with more protection. If you don't want to dig your root cellar into the ground, you can borrow the cold through a window or an exhaust pipe that you can close off. These options allow cold night air into the cellar but should be turned off during the day as temperatures rise.

Maintaining a temperature range of 32-40°F is ideal for food storage. You can still use the root cellar as a short-term storage area for apples and root vegetables if your temperatures are between 40°F and 50°F. Tomatoes, peppers, and eggplant can be stored for about a month.

You must invest in a good thermometer to monitor your root cellar temperatures.

Dealing with Insects and Other Common Root Cellaring Problems

If your cellar is appropriately sealed at all joints and vulnerable points, pests should not be a problem. However, the constant opening of the door will eventually let an unwanted guest in. We recommend simply using whatever pest-control methods you use in your house for your cellar. If you use mouse traps, put one or two in your cellar. If you use dryer sheets or spices to keep ants out of entry points, do the same for your cellar. Regular maintenance should be enough to keep your cellar free of pests.

Rodents

Mice and rats can be found anywhere there is food, including root cellars. The key to keeping them out is to prevent them from entering your root cellar in the first place, and the simplest way to do so is to seal off their entry points. Metal wire mesh is one of the best options for this. Place it over any entry points for these creatures, including vents. Consider elevating your storage if you're having trouble keeping mice out of your cellar. Remember that many rodents can climb; if their prize is your food, they will go to any length to get it. We'll look at some natural ways to keep rodents and other pests out of your root cellar later, but for now, keep it clean. You should also think about putting traps along the walls, which should be checked at least once a day and any dead rodents removed immediately.

Rot

Rot is an unavoidable problem in root cellars. You've probably heard the expression "one rotten apple spoils the barrel," which couldn't be truer. But how do you prevent this from happening? You cannot entirely prevent it, but you can significantly reduce its occurrence.

Take extra care when harvesting your vegetables. Before storing your produce, go through it and set aside anything damaged during the harvest, such as a fork cut or a space.

Set aside anything that has been bruised. If you drop something, such as an apple or a potato, it will almost certainly have an invisible bruise, even if it does not appear damaged. Set it aside, too.

Only foods that are undamaged and free of blemishes should be stored in your root cellar. Those damaged can be used immediately or stored in another way, such as freezing or canning.

Another common mistake is washing root vegetables before storing them—do not do this, no matter how tempting it may be. Root vegetables store much better when harvested with intact roots, stems, and soil. Washing vegetables removes moisture from them, hastening their decomposition.

Make sure that any canned or bottled foods have airtight lids. Before canning or bottling anything, the containers and lids must be sterilized—even the smallest amount of contamination can spoil the contents.

When storing produce, place the largest items at the back and the smallest items first—these are more likely to spoil quickly and should be used as soon as possible.

Check for condensation if your cellar is humid. When water drips from the ceiling or down the walls, it can get onto your produce and cause it to rot. Pretreat your cellar ceiling with a disinfectant, such as chlorine, before storing your food, as this slows the spread of diseases caused by dripping water.

As a cardinal rule, check your root cellar regularly. Any foods starting to wither, rot, or show signs of decomposition should be removed immediately.

Insects

This seems to be more of a problem where nuts and grains are stored, and since you have other food in your root cellar, you should never use chemical sprays or insecticides. The best way to keep insects out of your root cellar is to have a tight-fitting door, all cracks sealed up, and insect mesh over the vents and drainage. Alternatively, you can scatter bay leaves around—insects hate these with a passion—or other herbs with a strong smell.

Sprouting Vegetables

If you notice your root cellar vegetables sprouting, it means something is wrong, and it usually boils down to one of three things:

- **Ethylene Gas**: Look where you've stored the sprouting vegetables. What other ethylene-producing fruits and vegetables are nearby? If so, relocate them. Inspect your ventilation system as well—is it adequate? Is it functional? Is it in the correct location? If you answered "no" to any or all of these, it's a sign that something in your cellar needs to be adjusted.
- **Too Hot**: If the temperature is too high, it can force vegetables to grow, which you don't want in your cellar. When a plant begins to grow again, it must be consumed quickly. Check your ventilation system once more to prevent any more sprouting.
- **Too Much Light**: Do you visit your root cellar with the door open? Are the windows draped? Do you leave a light on for extended periods? The only way to prevent vegetables from growing again is to keep them as dark as possible.

Frozen Produce

If your root cellar produce is freezing, it simply means that the temperature is far too low. Check your thermometer first. If the temperature is below freezing, it must be raised. However, at this point, you may have already lost a significant portion of your stored foods. When most vegetable freeze, they become mushy and rot, rendering them useless. The second thing to look for is which vegetables have been frozen. If only those at the bottom are affected, the air coming in through the inlet is too cold, indicating that you did not dig your root cellar deep enough. There isn't much you can do about it except empty it and dig deeper. Remember that constant temperature stability is achieved at approximately ten feet or three meters underground.

Produce Going Off Too Quickly

Have you ever opened the door to your root cellar and been taken aback by the smell? Yes, your food is spoiling quickly, and the odor is strong. So, what would cause that to occur? Simply put, the climate in your root cellar is to blame. The main culprits are moisture, light, air, temperature, and microbial growth.

Damage caused by microorganisms such as yeast, mold, and bacteria is one of the most common causes of fresh food spoilage. However, this can only occur if the conditions are favorable—they require nutrients and water to grow and reproduce. Most fruits and vegetables have an average water content of 90%, making them an ideal target.

Light is a major adversary of fresh food in storage. Excessive exposure will cause the outer layer of the vegetable or fruit to spoil. This is known as photodegradation, and it causes discoloration as well as the loss of flavor, proteins, and vitamins.

The only thing you should never do is store vegetables or fruits wet or in an airtight container. A lack of air circulation does nothing but hasten decay. Water will pool on the produce if your humidity levels are too high, causing it to rot again.

Finally, the temperature is an important consideration that must be met. Keep in mind that some vegetables prefer it cool, while others prefer it hot. Temperature extremes can be problematic—cold to the point of freezing causes the food to form ice crystals inside, which expand and break through the cell walls, causing discoloration and, in some cases, a slimy texture.

One of the most important things to do is get your climate right on point before you start storing food. Once your cellar is full, use your thermometer and hygrometer to measure temperature and humidity. Using a notebook to record your results daily can give you an early warning when something is wrong.

Mold

When your root cellar is functioning properly, it will be cool all year, and the humidity level will be consistent. On the other hand, mold can affect all root cellars, whether underground, in a basement or garage, under the porch, or on a simple barrel in the ground. While you may believe you have properly sealed your cellar, construction flaws or inadequate maintenance can lead to mold growing in places you do not want.

Mold growth in your root cellar can harm the air you breathe if it is attached to or inside your home. Condensation is the cause of mold growth in a cellar or cold storage. It could be due to warmer air seeping into the room during the summer months, which happens when the door is not sealed correctly.

Condensation forms when warm air meets cold surfaces in your cellar, such as the roof or poorly insulated walls. This creates ideal conditions for mold to grow. That mold will quickly spread to your produce or onto the containers where your food is stored, and within a few days, your entire crop will be ruined—that is how quickly it can happen.

Your root cellar should have air vents, one of the best tools for controlling humidity. As a result, you can better control the environment and prevent mold growth—these air vents will keep fresh air moving through your cellar and keep it dry.

However, mold does not come from only one source. You can introduce it into your cellar through the food you bring in. No matter how well your root cellar works, the mold will grow and spread to other foods and the root cellar structure.

If you suspect or see mold growing in your root cellar, you need to do something about it immediately. If left unchecked, mold can quickly spread to other areas, especially if your root cellar is attached to your home. Professional help will be needed to remove the mold and repair the damage already done in some cases.

CHAPTER 2: WHAT CAN YOU STORE IN A ROOT CELLAR?

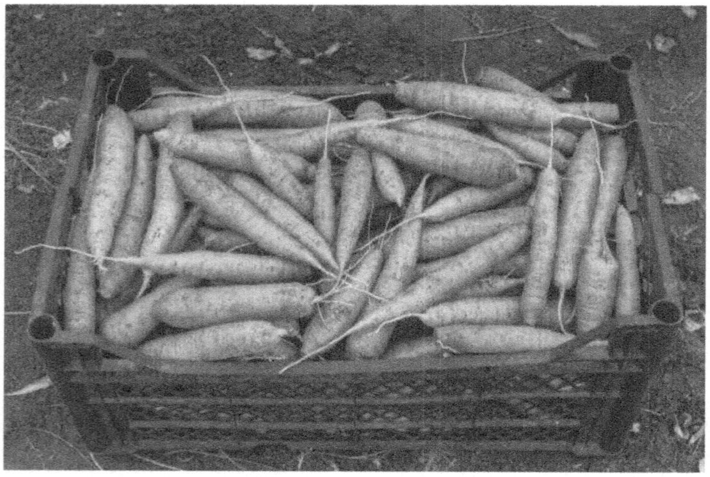

Because different vegetables have varying degrees of sensitivity, some will require more attention than others. Potatoes require little care and can be stored in a cellar for months at a time. Less hardy vegetables, such as tomatoes or apples, require frequent inspection and discarding any bad ones.

You can also keep cured meats and cheeses in the cellar, depending on the conditions you create.

While the temperature and humidity in your root cellar are ideal for vegetables and some fruits, metal containers should not be stored there. It will rust and spoil if you store canned food or anything with a metal lid in your cellar for an extended period. The same is true for flour, oatmeal, and any other cereal that needs to be kept dry. A root cellar is simply too humid for any food that absorbs moisture easily.

Having a root cellar allows you to enjoy vegetables and fruits that are out of season or produce that is not available at the grocery store unless sprayed and imported. You don't have to bottle, can, boil, or freeze anything to accomplish this.

Furthermore, you will no longer be limited to storing only certain vegetables—carrots, potatoes, and turnips. You can store nuts, fresh tomatoes, cantaloupes, sweet potatoes, and more if you carefully plan your root cellar program.

Don't worry if you find that you can't always fill your root cellar with what you grow. Visit the farmer's markets and purchase in-season or storage vegetables in the fall.

Here are some of the foods you can store along with useful indications:

Food	Temperature	Humidity	Shelf-Life
Apples	32°F	90 to 95%	Two to seven months, depending on the variety
Dried Beans	50 to 60°F	60 to 70%	One year
Beets	32°F	90 to 95%	Three to five months
Broccoli	32°F	90 to 95%	One to two weeks
Brussels Sprouts	32°F	90 to 95%	Three to five weeks
Cabbage	32°F	90 to 95%	Three to four months
Carrots	32°F	90 to 95%	Four to six months
Garlic	50 to 60°F	60 to 70%	Five to eight months
Jerusalem Artichokes	32°F	90 to 95%	One to two months
Leeks	32°F	90 to 95%	Three to four months
Onions	50 to 60°F	60 to 70%	Five to eight months
Parsnips	32°F	90 to 95%	One to two months
Pears	30°F	90 to 95%	Two to three months
Potatoes	40 to 45°F	90 to 95%	Four to six months
Pumpkins	50 to 60°F	60 to 70%	Five to six months
Rutabagas	32°F	90 to 95%	Two to four months
Squash	50 to 60°F	60 to 70%	Four to six months
Sweet Potatoes	55 to 60°F	60 to 70%	Four to six months
Tomatillos	50 to 60°F	60 to 70%	One to two months
Tomatoes	50 to 60°F	60 to 70%	One to two months—green tomatoes Four to six months for those varieties bred for winter storage
Turnips	32°F	90 to 95%	Four to six months

The above list gives you an idea of the temperatures and humidity levels at which certain foods must be stored.

As established, root cellars can be used to store just about anything these days. Traditionally, they were used to store root vegetables, mainly potatoes, turnips, and carrots. Today, people store other root vegetables, apples, pears, hard fruits, *etc.* In addition, you can store canned foods, medicines, salted meat and fish, and so much more. If you build one big enough, you can use it as an emergency shelter!

This will ensure that your food supplies last as long as possible without spoiling and losing flavor or nutritional value. Typically, you will have some food that needs to be stored in damp, cold environments and others that need a drier and warmer environment. In the list below, the produce has been sorted according to its temperature requirements, providing information on how to harvest and store it, along with a few good storage varieties.

All the fruits and vegetables listed must be stored at 32-40°F and 90-95% humidity.

CHAPTER 3: DIFFERENT DESIGN OPTIONS FOR ROOT CELLARS

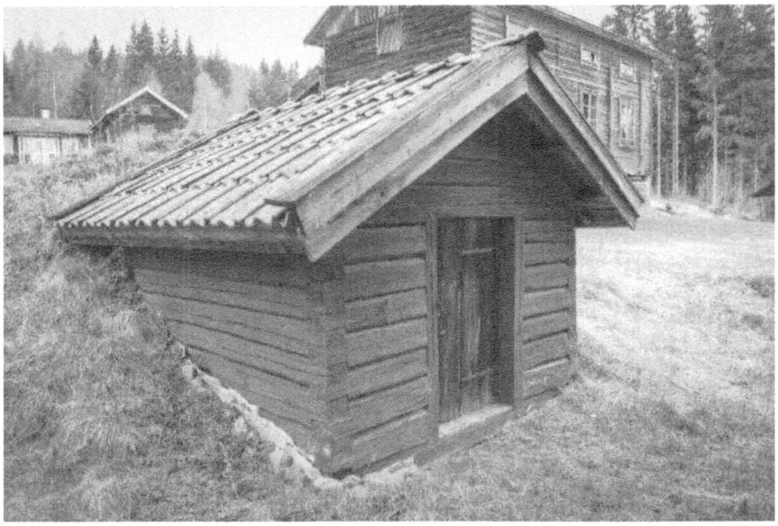

Earth Bag Root Cellar

This root cellar design is ideal for building into a hill or the ground and will save a significant amount of money on construction materials because it is built using earth bags, sturdy bags that come in various sizes and are then simply filled with dirt, as the name implies. The first step in this design is selecting the appropriate earth bags for your project.

Filling the earth bags is a laborious process made much easier with at least two people. One person should be in charge of filling the bags with usable dirt that is free of vegetation and stones and packed tightly, and another should take the filled bags and position them.

What You Require:

- Earthenware bags
- Door/window frames made of wood
- Gravel
- Barbed wire
- Baling Twine for PVC Pipe

What You Should Do:

1. Make room for at least an 8x8 rounded root cellar.
2. Drainage for the root cellar should be laid out using a 4-inch PVC pipe perforated to allow for proper drainage. Drainage will be adequate if the pipe is laid on a 4% grade down and out of the space.
3. Place one foot of gravel on top of the pipe and firmly tamp it down; this will be the root cellar's floor.
4. This earth bag root cellar will be perfectly round, as each ring of earth bags has a smaller diameter than the previous one until it closes at the top. To determine the starting point, use a compass and ruler to take precise measurements.
5. Remove the door frame and decide where you want the ventilation to go.
6. Lay out the first level of earth bags, considering the doorway and additional walkways. To give the earth bags some extra weight, the first few levels should be filled with 20% concrete and 80% dirt. The remainder can be filled with dirt alone.
7. After that, each layer of bags must be tamped down and covered in two lengths of barbed wire across the course.

   Each layer of bags should naturally move closer to the center of the root cellar, resulting in each layer taking up less space. Do not rush this process because allowing it to happen naturally will result in a structure as solid as any traditionally built structure.

   If done correctly, your buttress walls will be little more than earth bags connected to the main structure at the door frame.

8. Fill in the rest of the displaced dirt around the structure with at least two layers of polyethylene.
9. Cover the inside with lime plaster to allow the walls to "breathe," which will act as a moisture barrier.
10. Consider shelving carefully as round root cellars tend to have less space, allowing each shelf a bit of breathing room.

Septic Tank Root Cellar

This root cellar design splits the difference between the first two by taking a prefabricated item and burying it outside. Remember, only an unused septic tank would be appropriate for storing food. A great way to find a cheap future root cellar for cheap is to find septic tank whole sellers in your area and see if they are willing to sell any tanks they have which might have defects rendering them unusable for their intended purpose.

A 1500-gallon tank averages about five and a half feet wide, tall, and ten feet long, while a 2500-gallon tank provides an extra foot of headroom. New undamaged 2500-gallon tanks cost around $1600, while otherwise unusable tanks cost about half that. When buying a tank, ask the seller to remove the partition that is almost certainly inside, though it can be punched through manually if necessary.

Converting a Septic Tank into a Root Cellar

Once you've located a septic tank and dug out a location for it, it's time to spread a layer of crushed stone beneath the final resting place to support what's to come. Ensure that your layer of stone will keep the tank level once it is in place.

After the tank has been installed, it is time to construct a door and ventilation points. This is most easily accomplished with a concrete-cutoff saw. Begin by marking a four-inch spot four inches from the bottom of the tank on the side facing out of the hole that does not have an effluent pipe hole. This is the bottom of your door.

Cut out the space for the door and ventilation holes with a concrete-cutoff saw, wearing eye and ear protection. As needed, use a sledgehammer.

You can build your door, but getting it to seal is difficult; instead, consider an insulated steel door in a pre-hung frame. Before you cut the hole, look for a door.

When cutting vent holes, ensure they are at least four inches in diameter. Because the effluent pipe hole is already a four-inch hole leading out of the tank's top, you will likely only need to cut an entry air hole and use that for the exit pipe. Make an additional drainage hole in the center of the tank at the bottom for easy cleaning.

All that is left is to fill in the hole where your new root cellar sits. Before you do that, however, be sure to seal the access hatch at the top of the tank. Next, cover the top of the tank with a few layers of polyethylene to ensure the roof is waterproof.

Once the tank is buried, construct a retaining wall at the doorway to prevent dirt from getting inside.

In-Ground Root Cellar

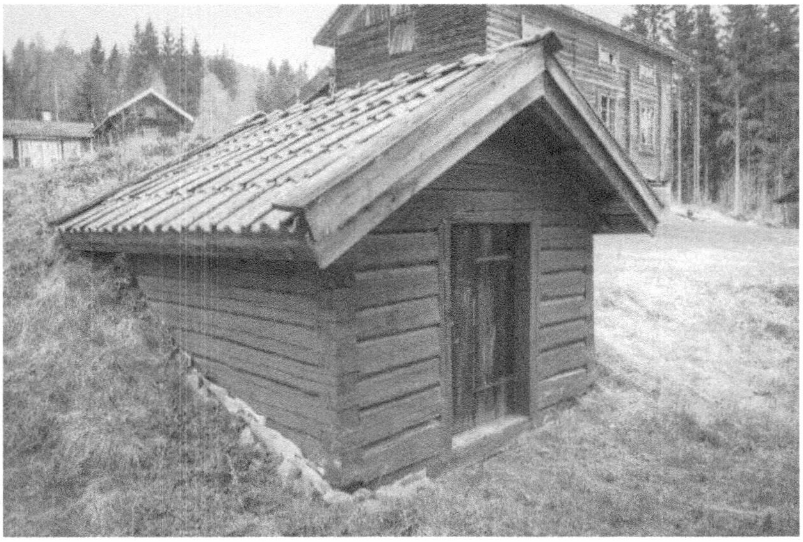

Building an underground root cellar takes a lot of time and commitment, so if you don't have either, you should look into another type of root cellar. If you are not skilled at construction or do not have the necessary tools, consider hiring a professional contractor to assist you.

First and foremost, you must select the materials from which your root cellar will be constructed. Among the options are:

- Natural stone
- Block of cinder/concrete
- Logs of cedar
- Tires stacked with dirt

Most people prefer cinder blocks because they are inexpensive and readily available in most builders' yards or DIY stores.

You could use a fiberglass water tank if you want to take a different approach and let your creative side run wild. These are easily adaptable to your needs and are easier to bury than digging out an entire room and constructing walls. Simply ensure that it is well-ventilated and has at least one foot of soil.

Consider your flooring options for the in-ground root cellar. Most people lay concrete, flat stones, or a packed earth floor with a layer of gravel. This is the cheapest and often best option because it ensures humidity can be better controlled.

Take into account the location of your root cellar. It must be located in a well-drained area—the last thing you want is water running in. You must also consider the water table; an in-ground root cellar cannot be built where the water table is high. Finally, ensure the opening faces north to limit exposure to the hot sun during the day. Consider ventilation, temperature, and humidity wherever your root cellar is located.

The first step to constructing your root cellar is making a hole. Depending on the size of your root cellar, you may need to use a backhoe or hire a contractor who owns one to assist you in digging it.

Dig deeper for footings around the cellar, then pour in the concrete. You must now wait at least twenty-four to forty-eight hours for this to harden.

When the concrete has hardened, you can start constructing your walls. Take your time with this step—it's a big job, and attempting to lay all the bricks at once will lead to disaster. Again, if you are not confident in your bricklaying abilities, consider hiring someone to do it for you.

You should also check your ventilation at this point. A 3 to 4 inches diameter PVC pipe should be inserted at the cellar's bottom to draw in colder air. A second one of the same size must be installed near the top to vent the hot air and ethylene gas. Ensure your vent pipes are covered with breathable screens so air can flow while keeping pests out.

Frame your entrance as you build the wall. After all, you'll need a way in! Build the footings for the door five brick rows high.

Make your roof. You could pour a flat concrete slab for the top, but condensation would be a major issue. As a result, the best option is to construct an arched roof. This necessitates excellent carpentry skills (or hiring someone to do the job for you!).

To build a strong enough structure, you will need 12-inch plywood and 2x4s; it will need to be built, disassembled, and reassembled on your cellar walls.

First, construct your skeleton out of 2x4s and plywood, as shown below:

Next, cover the roof of your structure with plywood.

Put it back together on the cellar walls.

Before covering the entire roof with rebar, place the plywood cover on top, cover it with a tight plastic sheet, and affix it to the structure.

Pour your concrete now. It should be 6 inches thick and cover the entire structure and the wall bricks. Unless you have a contractor on hand, you will most likely need to do this in sections.

Now is the time to be patient! Before removing the wooden form from the inside, the concrete must cure and dry. Allow two to three days before attempting to remove the form. A waterproof sealant should also be brushed over the concrete.

The next step is to construct your stairs. This is best done with concrete, though wooden ones can be built if desired. Add a top and bottom door, and your root cellar is complete.

Two doors are recommended because they keep creatures out and cooler air in—just remember to close the top door before opening the bottom one. You'll also need light atop the stairs to see your way down.

If you want to keep your cellar floor as packed earth, you can layer gravel on top of it.

To organize your cellar, use wooden shelves on your walls; these are not so fast to conduct heat and cold and can help you regulate your temperatures.

Container Root Cellar

Zoning

Before you can even think of using a steel container as a root cellar, you need to check if any zoning laws (city, county, or state) stop you from doing it or restrict where or how you do it.

Placement

Chances are you already decided this when you checked out the zoning laws. When you decide this, think carefully about how you will use your container. If you build it into a hill, you will want a door and steps to access it.

Structure

If you choose to bury your container, you need to think carefully about how it will stand the pressure on it from the earth. Containers are not exactly designed to be buried; they were designed to be stacked on a ship or at the docks. The only load-bearing parts of a container are the four corner posts—the sides are strong enough to support the roof, and that is it. You may need to plan on erecting a retaining wall around where your container is located without forgetting to include drainage. If you do, heavy downpours could submerge your container, fully or partially. If you are entirely burying your container, you will need a platform that pushes the earth's weight onto the four corner posts. The one thing you should never do is dig your hole and bury the container without planning—it will most certainly collapse.

Moisture

While containers are watertight and windproof, you need to consider how you will stop the earth's moisture from getting in. The floor is built of steel cross-members with treated plywood on top. You need to think about sealing underneath the floor and possibly pouring a cement base first. Your container must also be sealed with plastic tarps, roofing tar, or truck bed liners. Do your research and find the most cost-effective way of sealing your container for optimum results.

Ventilation

Your container cellar must have good ventilation and air circulation; otherwise, anything you store in it will be destroyed. The principle here is the same as any other type of root cellar.

Once your container root cellar is in place, you can follow the same rules for any type of root cellar. You can add an extra door and use it as a storm shelter—at least it will have food!

The 'Cave' Cellar

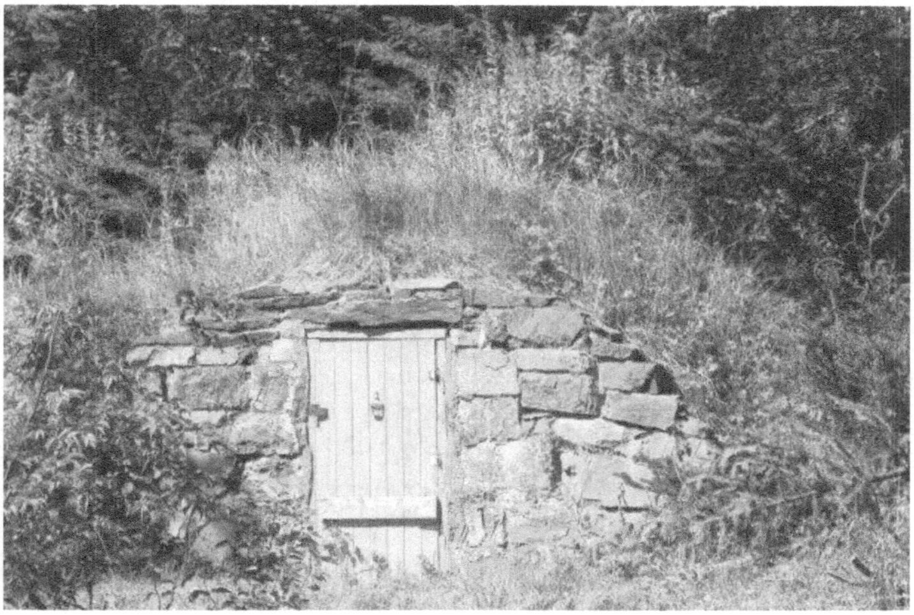

The term 'cave' simply comes from the fact that it is usually built into a sloping hillside, leaving only the front entrance visible. The rest of the building is covered with soil to a depth of at least 36 inches over the roof.

Of course, there are times when it takes up residence in a cave, with some modifications to make it fit for its purpose.

This is undoubtedly the most expensive type of root cellar (unless you have a cave!), and, of course, it depends on you having a hillside to build it into. A similar type, however, can be built by utilizing a dip in the ground to minimize excavation.

Depending on your specific circumstances, it can also be built on level ground and hidden beneath a mound of soil.

An early example of an old Root Cellar is one dug into a hillside and turfed over.

Depending on ground conditions, permanency, and other factors, there are numerous ways to build a cave-style root cellar.

The materials used can range from concrete blocks to lumber to straw bales! A temporary cellar can be built with straw bale walls and a strong timber roof to hold a few inches of soil or sod to insulate it.

However, in this case, we will look at a permanent structure that involves building into the hillside. However, the same construction methods can be used in various situations.

Caution: Imagination is required!

Material List (15 feet by 8 feet by 8 feet):

- Concrete block (CMU) 16 x 9 x 8 - 390 blocks
- 1.5 cubic yards of pre-mixed concrete for footings
- 2.15 cubic yards of pre-mixed roof concrete
- 4 - 8x4 insulating roof sheets (choose thickness), sand, and cement for mortar
- Rear vent pipe (minimum 4") long enough to reach from the floor to the finished ground level
- Front door, window (if applicable), and vent pipe
- Rough sand or gravel for the inside base
- Screws and fasteners

Note: These are all estimated measurements.

Construction Procedures:

- Step 1 - Equipment: Unless you intend to work on it for months or years, hire a backhoe and a driver. This is back-breaking work to do by hand.
- Step 2 - Digging: Dig into the hillside 18 feet deep by 13 feet wide for a cellar 15 feet deep by 8 feet wide by 8 feet high (internal). This is to allow for the width of the two walls to be 16 inches and access around the construction to apply a damp-proof membrane before backfilling.
- Step 3 - Foundations: Measure the internal width of the cellar, then mark and dig out a foundation area that is the center of the walls, as shown in the diagram below.

- Step 4 - Walls: After pouring the foundations and allowing them to set, build the walls with concrete blocks according to the diagram, and let them set for two days or so.
- Step 5 - Roof: Keep in mind that the roof is load-bearing and thus must be both strong and waterproof. This is accomplished by building a framework of 4x2 timbers topped by a 34-inch ply board.

  The timbers are secured to the inside of the wall with appropriate wall screws or nails. The 4 x 2 timbers are spaced at 24-inch intervals, just like you would when building a floor.

  This will support the concrete while it sets and will be left in place to form the cellar ceiling - minus the vertical supports, which will be knocked away once the concrete has fully cured.

  A vent pipe, consisting of one 4-inch pipe at the back of the cellar, leading from the floor level up through the roof, must be installed before this stage. Fit insect mesh to the outside cap to keep flies and bugs away.

  A second vent will be installed on the front wall near the ceiling level to allow warm air to escape and create an air flow.

  The reinforcing steel mesh is then laid on 'lifts' of stone or slate so that it is roughly in the center of the concrete when it is poured.

  The timberwork has been shuttered at 6 inches high, allowing the poured concrete to cover the wall head completely.

  The plywood extends to the inside edge, level with the wall head.

  Tip: If you use concrete blocks without reinforcing the walls, the tops can be covered with slate or other material to keep the concrete from pouring down the inside cavity.

  Before pouring concrete, a polythene sheet is laid over the timber in the preceding example. This is a good precaution because it prevents water from soaking into the woodwork below. This water-logged wood can cause the concrete to dry out too quickly, leading to mold growth later on.

  The Damp-Proof Membrane (DPM) completely covers the roof and walls. This can be a polythene membrane or a good tar-based coating, especially on the walls - follow the manufacturer's application instructions.

  I prefer to cover the roof area with a high-quality pond liner, such as EPDM. This is very flexible, will not tear easily, and is reasonably priced for the roof area (it should cost less than $100).

  Make sure that the membrane is tucked OVER the membrane on the walls. This ensures that the joint is waterproof.

- Step 6 - Front Door: I have assumed up to this point that you are aware of the need for a front door. Yes? Good! How difficult can it be to build a wall with a door?

  Although this is 'good enough,' it can be improved by including a second door inside the first - even if it is at the end of a short corridor. This improves the insulative qualities and is a great barrier against heat and cold when you access your cellar.

  In addition, a 2-inch builder insulating board on the inside of the door and front wall area, which are the only areas exposed to the elements, is an excellent idea for insulation.

- Step 7 - Infilling: Before filling the area to the side of the cellar, protect your DPM with a thin fiberboard to prevent it from being torn.

  Depending on whether you have enough roof covering, the roof is covered with 2–4-inch builders insulating board at this stage (at least 3 feet of soil). While covering over with earth will insulate your cellar and protect the DPM.

- Step 8 – Cellar Interior: Because your root cellar must have high relative humidity, no attempt is made to prevent ALL water from entering.

  For example, the floor is best finished with fine gravel or sand over the dirt itself. In most cases, this should provide just the right amount of moisture.

  If timber racking is used, some people prefer to run a border of concrete or slabs around the edge for the legs to stand, leaving only a 4-foot-wide channel of gravel down the center.

  A Front Vent (4-inch pipe) must be installed on the front wall, high up near the ceiling. This allows warmer air to escape while the rear vent draws in cooler air, resulting in an ideal air flow in your Cellar.

  If possible, an opening window should be included in the front wall construction to allow for better air flow when conditions call for it.

As previously stated, humidity is essential in your roof cellar because it prevents the vegetables from drying out and wrinkling. However, too much water can cause other issues, such as moldy vegetables and walls, which is not good.

The loose-fill flooring should provide enough natural humidity to meet your needs; if not, keep some water in an open trough or basin to help with humidity levels.

However, if the ground water rises during heavy rainfall and your cellar becomes inundated, you may need to install a lift pump in a suitable location.

This is more of an issue in a basement cellar or another cellar buried below ground level.

When the water level rises, a floatation switch in the pump activates automatically, clearing away the water before it becomes a problem.

It only requires a suitable hole dug in the floor and lined with brick or concrete – a sunken barrel or bucket will suffice. This should be at the bottom of a slope so that any water that falls on it is directed to it, possibly with the help of a simple gutter.

When the hole begins to fill, the pump is activated, and the water is pumped to the location you specify.

A perforated barrel is another option. Make the hole larger than the barrel and fill the surrounding space with pea gravel. If the water table is a problem, this will collect water seepage from the surrounding soil.

Keep this in mind when selecting building materials and consider using heavy timber in dry climates where wood rot is less of an issue (timber is an excellent insulator).

Excess water affects the damp-proofing methods used to protect the structure and the measures required to prevent mold in wet climates.

CHAPTER 4: ROOT CELLAR IN WINTER

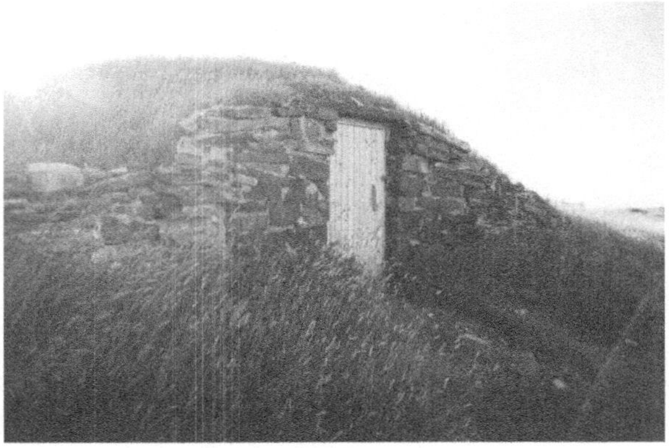

Depending on your physical location, your root cellar may be predisposed more towards one type of produce or storage method than the others. Suppose the area you live in is known for having mild winters. In that case, it may not be possible to get the low temperatures required for storing fruits and vegetables, and the most you might be able to get away with is storing things like grains, nuts, and dried fruit, much the way the ancient Egyptians did.

On the other hand, if the area where you are building your root cellar is known to be extremely cold, then your main goal will be to keep what you have stored from freezing. Cold-weather root cellars typically need extra layers of insulation and constructed air vents so that the sun warms the air as it travels down. Large barrels of water or a few hanging light bulbs powered by a generator can also keep the space warm.

In most places, root cellars will likely not be listed among the types of projects requiring permits. Unfortunately, this is mainly because they have fallen out of fashion, not because they do not require any sort of permit. This is occasionally not the case in predominantly rural areas where they are considered sheds for storing agriculture and exempt from regulation. Several other types of additional construction can also require additional permits. These include:

For a root shelter, the general idea is to create a cool space where the temperature stays at 32-40°F (0-4.4 C) with a humidity level of between 85-95%.

The reason for the cool temperature is that it slows the release of ethylene gas and stops microorganisms from growing, which causes the vegetables to decompose.

The humidity level is crucial because it stops your vegetables from drying out through evaporation, leading to withered-looking veggies!

This is the ideal temperature and humidity level to store a range of root vegetables, such as carrots, turnips, beets, parsnips, potatoes, and many other vegetables throughout the winter.

Ventilation is another important consideration for a successful root cellar. It removes excess water or condensation and replenishes the oxygen supply keeping the area fresh and reducing the chances of mold.

However, do not be fooled into thinking that a root cellar is only for winter use! During hot summer, the cooler interior of your root cellar will also double up as a free-to-use (no electric bills) temporary storage area for most kinds of vegetables and other food products.

Though not as cold as your refrigerator, it will keep most vegetables fresh and free-up the fridge for items such as dairy products – depending on your local weather conditions.

Tips on Keeping Your Root Cellar Cool

You must consider these aspects to store your vegetables effectively over the winter months. Creating the optimum atmosphere can be done by following these simple tips:

- Your root cellar should be dug about ten feet (or three meters), where temperature stability is reached.
- Do not site a dug-in root cellar near large trees. Not only will you find digging through the roots challenging, but they will eventually grow through your cellar walls.
- Use wooden platforms, bins, and shelves to store your produce on and in. Wood does not conduct the cold or heat as quickly as metal does, and plastic may turn brittle.
- Ensure your shelves are between 1 and 3 inches from the walls—this ensures good air circulation, minimizing the chances of airborne mold.
- If your root cellar is outdoors, the best flooring is packed earth, whereas, in a basement cellar, concrete is more practical and works better.
- Make sure you have a handy hygrometer and thermometer and check them daily.
- Use inlets and outlets to regulate heat and cold into and out of the root cellar.

More Tips on Storage and Root Cellar Conditions

If you need to preserve moisture in your cellar and create a humid microclimate, place the vegetables that need that climate in individual bags with holes. Alternatively, you can use perforated, sealed plastic containers. Avoid regular plastic containers—although they do work for some things.

On the other hand, dry microclimates can be created using sealed containers containing moisture-absorbing materials. A cup of rice, for example, absorbs air moisture while keeping the rice away from your vegetables.

Begin planning your root cellar storage as soon as the planting season begins. Choose varieties designed for long-term storage.

When harvesting vegetables, avoid washing them before storing them. The cellar will be disease-fighting, and washing it off may be harmful.

Do your homework—some vegetables must be cured before storing, while others store better if exposed to frost. Proper research ensures that your produce has the longest possible shelf life.

Nothing diseased or damaged should be stored. If you bruise or cut any vegetable or fruit while harvesting, set it aside—it should be eaten first.

Check your storage every couple of weeks to ensure nothing is going bad. If anything is, get rid of it right away before it ruins the rest of your harvest.

CHAPTER 5: STEP-BY-STEP CONSTRUCTION PLAN

Step 1: Get a Permit

Building permits are required in most US states for any new construction, including root cellars. Permits are typically issued at the county or local level, so get in touch with your local governing body.

Furthermore, zoning laws or neighborhood uniformity rules may limit where and how you can build your root cellar. It is critical to conduct all of this due diligence ahead of time, well before you begin digging, to avoid fines or other penalties.

If you must get some food into the ground and don't have time to consider a proper design fully, a metal garbage can buried in the ground can provide you with a temporary refuge.

Begin by digging a hole slightly larger than the diameter of the can and deep enough to allow the can to sit about four inches below the soil line.

Place the garbage can in the hole and fill the space around it with excess straw to insulate it. When you're finished, replace the lid, wrap it in plastic, and add more straw or mulch to help the contents maintain a consistent temperature.

This method works well for storing root vegetables especially, and they will keep in this fashion all winter long

Step 2: Choose a Design

While the traditional root cellar dug into the side of a hill may still be suitable for some, most modern root cellars are built straight down with stairs eventually leading down to the door. Colder climates will almost certainly necessitate the installation of a second door as a form of extra insulation. Root cellars have also been built using metal culverts or simple materials such as barrels, packing crates, or pallets to store an underground cache of food and supplies.

Regardless of style, the true value of any root cellar is the extra insulation it receives from the soil surrounding it. One foot underground can provide a temperature drop of up to 20 degrees compared to summertime temperatures above ground. A minimum of three or four feet of soil above the top of your root cellar is required to make it worthwhile, and a full ten feet of dirt between your root cellar and the outside world (both above and on either side) allows for the most insulation and temperature control. Remember, to get the most out of your root cellar, keep the temperature between 32°F and 40°F and the humidity between 70% and 85%. Temperatures up to 50°F can also be effective, though anything above that will not significantly slow the rate at which fruit rots.

When deciding on a location for your root cellar, take special care to ensure that any part of the finished structure that is directly exposed to the outside world never receives (or only minimally) direct sunlight. To maximize temperature control for future space, always build on the north side of a hill or in the shade.

Likewise, it is vital to ensure that any exposed parts of the root cellar will not be subject to rain runoff or leaks. Preventing such weather hazards is as simple as adding sloped doors or other drainage options but requires planning and foresight to attempt correctly.

Step 3: Root Cellar Placement

Before viewing root cellar designs, here are a few more things to consider when deciding where to place your root cellar for maximum efficiency and convenience. If you are planning to build your root cellar in your basement:

It may be easiest to provide two sides of the root cellar using the northeast corner of the house. After this, the other two sides can be filled in with board and stud.

Insulation is essential for keeping ambient house heat out.

The root cellar will still require its ventilation system.

If you intend to build your root cellar directly into the ground, scout the area for roots ahead of time; an abundance of roots will make digging the cellar more difficult and result in a less stable finished product.

Check for proper drainage. Sandy soil is ideal for this, as is building the cellar on a slope.

If the temperature in your area regularly falls below 25°F, ensure your cellar is dug deep enough to be below the frost line.

An easy alternative to modern insulation is straw and dried leaves; in cold climates, the dirt itself will not be enough.

Step 4: Materials

Tools:

- One or two long-handed shovels, plus a trench shovel for squaring off the hole you dig
- A hoe or something to spread concrete, plus a wooden float to smooth it
- A wheelbarrow
- Mortarboard, trowel, and jointer tool
- A level and a tape measure
- A plumb bob
- A hammer and a masonry chisel
- A saw to cut any lumber
- A keyhole saw for specialized cutting
- A plane for trimming rafters
- A set of screwdrivers and wrenches
- A caulking gun

Materials for the Floor:

- Stakes to mark off the area
- String
- Boards to establish the floor's perimeter
- Ready-mix concrete

- Materials for the walls:
- Hollow concrete blocks
- Masonry cement
- Wood

Note: You will be building a ceiling, a door with a frame, and a set of stairs. Consult with someone knowledgeable at your building supply store regarding the amount of wood necessary for your root cellar. Please note that you will have to treat all the wood in advance to protect it against your root cellar's high humidity levels.

Materials for Drainage and Ventilation:

- Drainage tiles
- Metal ventilation pipe, at least three feet long, plus a mesh screen to cover it
- Pipe covers to seal off ventilation when necessary

Additional Materials:

- A hatch door
- Spray foam insulation
- Extra weatherproofing for your doors
- Gravel

Step 5: Digging In

Note: Before you stab anything into the ground, you must first contact your local power supplier to check whether any power lines are buried in the ground.

You must first dig out or excavate a location for your root cellar. This can be done with a shovel or professional excavation equipment, depending on the size of the planned cellar and the soil. This is best done in early spring after the ground has thawed. If you need professional contractors to assist you with this project, you should hire them in early spring before their schedules fill up. However, before you dig, check the weather forecast; early spring rains could be disastrous.

When defining the dig area, leave more space around the perimeter than the actual floor area you intend to dig. For example, if your cellar is 8 feet by 8 feet, you should excavate a 10-foot by 10-foot section. This allows for the cellar walls and the soil that will be backfilled later.

The hole should be 4 feet deep to get your cellar below the frost line. Create a slope corresponding to the stairs on the side of the hole where you intend to put the entrance. You will almost certainly be constructing a doorway at the top and bottom of these stairs.

Be sure not to haul the soil you dig out too far away. You will be using it again.

Step 6: Foundations and Support Structures

A footing is necessary to support your root cellar, especially once it is well-stocked and covered with soil. Unless you have experience pouring footings and foundations, it is highly advised you consult a concrete specialist.

Stake out the surface area of your floor, then dig an even footing around the perimeter. This corresponds to the width of the walls and aids in weight distribution. You can then pour your footing. Allow the new concrete to harden for the required time before constructing the first level of mortar blocks on top of the footing to form the foundation of your wall.

However, you must first install your drainage tiles before building a wall. Pour two inches of gravel around the perimeter of the footing and slope it toward the door. Lay the tiles around the entire perimeter of the gravel bed, with the holes pointing downward. Both ends of the drainage tile should point toward the front of the structure and drain into three-foot-wide, three-foot-deep holes. After that, cover the tiles with about a foot of extra gravel to support the weight of the backfilled soil.

The masonry blocks can be used to construct the supporting walls. If you've never built a masonry wall before, seek the advice of a guide or an expert who can show you how to cut the blocks so that the patterns alternate and keep your lines straight. It is probably a good idea to pour sawdust or another type of insulation down the holes before the final course of masonry blocks. Do this on the front wall, if not all of them.

When your walls are complete, it's time to install the roof. There are numerous options for root cellar roofs but remember that it will have to bear a significant load once much of the structure has been covered with soil. Consult a roofing expert to determine which designs can withstand the load that your cellar will require, but in general, you will need strong support rafters, and you will need to build the roof at an angle that takes the pressure off the walls once the soil is on top. The advantage of building a cellar roof is that it only needs to be functional; no one will see it.

Note: If you are going to finish off your roof with concrete or tar, save that step for now. We will be going over ventilation shortly. After you have created a way to ventilate your root cellar, you can finish off the roof.

Step 7: An Entrance

Now that your doorway is in place, you must make entry and exit simple and convenient. First, construct a wall corresponding to the doorway and slope upward with the ground to accommodate the hatch door. Make sure to treat the wood you use to construct this wall. You'll need to build a small flight of stairs along the slope that leads to the doorway. You can get creative here but using a prefabricated set of stairs that line up with your doorway is the simplest option.

A hatch door may not be enough to keep the cold air out in colder climates. Consider fitting a second door into the frame you built in such cases. The most important thing, however, is to insulate the entrance. That is why you purchased spray foam insulation.

Line the hatch doorway's perimeter with spray foam insulation with care. It will start as a liquid but quickly expand into a thick, airtight foam. This type of insulation around doorways and joints is somewhat pricey, but it is well worth it because it effectively keeps air out.

Furthermore, insects or rodents certainly could not if air could not pass through those spaces. This foam insulation will be your first line of defense against pests that can smell all the good food in your cellar.

Step 8: Ventilation

You now have a standing structure with a functional door and a nearly finished roof. It's time to build a ventilation pipe so that controlling temperature and humidity will be much easier in the future.

To begin, use your keyhole saw to cut a hole in your roof between any two rafters that are the width of your metal ventilation pipe. We recommended making this pipe at least three feet long so it can protrude well above the backfilled soil you will soon cover this cellar with. Pass the pipe through the hole you created and secure it tightly. More foam insulation is needed here to make the seam around the pipe waterproof.

You'll need two covers at the top of the ventilation pipe: one conical in shape to keep out rain and large objects and one mesh screen fixed across the opening to keep out any insects or rodents falling down that pipe.

Finally, you need to create some kind of air-tight stopper for the cellar side of the ventilation pipe for airflow regulation. A simple rubber stopper that corresponds to the pipe's opening would be sufficient, but feel free to get more sophisticated.

Step 9: Electricity

Now is the right time to install any electricity if you choose and have been granted permission. Please note that the installation of electricity is an expert-only project. Unless you have lots of experience running electricity lines and installing electrical systems, hire a professional for this job.

Step 10: Backfilling

It's time to bury your root cellar so it can benefit from the earth's temperature-regulating abilities. Remember all that soil you dug up to make room for your cellar? This is where it comes in handy. Backfilling the soil around your root cellar is as simple as using a shovel and a wheelbarrow. Make sure the cellar's structure is completely sealed, the roof is complete, and all the walls have hardened sufficiently to withstand the weight of all this soil.

Spread the first layer of soil around the perimeter with caution to avoid crushing the drainage tiles. Continue to build up around the perimeter until the soil reaches the height of the walls. Increase the soil around the entrance so that only the hatch door remains. After that, start mounding up the soil on the roof, taking care not to cover the ventilation pipe.

Once your root cellar is covered, seed or sod the soil and let grass begin to grow. Within a few weeks, it will look naturally integrated into the surrounding terrain, and you will be ready to start storing produce.

CHAPTER 6: ROOT CELLAR INTERIOR TIPS AND TRICKS FOR FURNITURE, STORAGE SPACE, AND UTILITIES

Once your root cellar has been set up, the actual effective operation of the cellar is pretty simple. It centers around keeping the humidity and the temperature from any severe fluctuations.

Lack of humidity can be countered by simply putting an open bucket of water in the corner if your cellar is too dry or sprinkling water on the floor.

If the cellar is too humid, increase the airflow and check that the interior is not troubled with water seepage and other wet problems.

Food Storage Shelves

You can build a food storage system with spare walls in your pantry or an extra room in your house. Fruit, some vegetables, and canned and dried foods can all be stored here as long as your shelves are kept in a dark, cool place.

You will later read step-by-step instructions for building shelving units.

Crawlspace

You can certainly convert your crawlspace, or a portion of it, into a storage room. Choose a location away from furnaces, water heaters, and other heat sources. Add sturdy shelving to make more space; if it has a dirt floor, that's even better because dirt floors are the best at regulating humidity. Although concrete floors are not ideal, they provide a longer lifespan for most vegetables. Bring out your creative side while keeping adequate ventilation in mind.

Plastic Tote

Plastic totes are an inexpensive way to extend the life of your root crops. All you have to do is partially bury the vegetables in sawdust, which will help with moisture regulation and keep the vegetables from touching each other. Using a tote, you can also keep your vegetables in the dark. This method works well for potatoes, beets, and carrots, and if you can't find sawdust, you can use a straw instead—while it will need to dry out, you can reuse sawdust or straw the following year.

Under Your Porch

You can use the space beneath your porch if you're exceptionally clever and inventive. A hole in the basement wall leading to the under-porch space is one design. The entrance is lined with rigid foam, which adds insulation from outside temperatures and is designed to blend in with the room from which it came.

These spaces are not large, but they can be used to store several pounds of potatoes or other root vegetables in an otherwise unutilized space.

Window Well in the Basement

If you don't have any extra space but have a basement window well, you can convert it into a mini-root cellar.

Your window well should ideally be on a north wall. Cover it with a layer of straw bales and orientated strand board (OSB). This keeps it cool but does not cause it to freeze. And if the bottom of your window well is layered with gravel, it will help regulate humidity levels.

You can stack milk crates to hold your vegetables; because these stacks well, you can make the most of your space. You can also hang dark curtains at the window to keep the light out.

This method of storing winter squash and potatoes works well. However, it is not suitable for those who are not mobile, as accessing it can be difficult.

Earth Pit

This was another popular method for storing root vegetables, similar to clamp storage. All you have to do is dig a shady and well-drained pit, ensuring that water drains away rather than into it.

Cover the bottom of the pit with sawdust or sand, then add your root vegetables and cover them with more sawdust or sand and a thick layer of straw or leaves. Weigh down a black plastic sheet with logs, rocks, bricks, or other heavy items.

Making Use of Cardboard Boxes

You can store your vegetables in cardboard boxes if you have space in a room or under your bed. The idea is straightforward: Put your vegetables in the box and cover them with something damp but not soaking wet. This gives the impression that your vegetables are resting beneath the ground, waiting to be picked.

You can use any size cardboard box appropriate for storing the vegetables. For most vegetables, the filling should be sand, peat moss, wood chips (make sure the wood chips are not toxic), or newspaper for potatoes.

Most vegetables do not need to be washed before storing; simply rub dirt off potatoes, but most other items can be stored dirty. They should be because the soil can help fight disease and protect the vegetables. Picking your vegetables or digging them up and placing them directly in the boxes is the best method.

All root vegetables should be trimmed to prevent deterioration and drying, leaving a couple of inches of top greenery on them.

For Potatoes:

1. Fill the bottoms of the boxes with newspaper sheets.
2. Dig up your potatoes, sort them into storage bags, and rub off the dirt. Take care not to harm the skin.
3. Sort your potatoes by size or variety and layer them in the bottom of the box in a single layer. Add another layer of newspaper, followed by another layer of potatoes. Repeat until the box is full.

For Additional Root Vegetables:

Apply a thin layer of filler material to the bottom of the box before adding your vegetables. Try to arrange them so that the carrots are horizontal and the turnips are upright. Place a layer of filler on top, followed by another layer of vegetables, and so on. Make sure the filler is moist—it will serve as a humidifier. Place the box in storage after closing it.

Check your vegetables regularly and discard any that are deteriorating or drying out. Beets are notorious for drying out quickly, but if you get to them quickly enough, you can still use them. Simply place them in a pan of simmering water to bring them back to life.

If you dry the filler out thoroughly, you can reuse it many times.

Organizing Your Space

How you design your space mainly depends on what you are storing. If you only keep one type of produce, ensure the humidity and temperature levels are even throughout the cellar.

Build shelves for the walls and other storage units using wood—they will not conduct the heat or cold the same way metal does and ensure the temperatures remain steady. Also, ensure your storage options are a couple of inches away from the walls to keep them dry. Using shelving means storing foods that need different temperatures, too—colder at the bottom, warmer at the top.

Lastly, load your products, and don't forget to check them weekly. Discard anything going bad and reap the rewards of all your hard work.

Organizing your root cellar depends entirely on your wishes, budget, tastes, and what you want to store. You can opt to buy multiple storage bins and fill them with straw or sawdust, or you can just use old crates and boxes to place upon any shelves you create. Just remember to think vertically, *i.e.,* build-up. You won't be living in your cellar, so you should use as much space as possible for storage. This includes building tall shelves, which then give you flexibility regarding humidity (remember, the area close to the ceiling will be warmer and more humid).

Storing Vegetables in Sand

You can do this with just about any container on hand and a supply of fine sand (the type used in kids' sandboxes).

Put a few inches of play sand and tuck in your root vegetables. You can also use this method for firm fruits like pears or apples. Cover with more sand, leaving space between the fruits/vegetables so they can breathe and the air circulate. You should leave about an inch between fruits.

Ensure you do not wash anything you store this way, which hastens the decomposition process. Simply brush the dirt off and cut off green bits, like carrot tops or beet greens.

Another way is to add sand to wooden or cardboard boxes and store them in basements, cellars, or even a garage—so long as it is not heated. It does not matter where as long as the temperature doesn't go below freezing.

The same procedure applies to the crisper drawer. Keep your fruits and vegetables separate, especially those that give off ethylene gas, such as apples. This gas speeds up ripening and can taint other vegetables and fruits. Store root vegetables vertically in the sand and the rest lying down.

In-Place Storage

There are several methods for in-place storage; just pick which one suits you.

Garden Rows

Carrots and beets will keep perfectly through the winter, and their flavor may even improve over time.

The idea is to insulate the rows against sub-zero temperatures. To accomplish this, poke holes in a black garbage bag and fill it with wet leaves. When ready to harvest your vegetables, simply place them over the top and lift them off. Harvest enough to last a few weeks, so you don't have to keep disturbing the rows and exposing them to the cold air. Furthermore, when spring arrives, those leaves are ideal for adding to your compost heap.

Another option is to remove the carrot tops. Freeze, bottle, or otherwise use the carrots. As insulation, the carrot tops can be piled on top of another row of vegetables. Then, cover it with black plastic and weigh it down with bricks.

Mounding

This is another technique. Several pockets are dug into the earth and vented to allow air to circulate. A drainage trench will direct water away from the pockets. The disadvantage is that all the food in a pocket must be harvested all at once, so it is best to make several small ones. The pockets are insulated with straw and dirt layers, and this method works for onions, potatoes, and any other food that needs to be stored in dry conditions.

Hay Bale Storage

This necessitates constructing a hay bale structure around your vegetable rows. This is finished with a large sheet of plexiglass or a recycled storm door, transforming it into a cold frame. A blanket or tarp can be used for extra insulation in freezing weather. This method allows you to harvest food as needed rather than all at once, and it works well with crops that prefer moist conditions, such as carrots, winter radishes, and beets.

Mini Hoop-Houses

The final method involves building mini hoop-houses over your rows. These are made from lengths of PVC piping and clear plastic sheeting. You can find many different ways of doing this online, and they are pretty easy to construct and allow your crops to be harvested as you want them.

Basic Tips

All households have different eating habits, and the design and contents of all root cellars will vary wildly depending on the household's needs. For most people, root cellars offer a great place to store root vegetables and tubers, such as carrots, potatoes, parsnips, beets, and so on.

You might ask why you cannot just go and buy these as you need them. Well, you can if you want; however, take a careful look at the quality of the vegetables in your grocery store. They are often damaged and bruised; some already go off and are generally tasteless.

As such, these are the basic principles you must follow to successfully plan and build your root cellar.

- **Check with Your Local Building Department**: The last thing you want is to violate any building codes. Before you start building your root cellar, check with your local building department to see if there are any requirements or regulations you must follow. Before you begin, you must follow all construction or building codes that apply to your project and ensure you have all the necessary permits.
- **Make a Plan**: Design your root cellar to meet your food storage needs, considering any physical limitations you may have. For example, if you have difficulty using a ladder or stairs, choose a more accessible root cellar design.
- **Choose Your Size**: Your root cellar must be large enough to hold all your food. For example, if you grow an acre of food, building a tiny root cellar that can only hold a fraction of what you harvest is pointless. If you only have a small amount to store, don't build a massive one. If you build underground, keep the following safety precautions in mind. Some potential hazards include structural failure, accumulated unwanted gases, cave-ins, etc. So, build your cellar from the ground up, ensuring it's safe, sound, and has enough ventilation.
- **Consider the Location:** You must consider every aspect of the land where you intend to build your root cellar. Some areas have extremely high water tables, while others have septic systems, which can be disastrous because the root cellar will flood and fail.

- **Consider the Critical Aspects:** When designing, consider controlling temperature, drainage, ventilation, and humidity. These factors are significant and will influence how long your food will last in storage. People frequently approach building a root cellar based on the type of food they intend to store. So, as you create your plan, ask yourself the following questions:
- **The Foundations:** Next, you must plan the foundations of your cellar. You must dig a minimum of ten feet to reach the ground level, where the temperature stabilizes.
- **Lining the Walls:** If possible, use cinder blocks—they are less expensive, more malleable, and excellent for lining your walls. Remember that your walls must be built on the foundation to ensure their stability; you'd be surprised at how many people put in the floor first, then build their walls to the sides!
- **Plan Your Floor:** While many believe pouring a cement floor is the best option, the best flooring for a root cellar is gravel and natural dirt. This works better than a concrete floor at retaining moisture. The goal is to maintain a high humidity level; the more moisture you can keep, the better.
- **The Roof**: Graded ceilings are far superior for keeping rain and other external elements out and preventing them from resting on the cellar roof. Heavy rain or snow piled on the roof can add significant weight, all of which bears down on your cellar foundations.
- **Ventilation**: This is important in constructing your root cellar because it prevents too much humidity and moisture from spoiling your crops. Excess moisture causes condensation, which, as you are aware, results in water running everywhere, causing your crops to rot and spoil.

If you want to convert an existing building or space, ensure you follow the same guidelines for location and make the right alterations to fit what you want.

CHAPTER 7: HARVESTING, STORING, TRACKING, AND PLANNING

Beets

Beets should be harvested after a few days of dry weather if the roots have a diameter of around 2 inches. Dig up the beets, remove the greens, leaving 1 to 2 inches on the root, and brush off the loose soil.

The beets should not be washed. Simply place them in a lidded bucket or a wooden box filled with damp sand, peat moss, or sawdust. Make sure your beets are not touching. If you're using a bucket, put the lid on to help retain moisture, but don't tighten it (you still need air circulation).

Check on your beets from time to time and remove any that appear to be going bad—like apples, one bad beet can ruin the lot.

Varieties:

The following varieties are ideal for long-term storage:

- Long Season
- Boltardy
- Lutz Green Leaf

Shelf Life: Beets will store anywhere between three and five months.

Broccoli

Broccoli is not well known for being a long-storage vegetable. You can make it last for a couple of weeks when stored correctly.

Dig up your broccoli and trim the stems. You can store it in perforated plastic bags or hang it upside down in the cellar. However you do it, ensure you do not store it near any fruit, such as apples, that releases ethylene gas, as this can dramatically shorten its storage life.

Varieties:

The following varieties are ideal for long-term storage:

- Green Comet
- Greenbelt

- Marathon
- Legacy
- Waltham 29

Shelf Life: Between one and two weeks at most.

Brussels Sprouts

Brussels sprouts, whether you like them or not, are good for storing—though they do not have a long shelf life. Before harvesting your sprouts for the best flavor, wait until several touches of frost have passed. If you have enough space in your cellar, carefully dig up the plant and plant it in a container. Place it in your cellar and continue to harvest it. Alternatively, hang it by the roots in the cellar. Harvest your sprouts and store them in perforated plastic bags if you don't have much space.

Varieties:

The following varieties are ideal for long-term storage:

- Long Island Improved
- Jade Cross

Shelf Life: Between three and five weeks.

Cabbage

Red cabbage varieties will store better than their green or white counterparts, and late varieties are better than early ones.

Harvest your cabbages when the first frost has passed. Pull or dig the plant up and trim the leaves off. Choose cabbages with solid, unblemished heads to store.

These are best stored in bins or outside pits—if you store them indoors, the cabbage odor will go right through the cellar or house and can severely impact how pears, apples, and celery taste. If you can only store them in the root cellar, each head should be wrapped in paper and stored on a shelf, with a few inches between each one.

Varieties:

The following varieties are ideal for long-term storage:

- Danish Ballhead
- Brunswick
- Red Acre
- Late Flat Dutch
- Storage No 4
- Red Drumhead

Shelf Life: Between three and four months, depending on the variety.

Carrots

Carrots are one of the best root crops for storing right in the garden, but only if you don't have any pest problems and can mulch the carrots with one to two feet of straw or hay.

If you need to store them indoors, harvest them before the ground freezes at the end of the season. Cut or snap the tops off as close to the carrot as possible, leaving just a tiny bit. Leaving too much green on the carrot will deplete its nutrients and moisture and will not last long.

Lay the carrots in peat, moss, or damp sandboxes.

Varieties:

The following varieties are ideal for long-term storage:

- Danvers
- Kingston
- Chantenay
- Carson

- Bolero
- Nigel
- Kurota Chantenay
- Royal Chantenay
- Red Core Chantenay
- St Valery

Shelf Life: Between four and six months, depending on the variety and storage conditions.

Jerusalem Artichokes

Jerusalem artichokes keep better in the ground than root cellars, lasting the entire winter if not frozen. If you choose to leave them in the ground, you must take precautions because frost and freezing temperatures will break down the starches. Their texture, color, and flavors will change, and any diseased or bruised will spoil quickly.

Dig them up, remove the tops, and brush off the soil if you want to store them in your root cellar. They should be kept in plastic bags or damp sand in containers. They should not be stored in places where they will dry out and shrivel, as they do not store as well as potatoes.

Varieties:

The following varieties are ideal for long-term storage:

- Fuseau (most common)
- Coris Bolton Haynes (less common)

Shelf Life: All winter in the ground, provided the ground does not freeze. Suppose stored in the root cellar for up to ten days in plastic bags and one to two months in the sand.

Leeks

Leeks are another vegetable that can survive in the ground over the winter or until the first hard frost. Mulch your leeks heavily and keep them that way until after the frost. Dig them up, making sure their roots stay intact.

Fill a deep bucket with soil or damp sand and plant the leeks upright.

Varieties:

The following varieties are ideal for long-term storage:

- Musselburgh
- Arena
- Elephant
- Nebraska
- Zermatt

Shelf Life: Between three and four months in the cellar, all winter in the ground, provided you do not get frost.

Parsnips

Parsnips, like carrots, can be left to grow in the ground over the winter. Cover them with thick mulch and harvest them as needed. However, parsnips dislike freeze/thaw cycles and should be harvested if your winters are cold.

Cut off the tops at the end of the season, before or just after the first frost. Store in sphagnum moss, damp sand, or peat-layered boxes.

Varieties:

The following varieties are ideal for long-term storage:

- Hollow Crown
- All-America
- Offenham

Shelf Life: Between one and two months.

Pears

Pears are incredibly sensitive to changes in temperature and should be stored at the lower end of 29-31°F. If you store them at higher temperatures or for too long, the pears do not ripen. Instead, they break down, turning brown and mushy inside while the outside still looks fine.

Like apples, you should store only the unbruised and unblemished fruits, preferably with their stems. Each pear should be wrapped in a paper bag or newspaper and stored in wooden or cardboard boxes with a perforated plastic lining. This allows air circulation while keeping moisture levels up.

Varieties:

The following varieties are ideal for long-term storage:

- D'anjou
- Comice
- Bosc

Shelf Life: Between two and three months.

Potatoes

Unsurprisingly, potatoes are one of the best root vegetables to store in a root cellar, given that they were the original reason root cellars were built.

Wait until the foliage has died before replanting the potatoes for another two weeks—this aids in the curing and hardening of the skin for storage. Sort through your potatoes after carefully digging them up.

Set aside any bruised or damaged potatoes to be used right away. If any of them have green spots, don't eat them because green is a chemical that can cause digestive and intestinal upset.

Sort the potatoes by size; keep the same-sized potatoes together and brush off any dirt. They should not be washed. Place the potatoes in a dark place at 45 to 60°F for ten to fourteen days to cure.

After that, the potatoes can be stored in bins, boxes, or burlap sacks. Shredded paper should be placed between each layer of potatoes in boxes or bins, and air holes should be cut into the sides.

Do not store potatoes near any fruits that give off ethylene; do not allow the temperature to rise, as this will prompt the potatoes to start sprouting.

Varieties:

Most late potato varieties will store just fine (early and second early varieties are not meant for storage). The following varieties are ideal for long-term storage:

- All Blue
- Red Pontiac
- Kennebec
- Sangre
- Katahdin
- Yukon Gold
- Sebago

Shelf Life: Between four and six months.

Rutabagas

Like most root vegetables, Rutabagas can survive the winter in the ground. To keep the ground from freezing, apply a layer of mulch 10 to 12 inches thick, extending it about 18 inches on either side of the row. Even if there is a couple of feet of snow, the roots are safe. They must be harvested before the spring, or else new growth will sprout from the tops.

If you can't leave them in the ground all winter, lift them at the end of the growing season, brush off the dirt, and twist off the tops to store them for longer. You should not wash them, but if you do, they must be completely dry before being stored.

Sort through the roots and set aside any damaged ones; these cannot be stored and must be consumed immediately.

Layer the good roots in a wooden box or bucket with sawdust, peat moss, or damp sand. The roots should be packed and covered but not touching one another, and the container should not be completely sealed to allow the moist air to circulate.

Varieties:

The following varieties are ideal for long-term storage:

- Laurentian
- American Purple Top

Shelf Life: Between two and six months, depending on the variety.

Turnips

These should be treated the same as carrots and kept moist. However, unlike carrots, turnips should be stored in an outdoor pit if possible. Otherwise, the smell permeates and taints the flavors of other foods.

Varieties:

The following varieties are ideal for long-term storage:

- Purple White Top Globe
- Navet des Vertus Marteau

Shelf Life: Between four and six months.

Winter Radishes

Winter radishes can withstand temperatures as low as 28°F and can be left in the ground if heavily mulched. However, if you must store them away from the ground, consider an outdoor ground pit or garbage bins, as they emit a strong odor indoors.

If you're storing them in a root cellar, cut the tops off, leaving an inch of stem, and layer them with sphagnum moss or sand in boxes or baskets.

Varieties:

The following varieties are ideal for long-term storage:

- Chinese White
- Black Spanish
- Violet de Gournay

Shelf Life: Between two and three months.

Onions

Lift the onions when the tops turn brown and fall. Dig them up during a dry day and spread them on hardware cloth, a screen, or a newspaper. Let them sit somewhere cool, dark, and well-ventilated for ten to fourteen days or until the roots have dried and the skin has turned papery.

Cut the tops off, leaving about an inch, and store them in paper bags, net bags, or even pantyhose. Do not use plastic containers or bags that are not breathable—if onions are not stored in dry conditions, they will begin sprouting.

Varieties:

The following varieties are ideal for long-term storage:

- Brunswick
- Australian Brown
- Copra
- Red Burgundy
- Bronze d'Amposta
- Newburg
- Red Creole
- Norstar

- Red Weathersfield
- Stuttgarter
- Rossa di Milano
- Yellow of Parma
- Yellow Globe
- Sweet varieties do not store very well.

Shelf Life: Between five and eight months.

Pumpkins

Pumpkins should be harvested before the first frost because they dislike cold weather and will be killed by frost. Leave about an inch of stem on the pumpkin to prevent spoilage.

Allow them to cure for about ten days at 80 to 85 degrees. You can leave them outside if the weather is warm and dry. The curing process hardens the skins, allowing them to be stored for a longer period. However, any bruised, damaged, or broken stems should not be stored.

The pumpkins can then be piled up in your root cellar, two or three deep, so long as they are in a dry area—off the floor may be best.

Varieties:

The following varieties are ideal for long-term storage:

- Winter Luxury
- Howdens

Shelf Life: Between five and six months.

Sweet Potatoes

Sweet potatoes should be harvested as soon as the vines have died, usually in late fall. Dig the potatoes carefully, putting damaged tubers to one side for immediate consumption. Brush the loose soil from undamaged tubers and cure them for five to ten days, at a temperature of 80-85°F and with 90% humidity.

After this time, you can move them into the root cellar, wrapping each tuber in paper and layering them in ventilated baskets or boxes.

Varieties:

The following varieties are ideal for long-term storage:

- Centennial
- Allgold
- Jewell

Shelf Life: Between four and six months.

Tomatoes

You are not required to wait for your tomatoes to ripen on the vine. You can pick them while they are still green and allow them to mature in storage, or choose varieties better suited to longer storage. Some tomatoes store much better than others if the conditions are favorable.

If you're storing green tomatoes, pull the entire vine from the ground and hang it upside down in the cellar. Alternatively, you can select the tomatoes and individually wrap each one in the paper. Store them at around 55°F to allow them to ripen slowly; do not store them below this temperature, or they will not ripen. Green tomatoes typically take ten to fourteen days to ripen at the ideal temperature.

Varieties:

The following varieties are ideal for long-term storage:

- Eva Purple Ball
- Green Thumb
- Fried Green Hybrid

- Old Fashioned Garen Peach
- Reverend Morrow's Long Keeper
- Red Siberian
- Red October
- Winter Keeper
- Ruby Treasure

Shelf Life: Between one and two months for standard green tomatoes; up to six months for long storage varieties.

CHAPTER 8: YEARLY MAINTENANCE (TIPS, TRICKS, MUST DO, LOG PLAN, CHECKLIST)

Cleaning and Sanitizing a Root Cellar

The last thing worth discussing is cleaning your root cellar. This should be done twice a year, the first time in March or April and the second before storing your next harvest.

Most of your remaining root crops will have passed their best storage limits by the spring. Whatever you didn't use must be consumed or discarded, depending on whether it's good or bad. While potatoes, garlic, and onions are probably still safe, you should eat them soon or plant them in the garden to produce a new crop.

If you have an abundance of good vegetables that you cannot use immediately, find another way to store them. A lovely pan of scalloped potatoes can be made with potatoes, garlic, and onion! Make a batch of meals with your vegetables that you can freeze for another day.

If you have vegetables that can be stored for a few months, remove them from the cellar. While doing your spring cleaning, keep them in burlap sacks or dark, ventilated containers. They won't be exposed to light, and the air will still circulate, keeping them fresh. Set aside canned and bottled foods.

Remove any storage bins, crates, and boxes once you've cleared out all of your food from the cellar. Cardboard boxes may be usable for another year; if not, throw them away. It is best to burn them if they have bacteria or mold growth spots.

Reusable containers should be scrubbed out thoroughly. Use a weak bleach solution to kill bacteria and wash them in boiling water. Leave them to dry naturally.

Back into the root cellar, give it a good sweep. Clear up any dust, dirt, and debris from the shelves and the floor.

Once your root cellar is cleared out, leave the doors open to air out for a few days. If the cellar still smells musty, run a fan there for a few days to help evacuate the stale air.

Before you store your next harvest in the autumn, go back in there, have a final sweep out, rewash your storage containers and close down your vents. You do not want the warmer summer air getting in. Now you are ready to start over.

As a side note, you can use your root cellar in the summer months to keep early fruits and vegetables cool when you don't have time to process them straight away. However, do not leave them there for more than a few days.

During spring cleaning, go through your root cellar and list any repairs, improvements, or upgrades needed. Check for rot or damage if you use wood in any structures; this must be replaced first.

Examine the seals around your ventilation pipes and replace them as needed. Do the same with doors and windows, and make sure any drainage issues are addressed immediately.

Make sure you have enough storage containers and bags—buy new ones if necessary. Check that your old ones are in good shape, with no nails or loose bits protruding.

Check that your ventilation covers are in place and replace them if necessary. When the temperature outside is low enough, open your vent covers.

While root cellars are relatively easy to maintain, you need to be on top of monitoring it, especially when yours is newly built at the start of the season. Two of the most important things you can invest in are a hygrometer and a thermometer. As established, you must maintain the following conditions in your cellar:

- Humidity — 90-95%
- Temperature — 32-40°F
- Ventilation — Constant and adequately installed

Keeping the temperature stable is possibly the hardest thing to do. Most root cellars rely on the soil temperature to keep the cellar cool. Based on your climate, you may need to consider digging your cellar in a bit deeper—this is why research is critical.

It is relatively simple to raise humidity levels—leave a few water bowls in the cellar. Then, experiment with humidity and see how many bowls you need to use to get the humidity at the right level. However, be mindful of ensuring your root cellar is secured; water can attract insects and other unwelcome creatures.

By contrast, if you need to lower the humidity level, make your ventilation a bit bigger or angle it to where the winds prevail from in your region. Ensure your ventilation is covered with a screen; otherwise, you will get insects, dirt, rain, and all sorts in your cellar.

Adequate ventilation will stop ethylene gas from building up and destroying your food or causing it to sprout too early. Ethylene is odorless and is typically associated with fruits like bananas and apples.

Canned and Bottled Foods

Anything stored in jars, bottles, or otherwise preserved must be handled differently. When you began with your root cellar, you should have started a notebook detailing the dates each item was preserved and placed into storage. You should also have labeled each container with the date of preservation.

Your first job is to go through everything. Check for anything that has expired or gone off, and discard it in the garbage. Go by the dates on your containers or in your notebook—the earliest products should have been used first, so all you should have in storage are those stored later. However, if your system went awry, you may be left with old food—you really should not eat this unless it has been pickled. Dairy products are way past their "best by" date by now unless they have only just been placed into storage.

Also, dispose of any rusted, dented, or bulging cans and foods with torn or broken packaging.

Now, you can deal with what is left.

Wipe down all jars, cans, bottles, etc., to eliminate any dirt, dust, or sticky residue.

Restock your cellar using a FIFO system—First In, First Out. The older stuff should be used first, or it will go off soon.

CONCLUSION

Thank you for reading this book. Once your root cellar is up and running, take a moment to reflect on how far you've come. Then, in January, take a big bite of one of your vegetables, either from the farmers' market or your garden. Consider the tasteless produce grown on other continents and now available on the shelves of your local supermarket. The difference will be enormous. What you have in your hands, in your root cellar, is a vegetable that tastes exactly as it should, a taste many of us have forgotten.

Root cellars were initially designed for root vegetables; hence the name—vegetables like potatoes, carrots, parsnips, beets, and turnips are ideal for this type of storage. People store much more, such as apples, flower bulbs, canned goods, pears, pickled vegetables, etc. Consider a root cellar to be a large extension of your pantry.

Root cellars use the earth to keep humidity, light, and temperature levels stable. The ideal temperature range is 32-40°F, and the ideal humidity range is 85-95%. A successful root cellar requires humidity, darkness, and good ventilation.

The temperature is critical. Temperature control allows vegetables and fruits to slowly release ethylene gas, allowing microorganisms to grow and halting the decomposition process. High humidity, on the other hand, prevents moisture from evaporating.

Good luck.

HOME DEFENSE FOR PREPPERS

Easy and Proven Techniques to Prevent House Invasion and Save your Family

Tyler Gordon

INTRODUCTION

Defending one's home from attack is known as home defense. Defense strategies are based on the defender's home's security, mobility, and versatility, as well as their weapons.

A person's home is the only place they feel safe and secure. As a result, a home should be the safest place on the planet. However, this is not always the case in today's world. To keep their family members safe and secure, one should take as much care of their home as possible.

Home security includes physical and psychological security because intruders often exploit flaws in human psychology when breaking into someone's home.

This book was written to prepare us to defend ourselves not only from the event and whatever happens but also from what comes after; from men looking for sustenance for themselves and their families, who bring violence to our doors and loot those we have provided for.

In this book, I'd like to devote a section to discuss how to protect your home not only from vandals but also how to return claiming back your property after a disaster by protecting windows, installing perimeter alarms, or training your dog (if you have one) to be on guard around your property. I'll also go over what to do if you or your family are in danger.

Your family comes first; protecting it is your responsibility; I will show you how to do so by arming you with the knowledge you need to deal with difficult situations.

Psychological security will mentally prepare you for any such incident, ensuring you do not lose your cool while defending your family, loved ones, or home. Fear, anger, and adrenaline rush are all psychological triggers that can lead to a negative outcome in any type of self-defense situation.

The protection of the home includes the outer walls, doors, windows, and, most importantly, the house itself.

We should plan our home defenses to have an efficient and quick response in case of any intrusion. Let's get started.

CHAPTER 1: SECURITY PLANNING (BASICS ETC.)

Setting up a good defense system can be much more challenging in a temporary shelter because your shelter will only provide minimal protection. A tent, tarpaulin, lean-to, or leaf hut will not offer much protection against human or animal intruders.

As a result, good planning and a weapon or two will be required. If you carry a gun or any other weapon, you should ensure you are adequately trained to use it. You do not want to injure another party member while defending yourself. Ensure you have enough ammo and always know where your weapon is, especially at night.

Even if your defenses are minimal, secure what you can before bed, this could include closing and tying shut a makeshift door, closing a tent and locking the zippers together, or simply spreading dry twigs around your shelter to increase the likelihood of being woken by an intruder approaching.

If you have a choice about where you camp, choose a sheltered location not too close to the water. Water attracts predators, and while you want to access it, being too close may be dangerous. Being hidden from paths and out of sight may help you stay safe from human intruders, so ensure your shelter is hidden. Consider covering the shelter with sticks, leaves, moss, or other debris to keep it hidden.

If you are staying in a temporary shelter for an extended period and are concerned about intruders, there are other things you can do to strengthen the area's defenses. If you have the tools and time, you could, for example, dig a trench around the shelter.

You may find yourself in the wilderness with few resources and options for defense. If this occurs, consider developing weapons out of natural resources. Sharpening sturdy sticks into weapons, longer branches into javelins, and using rocks as ammunition are all options. If you can find flint, you can shape it into a makeshift knife. Stock up on stones and sharpened tools, even if you have to make them yourself because you don't have any.

However, you should carry weapons whenever you go out in the wild, especially if you plan to stay away from home for an extended period.

The first step is comprehending why you require home defense and fortification knowledge. To properly fortify and protect your home, you must first understand why you should do so. The average American home is not built to be defensive. Yes, even though all houses have locks on their windows and doors, they are still vulnerable to criminals breaking in. This explains why approximately four million burglaries occur each year. This figure would be much lower if houses were more challenging to break into.

Individuals in desperate need of survival will go to any length to survive. When people are deprived of food and water, they begin to turn on each other and murder one another to obtain what they require. If you have stocked your house with food and supplies, raiding and looter parties will immediately target it. Even if you do not have such supplies, others may believe you do and plan an attack on your home regardless of whether you own them or not. People will turn on one another in the face of any type of crisis. Terrorist attacks, foreign invasions, financial meltdowns, E.M.P. attacks, nuclear attacks, nuclear power plant accidents, and so on...

Assume, for example, that a fully armed and well-coordinated raiding party of four or five hungry people has launched an assault on your home. Would you be taken aback? Be completely honest: Do you believe you have the resources and skills to repel this invading group if a disaster occurs tomorrow? It's important to remember that the average American home isn't built for defense. As things currently stand, that raiding party will have no trouble breaking into your home.

It's a given that your answer to the previous question will almost certainly be 'no,' or at the very least 'probably not.' There's nothing wrong with admitting it; the vast majority of people in this country, and the entire world, would react negatively.

The good news is that by adequately reinforcing your home in a defense-friendly manner and mastering basic defensive techniques, you will be far better prepared for disaster than 99% of the general population. This alone should bring you some relief.

Think of your home as a fortress or a castle. It is your haven, haven, and comfortable refuge, as well as a safe place to treasure your belongings and stockpile your food and water supplies. Which path are you going to take? Will you let an invading army take over this castle, killing its inhabitants (i.e., your family), or will you fight back and defend your home?

Why are you being asked to regard your home as your castle? Because castles are relatively simple to defend. There is a lot of fortification surrounding them, and they are well-supplied. So can your home, but only if you make the necessary changes, which is what this is all about. As a result, why should you learn the skills required to build and secure your home? It all comes down to the need to safeguard your loved ones.

In an emergency, it is your priority to ensure the safety and survival of your loved ones, and if you do not know how to protect your home, both there and your chances of survival are significantly reduced.

Preparedness is the key; no one is safe from danger or unforeseen incidents. So, you must remain prepared for all kinds of situations to easily deal with them when they arise. You should help your family members remain ready to react appropriately and safely in any danger or emergency.

Always keep your eyes open for any signs of trouble threatening your family and/or property. If you spot something unusual, take the proper steps to make things normal again. If you are not aware of anything, then you can always involve the appropriate authorities so that they can take care of things for you.

It is a Family Task

Home defense is vital; we must care for ourselves and our families. Nighttime, in particular, can bring added dangers, and the risk of an intruder trying to gain access to your family home worryingly could become a reality. You must prepare your family to protect the house and themselves by following the advice discussed in this book.

Arm Your Family

Although weapons are not recommended at home, in these cases, having access to one within designated parts of the house could save their lives. When you are locked in, staring danger in the face, you may feel like it's wrong to be armed, but it might be the key to your survival. Please ensure that younger household members do not have access to these.

A flashlight is an essential piece of equipment. Some will choose to have access to a loaded gun, ammunition, knives, or even a claw hammer, which would be beneficial to protect yourself should the need arise.

Also, having a well-stocked first aid kit in case you get hurt while locked in is vital to treat yourself or a family member so you can continue to protect yourself, your family, and your property from an unwanted intruder.

Educate Your Family Members

It is essential to educate every family member, starting at a young age, on the most effective steps to take in an emergency or other unforeseen occurrence. The phrase " hide, run, fight" should be discussed, and a predetermined meeting place should be chosen in case there is an escape. We saw "Home Alone" when our children were older, and we used it as a guide for putting together our family's routine. Ensure that everyone knows the security system's controls, how to use the alert button, how to contact the police even if there isn't an inside alert, and how to handle outsiders who access the property.

Keep a Bag with All Your Stuff Together

A designated bag for your weapons, emergency supplies, and medicines will help you prepare for an emergency.

There are also electric weapons that can disable someone without killing them. There are many weapons that you can have at hand to defend yourself without the need to kill someone.

You can also have a belt where you keep everything you need, in case you have to escape at night to avoid harm.

Flashlights for Everyone

You should have extra flashlights and batteries in full working order to protect yourself; now, choose the ones with a bright light, not the dim yellow light that barely illuminates.

You can have one of those flashlights on your forehead to free your hands from moving around.

The other must-have is binoculars that will help you identify any danger from a safe distance, see what's coming, and be ready to defend yourselves and your property.

For other house members, they could use pepper spray; with it, they can disable any potential attackers and knock them out.

Protecting Your Family and Children

Protecting your family and children from danger is of utmost importance. You should help them learn the correct way to defend themselves from any intruders or otherwise.

However, if you are in a situation where you have to leave home, you should teach them the following guidelines:

- Your children must be well aware of the dangers in your neighborhood. They must know not to talk with strangers and not to accept any gifts or candy from them.
- Familiarize them with their surroundings so they would quickly know where they are going, even if they are walking alone. Teach your children as early as now about safe places that they can go to, even at nighttime.
- Do not keep money on the table or your bedside table. Also, teach them to hide valuable things in their pockets and pack them in a backpack whenever they leave home.
- In case you have to go out of your home, teach them how to lock it securely so that it would not be possible for intruders to enter anytime soon. Also, teach them how to open the windows if they are locked.
- If they must bathe in the public bath, teach them to swim continuously with their clothes on.
- Ensure your children know not to talk with strangers or play in front of streets or roads. Also, ensure they will never talk about bad things as some people might have different intentions for them.
- Never allow anyone to enter your home without permission unless it is a visit from a relative. Teach them to always look for suspicious people in alleys or dark places. If you will be allowed them to play outside, teach them never to go near the fences of your home as many dangers are lurking in there.
- Give your children a list of significant phone numbers such as police department and contact numbers so they can call for help whenever they get lost while playing.
- Teach your children not to approach any vehicles that are parked or unattended. Also, tell them not to talk with strangers inside vehicles because they might be bad people who could use them for their motives.

Other Ways of Protecting Family and Children

- **Safety Training**: You should give your family members protective training to protect themselves in an emergency. You can teach your family members the following things:
- **Self-Defense**: This includes both physical and verbal. Every family member should be taught how to defend himself in an intruder attack; physical self-defense techniques, such as punching or kicking, will help your children be prepared for any situation. Techniques for verbal self-defense include:

- **Verbal Confrontation**: This is the most crucial technique to teach your family members. Always keep in mind that their safety comes first and foremost.
- **Technology**: Nowadays, even children have cell phones and tablets, so it is critical to teach them how to use these devices to alert the police in the event of an emergency or a criminal attack. They should be prepared to dial 911 without paying attention to themselves or their location. They should also be taught how to use their cell phones to call for help while hiding in a safe location.
- **Personal Protection Equipment**: Aside from teaching family members how to protect themselves, parents must protect their children from harm by providing them with protective equipment. Typical protective equipment includes the following:
- **Wear a Safety Helmet**: It is a vital piece of equipment that can assist your children and other family members protect themselves from any unexpected incident or awkward situation.
- **Products for Home Security**: These are various types of home security products that will assist you in protecting your home from intruders and burglars. Many security products available today can be used for various purposes, but there are always exceptions.

These critical factors can help protect your family and children from harm.

As a parent, it is vital to remember that you don't need to stress too much about protecting them because you need to ensure that you keep them busy with something positive so that they don't take things for granted and always remain relaxed to keep their guard up at all times.

Self-Defense for Kids

When you're young and hear a story about someone being hurt or killed by someone else, your first thoughts are that it won't happen to you. When it does occur, the shock and disbelief can be more damaging than the initial encounter. As a result, self-defense training can be highly beneficial for children interacting with strangers regularly. They are more likely to make bad decisions on their own than adults because their perception is still low and impulsive. When they are young, it is the best time to teach them how to defend themselves against an attacker or a violent criminal. Children nowadays are more likely to respond well to a simple self-defense session in which they learn how to move, think, and act faster so that if they ever come into contact with a dangerous person, the encounter will be over as soon as possible.

A self-defense class is not intended to teach children how to harm others. It's about ensuring your child understands the steps they can take to protect themselves. They may not be able to prevent an attack, but they can certainly learn how to end it sooner rather than later.

In this day and age of cell phones, violent television shows, and movies, your child must understand how to protect themselves. Children are especially vulnerable to copycat behavior because they quickly learn from what they see. Their learning ability is very high compared to adults because their brain has not yet fully developed. They can store a lot of information before developing the capacity for rational thinking and complicated reasoning.

It's best to start teaching them self-defense before they start school. This is the first sign of trouble when a child feels threatened by another child or sees something that makes him feel unsafe in public or at home. Even if your child never faces a physical attack, it's essential to encourage them to learn self-defense, so they're prepared to encounter a violent criminal.

Building self-esteem is one of the essential things you can do as a parent because not only does it help your child feel better about themselves in the long run, and helps them become more successful and able to defend themselves. It will also make them more confident about their actions and decisions, which will probably save them from the mistakes many others make after experiencing a violent crime.

Defend Yourself at All Costs

If danger strikes, protect your family, do not get yourself cornered. Develop a strategy to tackle any intruders and have weapons at home that you are confident in using to defend yourself.

Designing and installing a perimeter defense will help you protect yourself by preventing intruders from gaining immediate access to your property.

There is a good chance that attacks will reach your home, so you must know how to protect yourself.

Creating a perimeter barrier will allow you to defend yourself and others, ensuring your survival. A good prepper must have weapons and ammunition to handle whatever comes close to home. If people know you have resources, attacks could last an extended period, so it's up to you to defend yourself.

In a group, situational awareness involves good communication between the house members. You'll require a system to keep all family members informed of developments happening outside and around you.

It can be as simple as taking notes in a group notebook that all patrol members review before starting their shift. It would help if you considered mapping the area and paying attention to landmarks to guide them when they are out and about.

You can set this up on a board and make any necessary changes after each patrol. Collective awareness also extends to communicating with neighbors and other trusted people in the area.

A network of contacts throughout the region will significantly increase the information available to you and your family. Create a system with these contacts so that you can exchange information with them regularly. It can be done through regular meetings or simply passing information between you.

Drills are vital to any successful program, but this is often missing. The plan is nothing more than a theory waiting to be implemented. Drills allow you to modify your plan, see what works and doesn't, adjust accordingly, make adaptations, or provide additional training to a member.

Often during a crisis, people freeze if they are not taught what to do in the situation. However, people will naturally attempt to defend themselves with proper training and practice.

CHAPTER 2: STRUCTURAL DEFENSE (PERIMETER DEFENSE, SAFE ROOMS, SECURE/HIDDEN STORAGE)

Perimeter Defense

Making a perimeter defense is one of the best ways to secure an off-grid home and may help deter animals and people. Perimeter defense will generally take the form of a fence, although you can also use plants, rocks, or other materials to make it more difficult to approach your dwelling.

You can build your perimeter defense using the natural resources you have on hand or buy fencing and erect it. Some people dig mounds into the earth to make it harder to approach their off-grid homes from certain angles.

You can also scatter things like holly leaves, old bramble, thistles, and other sharp, spiky materials in the vicinity. However, ensure you keep pathways clear to easily enter and exit your dwelling. While it may seem valuable to close off all routes, this could trap you near your home, which may not be very safe.

You can create dead hedges from cut wood if you are short on spiky materials. This is easy to do; you just weave together old sticks, branches, and dead plants to form an impassable mesh. Even if someone or something does break through, they are likely to make a lot of noise, alerting you to their presence.

You should not create a perimeter defense designed to injure someone approaching. It is unsafe and illegal in many states, so doing so could get you into legal trouble, especially if it hurts someone. Digging and concealing pits, creating tripwires, or otherwise rigging the environment to make it unsafe for someone approaching is dangerous and illegal and should be avoided. Booby traps are not the solution to keeping your home safe.

You'll be the first to admit that a defensive perimeter would practically transform your home and yard into a battleground. Therefore, please don't put yourself in a position where calamity may strike. On the other hand, the advantage of these measures is that they will do a great deal to keep opponents away. They may even deter individuals from assaulting you in the first place!

Installing a barbed-wire fence is the most effective method of establishing a protective perimeter around your property. If you already have a fence around your property, you may put barbed wire over it during a crisis, making this task much easier.

If you don't already have a fence, you'll have to physically pound in tall stakes and stretch or wrap barbed wire between them.

Even a layer of barbed wire fence can do a great deal to keep intruders out. A barbed-wire fence will be tough for your foes to cross and may, hopefully, be demotivating enough. It will also enable you to shoot at your enemy from behind your sandbags while they attempt to cross the fence.

But what happens if your adversaries manage to breach the barbed wire fence? What should you do in such a situation?

To make a long story short, build another barbed wire fence! If you have the money and the time to put up two levels of barbed wire fence, it will be even more effective against an assault than one layer of barbed wire fencing alone.

In addition, you may place nail boards in between your barbed-wire fences. Essentially, nail boards are plywood boards with nails drilled in, then flipped upside down. They are really fast and easy to construct.

As a result, your adversaries must first breach the perimeter of the first barbed wire fence, then a row of nail beds, and finally another barbed wire fence. You may even install more rows of barbed wire fences and nail beds if necessary.

Yes, putting up all of this will take a LOT of time and effort, and it should only be done in the direst of crises expected to last for an extended time. However, this will also be the most effective D.I.Y. protection that you can put in place.

Safe Room

A safe room must be equipped with multiple communications networks and resist power outages, fire, and efforts to burn or gas you out. It's a good idea to stock it with guns, lighting, and medical supplies if you have to flee a violent confrontation.

Traps help capture games in the wild and as defense tools in a genuine TEOTWAWKI or SHTF scenario, but they have no role in a home-defense strategy.

Your final resort must be fortified to keep your family secure, whether you call it a safe room, a panic room, an escape room, or a bunker.

Keep the following suggestions when constructing a safe room in mind:

- Your safe room isn't a waiting room for death. It should be equipped with emergency supplies and provide the same level of security as your external doors.
- It should mix in and not stand out too much. A modified closet or walk-in space will suffice.
- It should be large enough to accommodate your entire family.
- Build it in a convenient location where each family member can evacuate swiftly.

Creating a hidden living space can be difficult if your home doesn't have a lot of space, so be creative and figure out what works best for you.

The unprepared will seek food, drink, and shelter when SHTF. To ensure your and your family's survival as a prepper, you must be able to defend what you own. And fortifying your home is one of the best ways to do it!

You need to stock your safe room with food and water, as you do not know how long you might be there. Have at least 3 gallons of water for each person in your family. Apart from that, you can also store some non-perishable food items within the safe room if you and your family feel hungry. Keep rotating the supplies within your safe over time to ensure that nothing expires and you can access fresh supplies during an emergency. Keep flashlights and other essentials in the room beforehand to avoid last-moment hassles.

Door Security

The average door in American homes is extraordinarily easy to break through. The locks are weak, and the doors themselves can be battered down by anyone who wants to get inside, even if your locks have been replaced with heavy-duty models.

With a sledgehammer or an ax, any burglar who wants to get into your home will make incredibly short work of the wooden door you currently have. Alternatively, they could pick the locks as well to get themselves through.

While inexperienced burglars may have difficulty breaking into the average home, any experienced burglar will have no trouble. Fortunately, you can thwart them by taking just a few crucial steps:

- Replace your door locks with metal strike plates and long-throw deadbolt locks
- Drill longer screws into the door frame to keep it more secure
- Replace all wooden doors leading outside with steel doors
- Replace the wooden frame for your door with a steel one
- Keep two locks at the same height and several more locks at different heights (for your doors leading outside)
- Don't leave any openings for them to exploit.

These tips can help you improve your door security:

- Install top-of-the-line deadbolt locks. Choose single-cylinder one-inch deadbolts instead of double-cylinder deadbolts. The latter could be dangerous if you're stuck in a burning building.
- The greatest locks in the world will be worthless if you utilize regular hollow-core doors, which even a 12-year-old can kick through. Replace them with insulated metal or wood doors.
- Use longer set screws for your strike plates and door hinges.
- Door jammers should be installed. During an attempted break-in, you can buy some time with door jammers.

When the world as we know it ends and lawlessness reigns, no deadbolt will be able to keep an intruder from forcing your doors open. Extra reinforcements, such as barriers, door stops, and flip locks, should be added to your doors.

Doors are easily the most obvious entry point into your home, so the locks for your doors and the doors themselves must be fortified at all costs.

Locks

Keeping locks on your doors and windows and all other exit points leading outside is excellent, but at the same time, you don't want to neglect to keep things locked in your home.

Your home likely has valuable items, and you must keep those protected. Examples of items you need to give extra security include electronics, firearms and ammunition, jewelry, personal documents, items of personal value, and any survival stockpiles you have made (food, water, etc.) One of the best defensive measures is keeping your valuables in a safe with a durable lock bolted to the floor. Burglars often take the whole safe with them if they can't break into it.

Also, keep locks on your jewelry boxes and other essential boxes. You won't be able to put a lock over your TV, so that's one risk you may have to take.

Locks are used to secure your doors and windows, which is no small task if you're in the wilderness. There are several types of locks one can choose from, each of which has its pros and cons that are suited for specific situations.

Secure Windows

Large windows provide lots of natural light inside. Unfortunately, if your windows aren't covered properly, the light won't be the only thing entering your home.

The weakest feature of a house is most likely the windows. It takes no genius to smash them with a bat or simply a large rock found in the driveway.

Bulletproof glass is the way to go if you want your windows to be entirely secure. It may be costly, but it's a little to pay to keep your loved ones and survival supplies safe from the golden horde.

But don't worry if that's too expensive for you. You can also use the following security tips:

- Use security film to reinforce windows. It prevents the glass from shattering entirely, requiring the attacker to break the entire window to gain access.
- Thorny shrubs can be planted below first-floor windows, making it even more difficult for intruders to break in.
- Install burglar bars on windows to keep intruders out even if the glass is smashed. They need a quick-release system that allows you to flee in the event of an earthquake or a fire. This should be placed far enough from the window that an intruder cannot lean in and engage the release.
- Window locks should be installed. Robbers usually try to avoid calling attention to themselves. When forced to break the glass, they'll have difficulty keeping the noise down.
- If more prepared invaders with ammo try to take over your home, be ready to throw up sandbags behind windows.
- Always keep the windows of your house closed. Sounds easy enough, doesn't it? Not everyone remembers to close the windows, but it is necessary to do it in these circumstances.
- Don't forget to use deadbolts or safety pins to lock and reinforce your home's windows. If you have sliding glass windows, you should install a bar on the guide where the window slides.
- Iron bars and grills have proven effective in protecting your home from intruders.
- Buy a residential window security fence if you want an inexpensive way to make windows more secure.

If you don't want those metal or iron strips to ruin the perfect aesthetics of your windows (which matters little in extreme situations), you can choose beautiful decorative strips that can be customized to match your home's decor.

You can secure the underlying windows by strengthening the window glass. Therefore, those intruders will not be able to break the glass so easily.

Additional Tips

In extreme cases, you can put a thick wood or metal sheeting as a protective film on the window and lock yourself in. You have everything you need outside to identify the intruders, and they will not be able to see what you are doing inside.

The advantages of doing this are:

1. Security window films have the double advantage of protecting and, at the same time, hardening the window glass.

2. Protect your windows from being easily broken by intruders. Makes your single or double pane windows or any type of window burglar-proof.
3. Clear and tinted films keep burglars from looking directly into your home, making it an unwanted target.

You can also use shatter-resistant or burglar-resistant glass to make your windows more secure. Intruders can easily break ordinary window glass, so these security glasses allow you to reinforce windows and make your home a more difficult target for break-ins. Once burglars realize it is difficult to break into your home, they tend to look for easier targets, or at least you can defend yourself from the inside and keep them away.

CHAPTER 3: BUNKER OPTION

There are numerous advantages to constructing your underground bunker. These include increased security, more space, and lower construction costs. Choosing the right materials is also essential. Shipping containers are an excellent choice for building on private property. They are usually 8 feet wide and 8.5 feet tall. Depending on the length and width of the bunker, you can choose between 20 and 40-foot versions. Before purchasing shipping containers, check with your landlord or landowner.

Those who want to build their bunkers should be aware of the various factors that must be considered. To begin with, building a bunker necessitates specialized equipment and a solid foundation. The ideal materials for a bunker foundation are crushed stone pillow and concrete with M-200 strength. However, if a concrete foundation is not possible, temporary bunkers with a wooden base can be built.

Many wealthy people prepare for disasters and their homes for an impending emergency. Some are bracing for nuclear war, while others are concerned about riots over toilet paper or food. These structures typically cost over a million dollars to construct, regardless of the reason for building an underground bunker. Despite the high cost, the underground bunker industry is thriving. Some wealthy individuals have constructed these fortified homes, which include swimming pools, bowling alleys, and shooting galleries.

In addition to the necessary equipment, the bunker's exterior must be protected from corrosion. A fake wall is usually constructed to conceal the exit hatch, but the entrance is concealed behind a sheet steel door. The false wall serves a dual purpose: it only opens when a secret mechanism is activated. In a natural disaster, the bunker owner can lock the entrance door with a heavy bolt lock and prevent anyone from breaking in.

Bunker Capacity

Even though a long-term shelter is designed to meet only the bare minimum requirements to keep its occupants alive, the bulk of your focus must be on creating a strong structure to withstand disastrous situations. Size is also an important consideration, especially when designing a shelter for long-term accommodation. It needs to be large enough for people to live there as opposed to a temporary dugout that is only meant to be a place to hide during a storm.

People will have different requirements, and you need to have enough space to cater to these things.

Ideally, you should have a defined number of people you are looking to create the shelter. If you feel the need for it, you can create extra space for one or two additional people, but it is crucial to know how many people are there right from the start. According to the US Federal Emergency Management Agency (FEMA), shelters should follow the following guidelines:

- For short-term shelters, such as hurricane shelters (12-48 hours), shelters should have a minimum of 10 square feet per person.
- For medium-term shelters (5-15 days), shelters should have 20 square feet per person.
- Long-term shelters (several weeks) should have at least 40 square feet per person.

As you can see, long-term shelter size increases exponentially with time. This means that not only are they far more expensive to build, but due to their size, some homes might not even be able to create such an ample space underground for 5 or 10 people.

Location of the Bunker

This will depend on the bunker's purpose, but generally, you have the choice to either build a bunker inside your home, in the basement, or outside your home. Different situations will require different kinds of protection. If you want to protect yourself from tornadoes and hurricanes, you might be better off building a bunker within your home, as the house will serve as a second layer of protection. There are also different costs associated with each type. Depending on the construction and style of your home, it might cost you more to build a bunker inside your home than outside. To better understand each situation, research the pros and cons of both types of buildings.

Position of the Bunker

When creating a survival bunker, you have the option to build one that is underground or one that is above ground. If you go the underground route, you could consider using the basement of the house if you don't want to take a completely fresh start. In terms of security, underground shelters are the best options, and they are also ideal if you want to use this as long-term accommodation.

However, converting a basement into a shelter can be long and expensive. If you want to make a new shelter in the backyard or have some extra land that you want to use for this purpose, then ensure you get a geotechnical analysis of the area beforehand. This will tell you everything you need to know about the ground, and then you can take construction measures according to this report. It might not be possible to build an underground shelter in some areas due to a high water table, but the geotechnical analysis will also tell you about this. Also, you want to consider your surrounding area and whether or not an underground shelter will be appropriate. For instance, if you live in an area that is prone to flooding, or an area on a tectonic plate, this is not going to be the best option for you.

How to Build Your Bunker

Make a Structural Plan

Because building a bunker can be costly, you might not want to build a large one. While you can buy a ready-made bunker that only needs to be placed in the ground, it is more expensive. You could aim for a smaller space and use certain tricks to maximize your available space. Consider your bunker a trailer home where vertical storage is the best way to maximize space.

Make sure you have the correct measurements when creating a blueprint for your bunker. Include only the bunker's area, excluding trees and utility lines. Knowing the exact square footage of the area will assist you in accurately creating the blueprint you'll need before applying for permits.

You should have enough room to move around in the bunker without too much room. You can save space by using furniture that folds against the wall and vertical cabinets for storage. An open area will make your space larger, so don't consider compartmentalizing rooms. If you plan to stay in the bunker with other people, you can add curtains for privacy instead of doors and separate rooms.

No matter the design you are planning to have, you need to plan for comfort and efficiency in case you have to spend a lot of time in the bunker in extreme situations. The minimum recommendation for the indoor area of a bunker per person is 5 to 10 square feet. Use this guideline to plan your space depending on the number of people who might share your bunker with you.

Materials

The construction materials used for an underground bunker can vary widely. You can use tempered steel or a cheap alternative like metal sheeting. Both materials are durable and can withstand high loads. You can also use concrete or rebar for strength. Concrete is the least expensive and easiest to install of all the materials for an underground bunker. It is important to remember that the lining material must be waterproof as moisture is the biggest threat to your survival supplies.

Before constructing the bunker, it is important to check zoning regulations in your area. Make sure that you don't disturb underground utilities. You don't want to cause any damage or risk destroying the bunker if you accidentally dig into them. Also, check the building codes in your area to ensure that you can legally construct an underground bunker. You can also use the local government's resources to research the construction process.

Shipping containers can be used for bunkers. They are typically 8 feet wide and 8.5 feet tall. However, you must consider the soil and moisture content around the bunker. You should consider using dry soil instead of moist soil in arid desert regions. Alternatively, you can use shipping containers if you have a limited budget. Make sure to check with the landowner before purchasing these materials. A shipping container can be a relatively inexpensive alternative to building an underground bunker.

Permits

Depending on where you are and what kind of shelter you are planning to make, you might need several different permits, or you might not need any at all. If you are unsure about your local building regulations and whether or not you need permission from the local authorities to carry out shelter construction, get in touch with an expert and find out. Many cities already have permits specially designed for survival shelters. Building survival shelters and bunkers have become common, and government authorities have taken the necessary steps accordingly. One of the main problems people face and why they need a permit is that building an underground bunker can interfere with gas lines, sewage lines, electrical lines, and many other underground utilities.

Moreover, local authorities have usually already conducted a thorough ground evaluation. Before you decide to dig into the ground, they can tell you everything you need to know when you apply for a permit. Also, building additional accommodation might be illegal without a proper permit, so make sure you get in touch with the authorities and follow legal procedures to save yourself from any hassles down the line.

Construction

The construction of the bunker or shelter can be broken down into several stages. Namely, you need to source materials, prep the area, build the actual accommodation, develop utility solutions, and close everything up. If you are building an above-ground solution, you don't need to worry about landfilling, but the rest remains the same.

The primary materials used in most bunker constructions are concrete and steel, though bricks can also be used for above-ground solutions. However, bricks require more labor, making them more expensive. Whatever material you choose, ensure it can withstand all types of weather. These three options are excellent unless you live in a particular climate, but you could also use wood for colder climates. Even in colder weather, however, wood is susceptible to moisture, which can compromise the shelter's integrity. The last thing you want to do in a life-or-death situation is to repair your bunker.

Your contractor will almost certainly use machinery extensively during construction. For example, machines must dig out the land to make room for the shelter, fill walls with concrete, and then refill the bunker to conceal it. Having a good contractor will give you access to all this machinery without having to do anything yourself or manage third-party machinery rentals. Also, whether you have an underground solution or one above ground, you should leave plenty of space around the area. When construction begins, a large area around the actual build site will be used to accommodate the removed sand, store items, stand machinery during construction, and perform various other tasks. You don't want it so close to your house that you damage both the house and the machines, and you have a small workspace.

Creating the air vents, water lines, and sewage disposal system is critical to the construction process. You should use high-quality materials in this process, and it's also a good idea to have them extra insulated so that if a pipe does spring a leak, you can still use it until much later when you're finally able to repair it. If possible, have two or more air vents, multiple water lines, and multiple sewage lines. This way, if one fails, you have a backup option. It will increase the initial cost slightly, but it is a lifesaving strategy you should consider strongly. Also, if you have access to fresh water on your property, such as a borehole, make sure you have a direct connection from that source to the bunker or shelter. Consider installing more than one motor in that borehole as a backup in the worst-case scenario.

Aside from air vents, you'll also need a dependable air filtration system to process the shelter's outside air and internal air. When you live in such a small space for an extended period and even cook in the shelter, you need an excellent solution to keep the air clean.

As you may have noticed, many of the services provided by the shelter will require electricity to function. In some cases, you may be able to perform certain tasks without electricity, but even in that case, you should have some kind of backup power supply. This could take the form of a UPS with large deep cycle batteries, or it could be an off-grid solar setup. Generators are not a good option because they require fuel, which you may not have easy access to in a survival situation.

With all of these things done and the construction complete, the last thing to do is to cover the shelter. In the case of an underground shelter, you can completely cover it and only leave the entrance and air vents exposed, though even with an above-the-ground solution, you can do a lot to camouflage it with the surroundings. If you have a lot of trees or hedges around, you can use these to cover the construction, or you can even plant some new vegetation on top of or around the structure to make it more discreet.

How to Sustain a Living in Your Bunker

It is critical for security to keep your underground bunkers hidden. You don't want your neighbors to notice and either give you a dirty look or steal your gathered supplies. And if you have neighbors, you don't want to keep everyone hidden from them because that would mean no one would survive. However, there are ways to keep your bunkers safe without being a nuisance.

Covering the entrance to your underground shelter with plants, gazebos, or other natural elements is one way to conceal it. You could even cover the door with plants. However, if concealment is difficult, you can conceal your entrance by placing carpet or sofas inside it. You could also conceal the entrance with a survival outhouse or an old barn. Consider constructing an underground hallway if you want to go even further.

While building an underground bunker is expensive, the security benefits are obvious. By burying it, you will be out of sight of your neighbors while maintaining your security. You'll not only be protected from the elements but also have a place to keep your food cache, ammo, and other essential supplies. Not to mention, by stockpiling supplies in the bunker, you'll be able to protect your family and prepare for a disaster.

You will require four essential items in an enclosed bunker to survive for a while until conditions allow you to escape. First and foremost, your bunker will require a high-quality ventilation and filter system. A good system will draw air from outside and filter it to remove radioactive, chemical, and biological materials, ensuring that you breathe clean air.

Electricity is the next most important aspect of survival. You will need to install a generator to provide enough power for your bunker. Determine the number of appliances you will be using, including lights, before selecting your generator to calculate the estimated amount of wattage you will be using. Installing a solar generator in addition to your regular generator is the best option if you have to stay longer than expected and run out of fuel to power your generator.

A clean water supply is one of the most critical aspects of your bunker. You will need to install a bunker-specific water filter, such as a UV filter. The UV light in the filter is powerful enough to kill bacteria and viruses found in water. The waste disposal system comes next. This is a critical component of your bunker because improper waste removal can be hazardous to your health in a closed bunker. Numerous options are available, so you must determine which type best meets your requirements.

You can use a structure similar to an outhouse, a closed room with a toilet, but the waste is disposed of in an underground trench. This option is not the most sanitary, but it is the cheapest and can last long if appropriately built. Another environmentally friendly option is to use a composting facility as a bathroom. It does not require running water, so it conserves water for drinking, cooking, and bathing. It also converts waste into organic fertilizer that you can use in your garden. However, it can be costly and may smell, particularly in an underground bunker.

A PVC pipe can be used to make a poop tube as a temporary solution. When mountain climbers are above ground, they use it as a toilet. However, because this tube is not intended to last, it may not be the best option for a lengthy stay, but it can serve as a backup. The most common option is installing a waste pump system, which uses water like a flushing toilet. The system also includes a lift transporting waste from lower to upper levels.

Nonperishable food such as dehydrated rice, canned foods, and ready-to-eat meals such as those used in the military or on camping trips are also required. You should keep nutritious foods that provide you with the necessary daily calories. Canned beans, fruits and vegetables, dried meats, nuts, peanut butter, dry milk, energy drink powder, grains, and protein bars are everyday items to keep in your bunker. These items must be replaced regularly to ensure that you only have fresh food on hand when the time comes to use the bunker.

Because you have a generator in the bunker, you should keep a heating source, such as a microwave, to cook your food and make it more palatable. Alternative heating tools, such as a small portable stove or the flameless ration heaters commonly found in military MREs, can be included. You don't know how long you'll be in the bunker, so you want to make it as comfortable as possible.

You should also make the interior design as pleasant as possible or risk developing cabin fever. It is caused by being confined in a small space and can leave you feeling irritated, depressed, and unable to concentrate. Keep a few personal photos around the bunker, a portable speaker or a sound system for music, a few dumbbells, and a yoga mat for exercise and meditation.

You should also keep some medicine and a first-aid kit in your bunker, including antibiotics, pain relievers, disinfectants, sterile gauze, and bandages in an emergency. It is also advisable to include any form of entertainment. It may seem insignificant, but having nothing to do all day in an underground bunker can become highly stressful and claustrophobic. Items such as board games, cards, and books should be included.

You can seek help from a professional to help you build and set up the bunker, but now you have the proper knowledge to oversee the entire process.

CHAPTER 4: ARMORY (FIREARMS, OTHER WEAPONS, HAND-TO-HAND FIGHTS)

Humans have used weapons to defend themselves since the dawn of time. Weapons come in various shapes and sizes, some designed to attack and others to defend, but the majority are versatile, and the wielder determines their purpose. For most of us, the mere thought of holding a firearm, let alone injuring someone with it, is terrifying; however, many people would shoot without hesitation. This already occurs; imagine what would happen if a disaster struck and society's common sense no longer prevailed.

You may believe that a baseball bat or other short-range weapon will suffice for defense, but they are unlikely to protect you against a firearm. To be truly prepared, you should obtain a long-distance weapon. You don't have to go out and get a sniper, but a handgun or something more discreet that you can take with you when you go outside to do chores is probably a better option.

Of course, the best type of defense weapon depends on the user. Every gun owner has different preferences; we will go over the various types of guns so you can make an informed decision. But, before we get there, it's essential to discuss the decision of when, if ever, to shoot. This is a tough decision; there are no guidelines on this subject, which entirely depends on the circumstances. However, some pointers may be helpful if the situation arises. First, determine your goal. Avoid pulling the trigger in low-light situations or when under intense stress because the mind can play many tricks in those situations. Always know who or what you're going to shoot at and what's behind the target; you don't want to shoot or hit the wrong person.

Another thing to consider when using a gun is that just because there is no rule of law at the time does not mean you should act lawlessly. Shoot only when necessary, and keep in mind that the law may be restored one day, and authorities may investigate crimes committed during those times of crisis. Finally, if you and your family or group are well and safe at the end of a confrontation, you have most likely made the right decision.

In some places, carrying weapons in open view can be considered illegal, so you need to carry your weapon concealed under regular daily clothes.

List of Recommended Firearms

Shotguns and Rifles

Many believe shotguns are perfect for protecting your home. They have great close-range abilities, and you don't necessarily have to worry about accuracy if you are using a shotgun shell and not a slug. This is because shotshells spread when you shoot, so if your aim is directed at the target, you will hit it.

However, pay attention to the ammunition required. If you are using birdshot ammunition (shotgun ammunition designed to shoot birds), your chances of over-penetrating are lower. Overpenetration is when you shoot a shotgun with a shotgun shell and penetrate through your target, putting other people at risk of getting shot. This is especially important if you use it inside your home, as you don't want to hit anyone in the next room. These guns are relatively cheap, and their ammunition is also cheap and found in many gun stores. Although these are not the lightest firearms, they are pretty easy to use.

More than any other firearm, handguns should be chosen by how they sit on your hand and how comfortable you are with them. This is because the better one sits, the more you will practice with it, and the better you will become at wielding it. So, when purchasing a handgun, you might need to try a few out first to see how they fit in your hand.

Handguns can be divided into two categories: revolvers and semi-automatic. The advantages and disadvantages all depend on the user. A revolver is usually easier to use than a semi-automatic; however, the latter has more rounds, meaning you won't need to reload as many times. Regarding calibers, the most used ones are .45, .40, 9mm, and .357. The less common the caliber of a gun is, the harder it is to find ammunition.

Handguns are the easiest firearms to carry and use, making it more comfortable to carry lots of ammunition. Handguns are usually medium-range and, compared to other types of guns, have less reach. Plus, the further the target is, the greater the chance you will miss. On the other hand, if you want to protect your home from an intruder, a handgun will do just fine.

Rifles are designed for long-distance shooting. If you want to use your firearm for big game hunting, this might be the best option; plus, you can add a scope and turn it into a sniper rifle. With a sniper rifle, you can camp on your home's roof and surveil and defend the land around you. For many, having a .22 rifle is the best choice for survival, mainly because of its versatility. It has cheap ammunition, is easy to handle, and is excellent for hunting. However, many other people say that .22 is too low-powered, but the higher the caliber, the more expensive the ammunition gets, so if you are on a budget, a .22 will do just fine.

These are long-range weapons. They do not allow you to shoot at a close range. This is one of the essential categories for preppers as these are ideal for self-defense and protection. You might not be able to defend yourself with a handgun or a handgun, but you can guarantee safety with any rifle. The only downside to using this kind of weapon is that you have to have a lot of ammunition to protect yourself at all times.

Appropriate models of shotguns and rifles will be listed in the book. Most shotguns are pump action, while most rifles are bolt action or semi-automatic. Some weapons, like the Ruger 10/22, were listed because they are highly recommended for first-time gun owners. Having a weapon that is easy to use will be an advantage if you ever find yourself in an emergency.

Handguns and carbines are the next best type of weapon after the rifle. They are also long-range weapons. Since these are of short stature, it does not allow you to go for long-distance shooting. But unlike the rifle, you can use your handgun to shoot quite close to your opponent. This will enable you to take as many shots as needed to neutralize any threat. You can go for a pistol or carbine in this category, but the carbine is ideal for self-defense.

Automatics and semi-automatic rifles have no limitation on how close you can shoot your target. You do not need to reload your weapon as often as a handgun, but you will still have more ammunition than any other type of rifle. The semi-automatic rifle is considered the best for preppers as it allows for a higher rate of fire, which means you can shoot more than twice a second.

Carbines

Some people mistake carbines for rifles, and they are not wrong. They are, however, very different from more common rifles. Carbines are essentially rifles with shorter barrels. Carbines have a bad reputation because they've been used to commit various atrocities, but one of their advantages is how intimidating they are. Aside from that, their large ammunition capacity is a significant advantage. However, they are expensive compared to other firearms, and their ammunition is equally so.

The AR-15, SKS carbine, and any variant of the AK are the two most popular carbines, primarily because they are reliable and last a long time, which would be useful in a survival situation.

Various handguns and carbines will be listed based on your budget and preferences. Depending on your preferences, you can purchase a weapon in three sizes: small, medium, and large.

Automatics and Semi-Automatic Rifles

Most rifles are listed as Bolt Action or Semi-Automatic. Buyers should consider their preferences when shopping for the ideal weapons model in this category. Those who prefer bolt action will have more options, but those who prefer semi-automatic rifles would have the advantage of shooting twice a second.

- **Accessories:** Buyers should consider buying some accessories for their firearms, such as magazine adapters, flashlights, scopes, and some basic tools that can come in handy during an emergency.
- **Ammunition**: Buyers should consider as many calibers as possible because ammo is an important factor in a firearm. The 9 mm, .223, and .308 are three of the most common calibers recommended for preppers.

List of Manufacturers

- **Smith & Wesson:** This company is well-known for producing high-quality firearms such as revolvers and rifles. They've been around since 1857 and have some of the most popular models for preppers. They have a large selection of revolvers and rifles, including the M&P15 and M&P15C, listed here with technical specifications. This is a good option for anyone looking for a dependable, simple weapon to use and maintain.
- **Ruger:** This company has been in operation since 1848, making it one of the oldest that is still in operation today. Ruger became a subsidiary of Colt after Colt purchased it in 1999. This company produces several rifle models, which are detailed in this book. It is an excellent choice for anyone looking for a high-quality weapon at a reasonable price.

Which Gun Should You Buy?

I recommend that you have a variety of guns at home, ranging from the most basic to some of the most powerful calibers.

These are some examples, and I'll give you some pointers for each:

- Although it is questioned, a.22 caliber rifle should not be underestimated. It is a potentially lethal weapon.
- A shotgun is excellent; it makes a stunning sound, and any enemy who is a little cowardly will flee because no one wants a shotgun hole in the chest.
- A Winchester .300 rifle is designed for defense but can also be used for hunting.
- Have revolvers such as the classic 9mm, .40, and .45; they are expensive but well worth it.
- Assault rifles, such as the AR-15, AK 47, Ruger mini-14, and others, are also essential because you will not be the only one armed in a war.
- You can never have enough ammunition; the 22 has about ten thousand cartridges; the shotgun has about a hundred cartridges; the firearms have about 1000 bullets; and so on.

Make sure to have cleaning kits and holsters for all of your firearms. You can even have reloading kits for you to prepare your bullets. You never know how long this chaos will last.

List of Calibers: 9 mm, .223, .308

- **Shotguns and Rifles:** These are not to be used for close-range shooting. They are ideal for hunting purposes and long-range shooting. Buyers should consider these elements before buying a shotgun or rifle to purchase the right one for them within their budget.
- **Handguns and Carbines:** Buyers should consider the caliber of their weapon because it will determine how far they can shoot a target. The 9 mm, .223, and .308 calibers are some of the most commonly used calibers in handguns and carbines.
- **Automatics and Semi-Automatic Rifles:** These are long-range weapons with no limitation to how close you can shoot your opponent. Therefore, buyers need to consider the different caliber options available to them. The .223, .30, and 9 mm are some of this category's most commonly used calibers.

Other Weaponry

Non-firearm weapons won't have a chance against firearms. However, they can come in handy as tools. Regarding knives, you should look for a blade of around 5 to 6 inches lengthwise and a full tang blade. This means that the knife's blade runs through the handle, giving it more stability. The thickness of the blade is also important. The thicker the blade, the fewer chances of it breaking.

A knife or a blade can be ideal for self-defense because it is portable and safe if used properly. The preferred way in self-defense is to be used as a last option because of its high risk. Don't ever use a knife to defend yourself against an intruder unless necessary or you are not sure what will happen next. Many incidents have occurred because of knife attacks, and many people have lost their lives in such attacks. Using a blade during stress creates an imbalance that can cause serious injuries or even loss of life.

When it comes to the handle, look for something with a good grip, even when wet. You will also need a sheath for the knife, especially if you want to carry it around. For this, a simple leather sheath might be sufficient. Make sure it is comfortable when walking around and doing chores. When purchasing knives, it all comes down to how comfortable it is in your hand, but two of the most purchased knives for survivalists are the CSP by Mission Knives and BOB by TOPS Knives. You might want to research and weigh all the available options.

CHAPTER 5: OTHER TYPES OF DEFENSE AND TIPS (GUARD DOGS, COMMUNICATIONS, MUTUAL AID AGREEMENTS, CHILDREN AND SECURITY)

Watch Dogs

A barking dog may be a good alarm for you and your family. It'll help you be aware and keep you safe from dangers since many burglaries occur when the house residents are present.

It is also a fantastic deterrent, and even something as easy as placing a sign that says "Beware of Dog" will make potential burglars think twice about choosing one house as their next target.

This is a simple home security hack that many people take already. There's a good reason: a dog is a much more effective home defensive measure than you're probably willing to give it credit for.

First and foremost, if you get a dog, it's probably to give your family a companion you can love and cherish. Purchasing a dog to serve as a guard dog is probably a secondary reason to own one for you.

The mere presence of a dog or the sound of one barking is sufficient to send many criminals out of your house or even out of your property in the first place.

In addition, a larger dog, such as a German Shepherd, could defend you by keeping you safe from an intruder once they've entered your home or general premises.

But by far, the biggest reason to have a guard dog is that they are simply one of the best alarm systems available. When a dog senses danger, it will bark loudly and rush to the danger site. You can then grab your home defense firearm, send your family to the panic room, call 911, and rush to investigate.

Having at least two guard dogs will be even better than one. Yes, it's more mouths to feed, but it will be more intimidating to intruders.

Finally, while a larger dog will always be better for home defense, if you have small dogs, they will at least be able to alert you to danger. Smaller dogs tend to be more alert than larger ones, and the very sound of them barking may be enough to send an intruder scurrying as well.

Having one or more dogs is a great way to keep yourself safe in the wilderness, especially if you choose large canine companions. A dog's senses are far sharper than a person's, so your dog may alert you to danger before you detect it yourself. A dog is also a great deterrent against people and many other animals, and dogs are fiercely protective of their owners. They will alert you to someone approaching your home or danger out in the brush, and they are powerful fighters.

Many people operating off the grid choose to take a dog or several dogs with them for safety. A dog may also be able to assist you in:

- Detecting intruders
- Frightening intruders
- Avoiding nearby animals
- Hunting and finding food
- Alerting you to nearby danger
- Fighting off animals/intruders in extreme circumstances

Some people also use "Beware of Dog" signs even if they don't have a dog – while this won't be effective against everyone, it may be enough to encourage intruders to pause or choose another location.

Of course, having dogs brings additional responsibilities and advantages; you must feed, care for, and protect your animals just as they protect you. You will need a reliable source of food and water for them, the ability to keep them warm, and the ability to keep them safe. You must make sure you control the dog when something unexpected happens so it doesn't attack something dangerous and get hurt or escalate a situation you might otherwise be able to walk away from. Teach your dog to recall to get it away from other animals, or it may prove a liability than an asset.

The nature of watchdogs is to bark loudly and alert the family about the intruders entering their house. But they will mostly not attack them, as they are not strongly trained to harm humans! On the other hand, guard dogs have a protective instinct toward their families and loved ones. Therefore, when they sense an invasion in the house, they might bite and do everything possible to the intruders to defend their owners and family members. When properly trained, some watchdogs can also be turned into guard dogs! Technically people consider both guard dogs and watchdogs as the same!

If you prefer to get warned or are seeking home defense from intruders or danger around the home, here are some of the best watchdog or guard dog breeds that you can prefer to get:

- Bullmastiff
- Rottweiler
- Doberman Pinscher
- Komondor
- Giant Schnauzer
- Puli
- German Shephard
- Rhodesian Ridgeback
- Belgian Sheepdog
- Weimaraner
- Airedale Terrier
- Tibetan Mastiff
- Akita
- American Staffordshire Terrier
- Beauceron
- Belgian Malinois

These are just a few guard dog breeds you can prefer to get for your home defense. But remember that, depending upon your house's location and society, getting all the breed options on hand becomes challenging. Therefore, you get to choose just from the available options. It is because not all dogs can be bred in all climatic conditions. Therefore, some breeds prefer to live in cold regions for which location-wise breeding is approached. This won't be a problem because there are proficient guard dogs for almost all regions and climatic conditions.

Lighting Systems

Motion-activated external lights are ideal for home defense as early warning devices. They can warn you of potential intruders and scare crooks passing by by robbing them of their most powerful weapon: hiding. When the refrigerator light turns on, most bad guys, such as cockroaches, will flee. Whatever lights you have should be aimed at removing potential hiding spots caused by dark areas just outside the light overflow. This can be accomplished by layering different lights or keeping the light close to the home's façade, making it impossible for evildoers to hide.

Installing lighting systems will be just as effective as installing cameras. Burglars and intruders will do everything possible to avoid detection while attempting to enter your home, but lights will ensure they cannot do so.

You can also install lights both inside and outside your home. Motion sensor lighting systems are ideal for use outside, such as at entrances, patios, garages, and front lawns. Solar-powered lighting, in particular, will be the most affordable option.

Use a light timer such as the kind you use during Christmas for indoor lighting, and keep it connected to your lamp. This will also create the illusion that you are home.

Cameras

Having cameras on your property will greatly reduce the chances of a break-in. The good news is that home security cameras, such as CCTV, are cheaper and more available than ever before.

Why are cameras helpful at reducing a break-in? The answer is that a burglar simply does not want to get caught. They may not want to take the risk even if they suspect your cameras are fake.

Another advantage to CCTV cameras is how high quality they are. They'll produce more than just blurry images, and police may be able to identify the burglar if the camera catches them.

Landscaping

By making your home appear looted, no one will think that it holds anything precious, and raiders may be enticed to go on to the next property in search of more valuable items. However, for this to work, your house must seem trashed.

A lawn with tall grass is a clear indicator to a burglar that either your home is possibly unoccupied or you aren't taking the defense of your home very seriously.

Besides, you shouldn't have tall grass on your lawn anyway… It looks bad.

If you're planning to go away on a long trip or vacation, you can hire a teenager in your neighborhood to help keep your lawn cut. It will do more than you think to make a burglar think twice about intruding.

Remove any trash you find in the yard. Place black tarps or trash bags over your windows to give the impression that the house is dark. Graffiti can be spray painted on the outside of your home. To fulfill your obligation, you may demolish elements of your home (such as the railing) if you feel compelled to do so.

Trim the bushes and trees around the property so intruders cannot use them as cover while attempting to enter the house. When a yard is left unattended, it communicates to potential intruders that the occupants are away. Planting prickly shrubs near the casement helps deter potential trespassers. Consider a barrier as an extra layer of security for your home. When thieves plan their escape, they have an additional obstacle to consider in the form of the fence. Cement bases can add stability, and it is preferable to use chain links or open metal rather than strong or rigid walls because solid walls can make it easier to get a footing and provide another area to hide.

Protect Your Garage

Anyone can enter your house through the garage, like a big door where you put the car. So, my advice is that in case of catastrophes, if you are not going to use it, you should place a well-secured door on the inside. You can also place some items to block the door. The plan is to keep burglars from breaking in.

Most people serious about home security recognize the need to fortify their doors and windows, but far fewer recognize they also need to fortify their garage.

In reality, numerous homes have been broken into because the intruders went through the garage rather than the doors or windows. You do not want to make the same mistake of leaving your garage vulnerable. Don't overlook it.

Remember that burglars may purposefully go for your garage rather than the rest of your home because they know that most garages contain valuable items, such as tools, important financial documents, and your car. And if they decide to get into the rest of your home, they'll have a clear point of access anyway.

There are several steps you can take to ensure that your garage remains protected, including:

- Replace your current garage door with a heavy-duty door
- Replace the door leading from your garage into your home with a steel door and heavy-duty locks
- Keep any particularly valuable possessions out of the garage and other belongings in it hidden
- Have a motion sensor light installed
- Have security cameras installed (even fake cameras will be better than nothing)
- Never leave your keys or any other valuable possessions in your vehicle

Keep aside the concern for protecting your vehicle from getting stolen or your random storeroom items getting vandalized. Your garage can give direct and easy access to your home. Today, most houses are constructed with an internal doorway connected with their garages. It is to give ease of entering and exiting the garage space! Therefore, if you miss out on securing the garage, you might not just compromise the contents stored in it but will eventually give easy access to your main home.

Therefore, garage defense and security planning are essential for preppers to work with all-around home defense. To ensure the garage's security, you can adapt preventative measures based on the budget and preference. You can plan on installing security cameras, motion sensor lights, alarm locks, and others. The motioned lights are accountable for being the best version of security for your garage. Make sure you connect one of the motion lights on the other side of the garage door within your residing home. Connect those lights parallel so that if the garage light turns on due to motion, the light within the house will also glow.

Hence, it will give you an indication that someone is trying to get into the house through the garage or is trying to steal your car or stored items. You can take proper action at the moment and call the police. Until the police arrive, you can rush to your safe room and wait till the help arrives. On the other hand, the alarm locks will raise a loud alert right from the time when someone tries to compromise the garage door from outside or inside. CCTV cameras should be a common security aspect to record the activities of intruders around your garage space.

Always Make It Seem Like Someone is Home

Will a burglar break into a home they know or have good reason to believe someone is inside? Very possibly, but the chances of them doing so are quite low.

The overwhelming majority of home break-ins happen when a person is not home, such as during the daytime when they figure the parents are at work and the children are in school.

Therefore, when you leave home each day, make it a habit to seem like someone is home. Examples of what you can do include keeping the radio and TV on or always having the lights on.

Use Warning Signs

The faster you detect an intruder, the greater your chances of neutralizing the threat or reacting effectively. Alarm systems are, therefore, extremely important. They could be as simple as a system of strings linked to bells or tin cans containing pebbles. Once the intruder touches one of the strings, it will make a sound and alert you.

You can opt for something less primitive and get battery-powered alarms like motion sensors. However, make sure you have enough batteries to use them through long periods in a survival situation, at least a few months' worth of batteries. If you do use battery-powered motion sensors, do your research, and find out the best locations for them around your perimeter.

You've likely driven by homes or properties before with signs outside such as "KEEP OUT!" or "BEWARE OF GUARD DOG!"

There's a good reason you commonly see these signs; they are effective at keeping burglars (particularly less experienced ones) at bay. The reason is that it tells them that you are someone who is taking the defense of your property and home very seriously.

If you're still not convinced that setting up warning signs is effective, just know that it is believed warning signs reduce the chances of having your home broken into by over fifty percent.

Situational Awareness

Being aware of your surroundings is crucial for staying safe off the grid. You should always be alert to what's happening in your local vicinity and whether it presents any dangers to you or others.

You should practice being aware of your situation whenever you have an opportunity, particularly in a new area with potential unknown threats. For example, if you are somewhere where you might run into dangerous animals, you should be careful and look for signs of what you might be dealing with.

Things like animal tracks, droppings, and damage to the local environment should help you establish what is likely to be in the local area. You might also pick up scents for certain creatures. If other people are in the area, you might find evidence of fires, dwellings, or debris (e.g., litter).

Developing situational awareness isn't easy, but you can do a few simple things to make a start, such as not listening to music while you are out and about and changing up your routine regularly so that you don't operate on autopilot.

Some people say that situational awareness involves perception, comprehension, and projection. Below is an example:

You are walking in a new area. You use your perception to assess the local environment and notice a pile of feathers under a bush. Your comprehension of the situation tells you that a predator must be nearby but that the bird was small and the only predators in this area hunt at night. You project that it is safe to keep walking, but you look for signs of fresh tracks and make sure that you have a weapon to hand.

Situational awareness is about taking in information, assessing the information, and acting accordingly. It could save your life if you make this your standard operating mode.

You should also work on this as a team effort, ensuring you involve others in your group. Practice identifying common threat signs and discussing how you would resolve the dangers that could arise from them. This group exercise is a great way to improve collective and individual awareness.

Too many people are burying their faces in their mobile phones and becoming completely unaware of their surroundings. This is the exact opposite of what you want in a survival situation. You want to know exactly when and from where someone might be approaching your home. You want to be hyper-aware of everything in your surroundings.

If any stranger tries to approach your perimeter, they shouldn't be left unchallenged, but you don't want to start shooting straight away. Use diplomacy and ask questions before you take further action. Another thing that you should be aware of, especially if someone approaches your home, is that they may be a diversion. In other words, they may be distracting you from someone else approaching your perimeter from another location. Ideally, you would have enough people in your group to rotate surveillance so that you are always aware of the goings on your perimeter.

You should consider getting a dog if you don't have enough people in your group to take shifts and rotate. Besides being great companions, a well-trained dog can do the job of several people when it comes to detecting intruders.

Alarms

When prepping for an emergency, alarms should be on your list. Alarms are used to alert you of any unwanted entry into your home, but they're also best used as a deterrent to said unwanted entry.

When it comes to alarms, you'll want to use two types: the audible and the automatic.

The audible alarm is a device that makes noise (typically with a siren) to alert you of intruders or other dangers. In most cases, you'll hear the siren go off before the intruder has managed to enter your house, but if they do manage to break in, an audible alarm will tell them that someone's home and might scare them off before things get more dangerous.

The automatic alarm is very similar, except instead of simply letting the intruder know that someone is home, it'll send a warning that something's wrong if the alarm goes off. This can be helpful for individuals who are elderly or otherwise disabled and don't have the means of communicating their presence to others.

Regarding where you should place your alarms, this depends on what needs to be protected, as discussed before, regarding your shelter/shelter. Suppose you're prepping for natural disasters or other situations where you need multiple shelters. In that case, alarms are usually best placed near your doorways so that they'll detect anyone attempting to enter simultaneously. If you're prepping for an invasion, alarms are best placed outside near your doors and windows to detect an intruder before they get too far.

Alarms don't have to be expensive, but they can still become a hassle if you don't know where to start.

Professionally installed house alarm systems are an excellent investment for protection and peacefulness since they may warn neighbors about a particular danger long before the cops arrive.

It would be pretty beneficial to speak with the neighbors about this subject in advance, for instance, to arrange mutual aid in the neighborhood and alarm system.

The alarm system should act immediately if an entrance or window is opened or two wrong password hashes are entered. An alarm is designed to wake you up and warn you somebody is entering the house. Secondly, they should frighten and scare off unwanted visitors by letting them know they are no longer imperceptible.

Chemical/Nuclear Defense Systems

There are many things that a person might need to worry about in times of emergency. One thing that comes to mind is defending oneself from other people. The saying goes, "a gun will only stop one bullet." Therefore, many different levels of defense systems can help with this problem and make a person feel safe when caught in the middle of something.

Chemical weapons include powerful gases such as mustard gas and physical objects like tear gas or mace (though these are typically found in non-lethal form). The same applies to chemical plants, bomb shelters, and various chemicals used for various time-sensitive functions.

Filtration systems can be beneficial when a shelter is created, and the priority is finding a water source. One of the most important reasons these filters are so handy is that they can be used as storage units for other items, such as water containers. The result is that fewer things are placed in the same space or volume used by these chemicals, and there is less risk of accidental poisoning.

Radiography can detect incoming radiation sources to prevent them from getting into shelters by accident. On the other hand, nuclear bombs and nuclear plants include radiation from the sun and radioactive substances such as plutonium or uranium. Then there is the very real threat of radiation poisoning.

To protect oneself from nuclear bombs, radiation, and accidental chemical spills, defensive systems include shielding buildings, non-lethal weapons such as rubber bullets and pepper spray, and anti-radiation devices.

Once again, many different types of systems can be used for this purpose, as well as various levels of protection. Tear gas cartridges have been designed to keep bombers out for 10 minutes without harming anyone inside a building or a car. Chemical bombs contain poison gas or fire-retardant chemicals that can keep someone out of a building for up to 40 minutes without causing damage. Pepper sprays are designed to disable attackers with irritating effects lasting around 30 seconds.

Several chemical defenses can be used in varied ways depending on the situation. The most important products are designed to get into someone's eyes, nose, or lungs. Most even have antidotes, making them useful as defense systems and first aid kits.

Anyone with a mask can use aerosol chemical spray to spray at a moving car or animal, thus keeping them from attacking the driver or traveler. They work like most other sprays but with a different effect. Depending on how high the concentration is sprayed, they'll cause temporary eye and respiratory irritation, making it hard for attackers to see what they're doing and even more difficult for them to breathe in harmful substances. One of the downsides is that they can also be sprayed to attack a car or person in defense and get into their mouths and eyes.

Chemical Foam is similar in that it's designed to use in confined spaces such as a car or tunnel. The main difference is that it forms an opaque blockage that can trap attackers inside the building or tunnel without allowing them to see who they're attacking. This can make fighting with them more difficult for both sides. Another difference is that it's more like foam than a spray, so it won't spread as much as a spray and has more stable properties for spraying at moving vehicles.

One of the most obvious defensive products is chemical relief masks and goggles. The masks are available to fit over glasses or goggles that are worn under a respirator if needed. They're designed to work by taking in less air through the nose and then releasing an amount of any of several chemicals that need to be inhaled at certain times when they're activated. If a person is attacked with a chemical in the air, their eyes will burn, their throats will be irritated, and their lungs will feel as if they've been crushed by concrete.

An eyewash or acid wash kit works similarly but uses sodium hydroxide and other materials. A special solution is sprayed into the eyes and then washed with a special cloth. This causes a painful burn to anyone who touches them, making them less effective as weapons. On the plus side, they can be used over and over again without requiring a special solution to be made, unlike many face masks.

Several chemical bomb suits protect people from gas and radioactive material. The first is more like a blanket than an actual bodysuit. It covers the body but isn't tight. It's designed to keep attackers at bay and also prevent them from harming you if you're in their way when they're shooting explosives or grenades at you. Since most of the damage from these attacks comes from debris, it's not as helpful in blocking radiation but can still help against fire and shrapnel.

The second type of suit is like a full-body cloak covering every body part. It's a lot more useful for long-term use. It doesn't protect from attack but could be worn under most types of clothing to shield radioactive material when escaping through nuclear zones or cleaning up after a nuclear accident. It's also very useful in dealing with diseases such as AIDS and SARS that spread through direct contact with bodily fluids since it will keep anything released inside the suit from getting out.

Chemical defense gear such as masks and suits can be used to prevent the spread of germs, and nuclear bomb suits can be used to keep you from being killed from the shockwaves of an attack. They can even protect you from fire, heat, and smoke for a short time. Other measures include having special vehicles that can either burrow through the ground or fly over the top of buildings to protect you from most attacks unless your enemy is particularly determined.

Another form of protection against nuclear attacks is time travel, which involves sending people to the future when they're in danger. This can be used for protection from bombs as well as other emergencies. The main idea is that people will hide in specially built bunkers until it's safe to come out again, which could occur months or years later. One way to survive the waiting period is to use hibernation chambers similar to those used for medical treatments and space travel, allowing people to sleep safely until the danger has passed.

Pack for Trips Unseen

Always pack your belongings for a trip or vacation out of sight. This indicates that you are leaving home to any potential burglar who is sneakily watching your neighborhood.

So, for example, if you're planning an outdoor trip, load up your bikes and coolers inside your garage rather than outside in your driveway. When packing your clothes, pack them inside a room where someone won't be able to peer through the window. You get the idea: you don't want burglars to know you are planning to leave.

It is not a good idea to announce your vacation plans over social media or spread the word around the entire neighborhood. If you are keen to plan security for your home and ensure that your valuables and property remain safe from home invasions without violence, then you need to act smart in certain situations. Most people add social media updates to any international vacation plans. Not just that, but they also mention the days they will be out from home, with the specific dates.

Social media is now easily accessible to genuine individuals, intruders, and potential burglars. You never know who might have sneaked into your profile to stalk your information. When you make your vacation plan public, they will start planning to enter your house and steal all your valuables without anyone interrupting them. And you would be on vacation, while the thieves would do their job finely without raising any kind of alert.

When the intruders know that you won't be at home with your family, they will take ample time to break through your security measures, such as CCTV, alarmed locks, and others. It will be very risky to defend your home from a vacation trip! Therefore, it is advised that you keep your vacation plans private and set up the house so that it feels like someone is living in it at all times. When you leave for the vacation, you should count on turning on the living room lights and a couple more lights. Keep the exterior lights turned on throughout the day and night.

Don't leave the house darkened at any corner of the property when you are not available on the spot. Let the intruders feel frightened upon even wandering around your property. But first, you need to understand the necessity of separating the topics that should or should not be shared publicly.

Asking for Help from the Neighbors

If you do not have any security measures implemented on your property, this planning measure would be the first. But let's consider that you have at least implemented a few of the above plans to ensure complete prepping of your home with defense systems and practices in hand. In that case, you might not have to ask for help from neighbors on priority, as they might say yes or no to take the risk!

The maximum help that a neighbor can do is inform the police on your behalf when you cannot make noise amidst the intruders from your safe room. Drop a text to them, and they will do the needful. If a group of people can come together from the neighborhood to counteract the measures of intruders, then you can get hold of the situation even before the police arrive. But not all neighbors are that courageous to take on the first approach to catch hold of the intruders if they have weapons in hand.

Therefore, the safest move is not to risk anyone's life and simply ask help to contact the police immediately or go to the station and bring them to the spot. This is the maximum help that you should seek from your neighbors.

Even though some crisis events are unpredictable, the impact is always known. For instance, the burglar's approach toward a house invasion is always predictable and known. They intend to get the family members hostage or asleep with toxic fumes to do their job. Therefore, the defense properties are important for adaption, for which you need proper security planning. All the points stated above are ideal for you to consider in your security plans and take measures upon executing them in a planned manner.

When you are done with your planning and execution, you can then move ahead to realize the other security essentials for a complete home defense prepping approach. So, make sure you follow this book till the end!

Security guards are stationed where criminals are most likely to infiltrate the community. Remember that some gangsters are cunning and may even have combat training; think about regularly having the patrols double back to the neighborhood perimeter. Finally, protecting your house against looters and criminals during social instability does not have to be expensive. A good home security system is more about concealing the defenses than your strategies.

Traps

Set booby traps within and around your home to give undesirable visitors a surprise they will never forget.

You can construct various things to prepare for SHTF, ranging from mild to lethal.

On the other hand, the fatal ones don't just look intimidating; they also execute their job... Too well. We don't endorse them since you're more likely to get into problems with the authorities for setting them up than you experience Armageddon.

Instead, try one of the booby traps listed below. They're almost innocuous, but they still can stun the bad guys. These traps will either make them flee or keep them occupied while you carry out the following step in your home security plan:

- Perimeter alarms
- Tripwires
- Corn flour explosive
- Pit traps

Fortifying Your Home

You should not only focus on strengthening your arsenal of weapons but also on fortifying your home. You can do many things to fortify your house without turning it into a bunker.

The first thing that you need to do is identify any weak points your house may have. The weak areas of your home are usually doors and windows, so you should look at options to increase their strength. When it comes to doors, there are two immediate things that you can do. Replace the screws on the hinges of your outside doors for longer ones. Normal screws are only to secure the door; by changing to longer screws, you are allowing the screw to get inside the door frame and make it more resistant to forced entries. Adding deadbolts to your doors will also increase their resistance.

Boarding your doors and windows can also increase their strength, although this is probably only a good solution for the doors and windows you do not use. Purchasing a couple of 2x6 boards and screwing them against any unused exterior door frames can increase security. You can also do this to your main door frames when you need to barricade yourself inside the house.

Windows can be a real problem, mainly because they are made of glass that can easily break. Boarding them is the best solution, even though it will block the sun. You can get a measured plywood board and attach it to the window frame with long screws. Add the plywood to the inside of the window, not the outside, because if a window gets broken, the glass will fall outside your house.

Go to your local gardening shop, purchase a few bags of sand, and place them around the house, for example, in front of your upper windows, to allow a temporary firing position. Sandbags can be highly resistant to bullets.

Don't waste time getting into devices such as large traps, dead drops, punji pits, etc., to trap people. These are very trying and time-consuming, and most don't work, so they are not cost-effective. And pulling out dead animals all the time can be distressing.

Yes, they are used in guerrilla warfare, but only because the groups are poor and have scarce resources; there is nothing else they can do. A good scout will find them easier than firing wired grenades. I recommend forgetting these primitive stick and stone methods when there are great alternative options.

First and foremost, and probably the cheapest, is a passive boundary far enough from your main compound/shelter that it is too far to fire or throw incendiary bombs easily, usually more than fifty meters, ideally around a hundred meters, with anti-intrusion alarms and obstacles.

Then add convoluted footings and strategic counter-defense areas that can be upgraded under challenging scenarios, with more effective counter-attack teams that you can create with legitimate supplies at home.

Another effective strategy is to increase the number of obstacles thrown in your adversary's path. The enemy's ability to progress and their morale will be hampered. It makes accomplishing their assault more difficult while making your defense more effective. Difficulties such as barbed wire fences and nail boards are two excellent examples of the kind of obstacles described before.

However, you may also be creative with the other sorts of barriers that you can build up, such as the following:

- Tripwire
- Obstacles and snares (make a hole, plant stakes in it, and cover it with foliage or tarp)
- Planting thorny bushes, stake trapping… Your imagination is the only limit!

CONCLUSION

Thank you for reading this book. In most cases, you can't precisely summon the police to your off-grid home, so that home defense will be up to you. Whether your intruders are humans or animals, you must be prepared with weapons and a defense strategy.

It is critical to prepare your home to defend it against potential threats. Everything changes when a disaster occurs. The normalcy we are familiar with vanishes; pharmacies, supermarkets, doctors, water, and everything else become valuable to those in need. Those who cannot access them will challenge you for supplies.

A firearm is generally a good idea for off-grid security if you are trained and have a license, even if you only intend to use it against animals. Consider bear spray, loud alarms, and bright lights to frighten off beasts. Not everyone can own or operate a gun, but whether you can or cannot, you should have some other weapons. A knife is an essential tool for many types of off-grid survival, and it will come in handy in home defense. A knife allows you to deal with an attacker less lethally, making it a good choice if you don't want to kill, but it may not be as effective against animals. A strong metal rod can also be helpful for self-defense and may have other applications around your off-grid home.

Consider other things that will make your home safer and less appealing to approaching humans or animals. Motion-activated lights, for example, are a significant deterrent because they alert the occupants to the intruder and startle animals. Humans are more likely to flee if they believe they will be discovered.

You should inspect your home's entry points for flaws that could lead to an attack. If possible, windows should be made of toughened glass or have retractable shutters, and doors should be reinforced. The strength of your structure will be determined by the materials used, but at the very least, ensure that all entry points, including windows, can be closed and locked. Even a weak lock is preferable to no lock.

If you have access to power, a good alarm system is also a plus, though you can build a makeshift alarm system by hanging things like cans and wind chimes in common walkways. These will be discussed further in the section on early warning systems.

Always begin your home defense planning by considering what intruders you might face and how they might approach you. Prepare not only for humans but also for the animals you may encounter. You may attract animals, including bears, if you keep food in your off-grid home. You should have a warning system and a strategy to deal with as many different scenarios as possible.

Good luck.

SURVIVAL ITEMS TO STOCKPILE FOR PREPPERS

50+ Essential Items Every Prepper Should Hoard Before the Collapse

Tyler Gordon

INTRODUCTION

Preparing for an emergency will allow you to manage your resources more strategically to ensure long-term survival in your community. Each of us should prepare for a year or more without outside help. This includes stockpiling essential everyday items, some less common supplies, and developing skills to put these items to use when times are tough.

There are numerous factors to consider. Some of these are more practical, but they should all be considered. The best preparedness plan is tailored to your specific needs and circumstances. Preparedness is a reaction to concerns about future adverse events, both natural and man-made, that may jeopardize well-being.

This informative guide is critical because it outlines simple steps to take in an emergency. Disaster strikes unexpectedly, but you shouldn't be too concerned when you have all the right information. All disasters may occur anytime, so you should be prepared for such an event. This beginners' guide to risk preparation and management provides you with basic survival tips that you can use during a natural disaster.

Maintaining the proper frame of mind is one of the most challenging aspects of dealing with a crisis. It will be much easier for you to deal with this procedure if you understand what needs to be done and recognize that fundamental stages must be completed. You are far less likely to find yourself in a difficult situation if you have a disaster preparation strategy. Remember that disasters can strike without warning and when you least expect it. Put another way, always hope for the best while bracing for the worst.

Whether your goal is to become more self-sufficient or weather a major disaster, both require preparation. To be well-prepared, you must learn everything you can about what will occur.

This survival gear list does not attempt to provide information on obtaining these items and does not recommend them to those looking to improve their survival skills. On the other hand, this list provides some general guidelines on where people should focus their efforts if they want to acquire these skills through training courses and books explicitly geared toward preppers.

This handbook is unique in that it has been meticulously compiled to include all the details about emergencies you should be aware of. It outlines various measures that can prepare you for any situation that may arise during a crisis. The workbook is simple to follow and ideal for those new to emergency preparedness.

Some have viewed the prepping movement as a means of preparing for the apocalypse and thus ensuring your and your family's survival. This is an extreme viewpoint, and it is unlikely that everyone who prepares is hoping for a lunar landing. Some people simply try to expand their skillset; others want to be more self-sufficient or make money from home. Let's get started.

CHAPTER 1: SURVIVAL STRATEGIES

You'll need several different survival strategies. This is the foundation of planning. You can't expect to get anywhere promptly if you don't have a road map. Your plans will tell you the following:

- How to get out of a burning house.
- How to perform a house safety check to protect yourself from everyday disasters.

Survival Strategies You and Your Family Should Know About

How do you decide what to do when there is a major disaster and your family is dispersed across the country? Where will you be meeting? What emergency contacts should you have on your phone?

To ensure your safety and those of the people you love, here's a list of things you should discuss during your monthly family meeting.

Water

Experts say you can't go more than three days without water, but many households use hundreds of gallons daily. You can't keep that much water indefinitely, so you'll need a water strategy. What should you save, and how much should you save? Yes, you should drink; yes, you should cook; no, you should not bathe as frequently as you believe.

A good rule of thumb is one gallon per person per day. There will be no extra if that is your plan! There are simple ways to gradually improve your water storage and have methods to store and purify your water on hand. Start thinking about water storage today.

Food

You can go for weeks without eating, but it will be unpleasant. Your food planning should include what you'll pack in your 72-hour bag if you have to leave out and what type of food you'll need on hand if you stay in without power.

A solid food storage strategy is considered a safe, self-sufficient, and cost-effective living.

Hygiene and Sanitation

You've completed your meal, you have your water, but now everyone is sick with the flu because you failed to prepare for sanitation and hygiene. It may not be pleasant to discuss, but it must be done!

Following a major earthquake, people in Christchurch, New Zealand, constructed dual bucket toilet systems. Perhaps it will work for your family as well. You'll also need antibacterial wipes and a way to keep surfaces clean without wasting water.

Communication

Have you ever been in a situation where you needed to contact your family to ensure they were safe? It's reassuring to know that you can communicate in an emergency. Large wind storms are common in the Pacific Northwest, and landslides and floods frequently accompany them. Mobile phones may not always work in an emergency due to overloaded lines.

In the event of an emergency, how do you intend to communicate? Long-distance calls frequently work, whereas local calls do not. Is there anyone in your family living out of state you can contact to let you know they're safe? Texting, Twitter, and Humanitarian Aid Apps that can post a message on the Facebook page are all possibilities.

Energy

If you have a camping family, you may have been practicing this all summer. Perhaps you live in a city apartment with few opportunities to rough it. Questions about energy requirements will include how you cook without electricity, stay warm, and whether you have a safe way to see in the dark.

You'll also need to understand how to safely store gasoline in an emergency.

Medical

It's natural to keep a basic first-aid kit in your home. You keep inexpensive dollar store bandages for the kids to "play with" while saving the more expensive ones for emergencies. Making a basic dollar store first aid kit, an advanced first aid kit, a suture kit, and a stockpile of splints, bandages, and medicines could be part of your medical supplies preparation.

It will also include information on how to apply stitches, CPR training, and basic first-aid skills. You can also add various herbal medicines on top of that.

Security

Only you can decide if firearms are appropriate for your family. If they are, ensure you have the necessary skills to stay safe. You must also learn how to disguise yourself and your supplies, as well as how to barricade your home.

Are you debt-free (or on your way there)? Do you have emergency savings and follow a budget? When you are financially prepared, you can relax. Being financially secure is vital to your family!

Spiritual and Mental Fortitude

Perhaps you are spiritual, or maybe you are not. But that's not the point. You will need all your spiritual and mental strength when things get tough!

You must have the personal confidence to adequately prepare to be safe and psychologically manage any difficulty that arises. Survivors do that, so go into survival mode and don't let anything stop you. Take expert advice on psychologically preparing for a big game, which also pertains to disaster preparation.

Prepare Your Family for When Disaster Strikes

Families need to have contingency plans. If children are involved, it is easier for them to know how to act and calm down.

1. Work together to find evacuation routes and meeting points for all household residents.
2. Find out which objects may be dangerous to drop in a disaster.

3. Find the safest place in your home to know where everyone will be in the event of an earthquake. Try to practice the drill at least once (this will help the whole family get a good idea of contingency planning).
4. Tell children, especially the young ones, the best place to be in case of an earthquake and explain that they will always have parental support.

It would help if you taught them to stay safe, know how to open food, and canned food, preserve, make good use of water, make the most of the bunker and even teach the older ones about first aid. In a catastrophe, they could heal themselves or you.

Bugging out

However, there are times when you must face danger because it is the only way out. For example, if the fire you want to escape occurs on the second floor and the only way to escape it is by jumping out a window, you must, unfortunately, risk your life to avoid being burned to death.

It's about weighing your options and deciding what's best for you.

The Bug Out Bag (B.O.B.), also known as the Go-To Bag, is a survival kit designed to keep you alive for at least three days. A bug-out bag is not intended for long-term survival but rather as an emergency bag if you need to flee quickly.

If a natural disaster, a chemical leak, or a terrorist assault threatens your home, you should be prepared to gather your bug-out bag and flee to safer ground as soon as possible. While bugging in at home is generally a safer approach than bugging out to unfamiliar locations, being prepared for any eventuality is a part of prepping. As a result, you should start your prepper life by assembling a bug-out pack to prepare for a home evacuation if necessary.

The idea of bug-out packs is trendy among survivalists. The size of the bag, the material it's made of, what it's designed for, and what you put inside it are all critical considerations.

What Bug-Out Bag You Should Get

Here are the steps you should take when selecting the best bug-out bag for you.

Support

After you've decided on the size of your bug-out bag, you'll need to determine the type of frame it will be mounted on. There are two kinds of backpack frames: internal and external.

Inside the backpack of internal frame, packs will be an aluminum frame. They are substantially more flexible than external frame backpacks because they shift the pack's weight from the shoulders to the hips. Furthermore, internal frame backpacks are slightly lighter and smaller than external frame backpacks, so if you need a pack with 90 liters of capacity to last you a week, an internal frame arrangement is probably not the ideal option for you. However, the vast majority of bug-out bags are only designed to last three days; thus, an internal frame backpack should be seriously considered in that regard.

External frame backpacks are larger, stronger, and heavier than internal frame backpacks. Rather than being installed within the pack, the frame supports the backpack from the outside, as the name implies. The ability to attach more gear and supplies to an external frame backpack is advantageous. Backpackers frequently use external frame backpacks to attach heavy-duty items such as sleeping bags, tents, coats, and so on. Another benefit of external frame backpacks is the extra space between your back and the actual pack, which reduces sweating while hiking.

Overall, the external frame backpack is the way to go if you want a pack that will last you a week or more. Because of its lighter weight, the internal frame is a better choice for a more typical three-day bug-out bag.

Capacity

The volume and capacity of the backpack are the first things to consider in a bug-out bag. Many preppers, however, are perplexed because, while some backpacks promise to hold the same capacity, not all backpacks can have the same amount of goods due to the arrangement and design of their compartments.

Look for backpacks with a variety of large and small compartments that can be easily closed with a zipper, Velcro, sealed pockets, and so on. This ensures that your bag can hold as much gear as possible while traveling without losing its capacity. If you need to last for three days, look for a backpack with a volume of 40 liters/2,500 cubic inches, or one with a capacity of 50 to 60 liters/4,000 cubic inches, which is what most bug-out bags are meant to do. Increase the capacity to 6,000 cubic inches/80 to 90 liters for a week's worth of rucksack meant. If you're looking for a backpack that can store enough supplies to last you more than a week, you're probably not being realistic about what your body can physically take.

High Quality

After deciding on the capacity and frame of your backpack, the next thing to think about is the construction quality. Your backpack should be made to withstand harsh conditions and be water-resistant, the zippers should work smoothly, and the straps should be thick and adaptable. If you purchase your backpack in person, you should be able to tell if the material is sturdy and durable simply by touching and holding it. If you're looking on an excellent deal on ebay or Amazon, it'll be a little more challenging to tell if the pack is durable. Still, online reviews and item descriptions should give you all the necessary information. Furthermore, if the backpack arrives in the mail and appears poorly constructed, you can easily return it. Military-grade packs, such as an Alice Pack or Three-Day Deployment Bags, are the ideal backpacks to seek.

The Right Equipment

With this information, you'll be able to choose the best bug-out bag for your needs. The following stage is the most pleasurable: filling it up! As a hint, acquire all of your goods BEFORE purchasing your bug-out bag so that you know the basic size and style of backpack you need.

When you've packed your bug-out bag, make sure it's well-organized, with the most vital goods in easy-to-reach places. Keep reading and follow this guide loosely, which means you can remove or add items as you see fit for survival in your specific location, but it is intended to serve as a basic guideline for what you need.

Bugging In

Suppose you opt to stay at home and batten down the hatches rather than bug out. In that case, you must learn how to enhance your chances of survival, especially when tragedy causes anarchy and turmoil until government troops can restore peace and order. This is especially essential when you consider that most of the country's population is located in cities and other densely populated areas, which means there will be a fierce rivalry for life supplies, which will mean more danger.

Strategies for Bugging In

Here below, you can find the main aspect of these strategies.

Self Defense

This will be your top priority if you and your family decide to stay and hold the fort. Because disasters have the power to neutralize the government's law enforcement, even if only for a short time, resulting in anarchy and mayhem - everyone for themselves. Expect criminality to be the order of the day in such survival scenarios. Those who are unprepared are always the targets of those who are. You can make some decisions to reduce your chances of encountering unsavory behavior from desperate people during calamities that can paralyze government operations. Please keep in mind, however, that these are only guidelines and ideas and should not be taken as absolute truths. You should use your best judgment in deciding how to apply this in your situation and area in the event of an urban disaster.

Fortify

Secure your home as much as possible to avoid drawing too much attention from the outside. Reinforce your home's entry and exit points with extra bolts, door jammers, chain locks, and barricades. If they don't deter invaders, they can at least slow them down long enough for you to escape by the back door or prepare to take them down.

Darkness is Your Friend

You can avoid attracting the attention and interest of looters and other criminal elements by barring your windows and turning off your lights at night to the greatest extent possible. When the entire metropolis is in darkness due to a lack of power, even the smallest of lights can attract the attention of unwanted elements.

Make a Group

Colaborate with your neighbors and neighborhood as much as possible to build a strong bond while there is no tragedy. Close relationships with your neighbors give you access to help when needed, better protection from unwanted people, and a lower risk of them targeting you for personal survival. It's also your best option for long-term disaster survival. To understand what I mean, consider how they come together in The Walking Dead!

Make Sure Your Home is Unappealing

Many supporters of the "beautiful home" principle may find this heretical but bear with me. Making your home appear unappealing or unassuming from the outside, i.e., not designed as a palace or a fortress, makes it less noticeable and an unattractive target for looters, gangs, or desperate people looking for food or other supplies.

Now I'm not wishing to turn your house into a dumpster or a scary abandoned house. Unattractive does not always imply ugly; it simply means that it does not draw notice.

CHAPTER 2: SURVIVAL PLANNING

Everyone needs survival skills. That has been the way with humanity since the beginning of time. Unfortunately, the ease of modern convenience and technology has taken us further and further away from those critical skills. It has resulted in a civilization that is no longer self-sufficient. The majority of our population is unaware and unprepared.

We don't need these skills because we've lost them. This is not to say that we are no longer confronted with problems, emergencies, or natural disasters. It means that when these situations arise, the vast majority will be caught off guard and succumb to the negative consequences of what has occurred. Most of the time, we cannot prevent every negative circumstance. That is the truth. We can arm ourselves mentally and physically with the necessary tools to deal with those situations when they arise.

Every day, we see people suffering due to forgotten knowledge and losing abilities that allow us to persevere under duress. Tragedy is still all too common around the world. According to the indicators, the conflict is widespread and frequently far more intense than it should be.

This is due to a single major factor. When disaster strikes, the general public is at a loss for what to do. The frightening thing is that we see these things happen to people on television every day. We are aware of the possibility. We are aware that it is commonplace. The obvious is right in front of us, but for some reason, many people choose to ignore it. This is a blunder.

Natural disasters happen on every part of Earth without exception. Every time, the majority of people are not prepared. Natural disasters have displaced an average of twenty-five million people in recent years. That number almost doubles if you factor in the people affected by conflict zones. Amidst all of this, most people will do little to ensure their safety. It is just not clear why this is so. It seems unreasonable.

Strategy and Planning for Preppers

The basic understanding of survival revolves around air, shelter, and water. Most of the preppers prefer to adopt the rule of 3s. There is a belief that you can survive 3 minutes without the availability of air, three hours without any shelter in bad conditions, three days without water availability, and finally, three weeks without any food. Therefore, the idea of prepping should execute upon these rules of 3s! When you have all of these settled and covered, you can move ahead of the layer of prepping and plan other important aspects. There is a specific pyramid of prepping that all preppers adapt to learn the basics of survival. The pyramid contents in the order from top to bottom are as follows:

- **Self-Actualization:** It is like achieving full potential with all creative activities.
- **Esteem Needs:** There should be a feeling and prestige of full accomplishment.
- **Love & Belongingness Needs:** It is about preparing for friends and all the intimate relationships.
- **Safety Needs:** This is about making arrangements for safety and security needs.
- **Physiological Needs:** You must make arrangements for the basic food, warmth, rest, and water needs!

All these needs combine to fulfill your self-fulfillment, psychological and basic needs! You must remember to impose self-actualization on priority, where you will learn to prioritize your hobbies and find yourself. These are the two essential frameworks to keep your preparations grounded and concerned.

Your priorities should be clear. You should be able to survive longer than to survive better for just a few days! For instance, you should count on storing four boring meals rather than having just 2 of your favorite meals at the same cost. Believe it or not, this mindset will help you make optimal preparations for dealing with catastrophic events.

For any crisis, be it environmental, natural, economic, financial, or other, the best time to prepare is now. It is because you never know when you will face an emergency crisis. Therefore, you need to be prepared at all times. All the preppers do the same. Even some people who are not preppers tend to prepare for emergencies. However, for a beginner, it can feel like a lot. The first thing that you need to do is relax. Just think of the small things. Everything that can help you with a crisis in the future counts as prepping, be it a savings account or insurance or installing a fire extinguisher. Everything is included in prepping. Some of the primary steps involved in prepping are listed below:

- Get yourself health and medical insurance and build a savings account.
- Prepare your home for a two-week emergency, stock it up with supplies and make it more secure.
- Have a bug-out plan and a bug-out bag ready so that you can evacuate the place at even short notice.
- Learn some skills to help you survive in the wild.

- Try to communicate with others. It will help you in your learning and growth.

Tips and Common Beginner Mistakes

Some of the tips and common mistakes that beginners make are as follows:

- Many preppers purchase emergency kits that are available online. It is best if you avoid them at all costs. The majority of them do not exercise.
- You should not base your decisions on assumptions. You never know what you'll encounter, so be prepared for anything.
- While prepping, you should be more realistic in your approach.
- Because you don't know when the crisis will strike, the best time to begin preparing is now. You should always be prepared.
- Don't get upset or stressed out about the prospect of a crisis while preparing. Just enjoy the moment and keep preparing.
- Contact other people who might be interested in prepping, or search for preppers online. It will be highly beneficial.
- Don't predetermine whether you're going to bug in or bug out. Prepare for both scenarios, and when the time comes, assess the situation and choose the one that appears more reasonable.
- It is not enough to simply purchase safety equipment. It is equally important to practice and learn how to use it.
- If you have a large budget, try buying high-quality rather than low-cost items. High-quality materials will be more durable and practical.
- Make a bug-out bag. This bag should contain everything you might need to leave the house.
- Always stay prepared. There is no time to relax during a crisis. It would help if you were always alert.
- If you are a beginner and consult with some professional prepper, the first thing they will ask you is what you are prepping for. You should know what you are prepping for. It can provide you with a good start.

Get Your Health and Finances in Order

Financial crises and medical emergencies are the most common type of disasters you can face. They can be very unexpected; therefore, you must be prepared for them. According to a survey, it was found that 50% of Americans are unable to afford a $500 emergency without paying through credit cards. It would be best if you had a backup plan for these emergencies so that you don't have to spend money. Similarly, you should have health insurance or a suitable fund saved for emergency medical situations to afford the treatment without spending your money.

Another thing that you should keep in mind is that these crises mostly come together. For example, you cannot go to work with a health emergency and thus start having financial problems. The savings and insurances are for these hard times so that you can focus on your health or other matters.

Learn, Practice, and Plan!

Even if you have the necessary supplies, you may still be unprepared for the crisis. It is because prepping is about learning new skills, planning and practicing, and stocking. Purchasing the necessary equipment and security weapons, as well as stockpiling supplies, is therefore insufficient. You must also learn and practice. Everything that you are storing should be familiar to you. You can do this while gathering supplies. You should also have all of your plans in place before the crisis. Following that, you must learn fundamental survival skills. Some examples might be:

- Compass techniques
- How to read a map
- How to light a fire
- How to care for a wound
- How to apply stitches
- Use of a tourniquet
- How to put up a tent
- How to sharpen a blade with random stuff

Stockpiling Necessary Supplies

Everyone needs at least water, food, and shelter to survive. In addition, during a long-term disaster or survival situation, individuals need a continual supply of these three things. Preppers know this and try to be prepared should a disruption in these supplies occur. They do this by stocking up on extra food or growing their garden.

Start with the home because it will be where you will spend most of your critical time. And home is possibly the best place to overcome any kind of emergency. Therefore, governments advise all citizens of their country to be in their homes in case of emergency. This step's primary or initial goal is to prepare yourself for survival in your home for the next two weeks without seeking help from outside or expecting government agencies to arrive anytime soon.

Learning Important Skills

True disaster preparation goes beyond storing food, water, and other emergency supplies; it involves regularly learning and practicing survival skills. There are plenty of things you can learn on your own at home or by taking courses.

For example, you can learn outdoor cooking methods, emergency first aid, hunting, fishing, or shelter building. The specific skills you learn will depend on where you live and what situations you are likely to face after a disaster occurs in your area.

Building A Community

Those who prepare for a disaster realize the importance of getting to know others with similar mindsets. You can learn from each other and help out if a disaster should happen. There is a chance that you won't be ready or prepared before a disaster occurs.

But if you know of some people (friends or neighbors) who have done their preparation, you can pool your skills and resources and work as a close-knit community or as a team where you contribute your skills and the "know-how" and survive the disaster.

The Rules of A Prepper

Never Reveal to Anyone that You are a Prepper

Never tell your neighbors, coworkers, or acquaintances that you are well stocked and supplied. Your extended family may be aware of your preparations. Perhaps a few trusted friends can find out.

People who appear nice now may not remain, so if things worsen. People will start looking elsewhere if food and supplies run out on store shelves and in their homes. You don't want people coming to your house looking for things.

Make a Plan and Know It

What are the most likely situations to affect you where you live? If you live below sea level, such as in New Orleans, you know that flooding is possible. Civil unrest, rioting, and supply shortages are all possible in highly stressed cities like Minneapolis.

These are things you should consider ahead of time. The disaster and the environment will determine your plan.

Do you have any children? They are also a part of the plan. They must be aware of the strategy. They must be able to tell you the plan at any time.

You practiced fire drills at school. Practice at home. How quickly can you leave the house with everything you need and everything in your truck or car?

Maintain Multiple Redundancies

Get one or two more of whatever you have. What do you do if your trenching shovel breaks? You may not be in a position where a quick trip to Home Depot will solve your problem.

Things fall apart. The batteries in flashlights run out. Medicine bottles are running out.

Preparing is an Ongoing Project, not a One-Time Event

This isn't about buying stuff, storing it in your basement, and forgetting about it. Even food with a long shelf life requires rotation and replacement. You must use and replace supplies regularly.

New products are constantly being released. Much of it is garbage or the same old stuff with a new label, but some are fantastic. You could use those items to supplement or replace other items.

Gardening will be a Daily Part of Your Life if You Have One

The same goes for knowledge. This book will cover many topics, but it simply cannot contain every possible piece of knowledge you might need for every situation. There is always more you can learn, more you can prepare for, and more you can train for. Read books. Watch videos on the internet. Take classes.

Things to Know Before Becoming a Prepper

Most people make mistakes when they start prepping. For most, it is because they rush in, not taking the time to think and plan; for others, it lacks decent information. So, here is a list of 21 things you need to know so you do not make the same mistakes, and waste time, energy, and money when you don't need to.

Live Within Your Means

Now, forget about using a credit card to buy all of your prepping supplies at once—find ways to cut your bills and save the money you have.

Don't Blow Every Penny in a Month

Prepping is a steady and slow business. You may believe you need that survival item immediately, but you should shop around for the best deal and wait—patience pays off when you find a lower price or have a substitute that will suffice.

Begin Storing Water

Water is more important than food, and a few liters won't get you very far. Begin storing it right away. Collect your own and store it in clean barrels and collapsible containers in your basement or garage—it can be kept for long periods if properly stored.

Don't use old milk jugs to store water. It may appear to be a good idea, but it is doomed from the start. You can never get all of the milk residues out of these jugs, which can lead to harmful bacteria colonizing your water. Furthermore, because it is made of plastic, the jug will degrade over time, creating a sloppy situation.

Don't Waste Money on Food That will Go Unused

You might think you got a good deal on a ton of canned spinach, but do people eat it? It wastes valuable resources like time, money, and storage space. Look for great deals, but if it doesn't get eaten, don't waste your time or money on it.

Don't Limit Yourself to Canned Foods

Some people believe they should only store canned goods. Wrong—a good diet requires a wide variety of foods, including canned, freeze-dried, and dry foods. Otherwise, you risk becoming bored with food. Not only that, but canned foods are high in sodium, which isn't good in excess.

Make Certain That Your Storage Shelves Are Sturdy

You may believe you got a good deal on those particleboard shelves, but they won't last long once you start piling things on them. Make your sturdy wood or metal shelving, or use wire shelving.

Don't Keep Everything in One Location

A single untimely disaster could deplete your entire supply of food and other supplies. Separate your food and water into multiple caches, keep a bag on hand (one in each vehicle), and keep a few supplies at your bug-out shelter location.

Preparation is about more than just how much you store. It is all about developing skills and knowledge to help you survive. You'll need some training and a lot of hands-on experience—a list of those skills can be found at the end of this section.

Hygiene and Sanitation are also Essential

Food and water are important but don't forget soap and toilet paper. Cleanliness is vital for avoiding illness—the last thing you want in a survival situation is to become ill, especially when hospitals are overcrowded or closed entirely.

Don't Forget About Special Needs!

People who require wheelchairs, oxygen, insulin, and other medical supplies should be included in your planning.

Do You Have Pets? Don't Forget About Them

You have two options for pets in a survival situation: abandon them or care for them. Most people will opt for the latter but make your decision now. Then begin stockpiling food and other necessities for them—and remember to include them in your water calculations.

Recruit Family Members

Everyone must be involved; they do not need to be as enthusiastic as you, but they must know how to do things and have a certain level of knowledge. Get them involved right away.

Don't Tell Everyone About Your Plans

You don't need everyone to know what you're up to or what you have in stock. If the SHTF, you don't want the entire neighborhood knocking on your door; you can't help your own family and everyone else simultaneously. Keep your plans to yourself, your family, and a few close friends.

Maintain Your Fitness

If you don't, the first day of any disaster scenario will exhaust you. You'll be hiking around, transporting supplies, repairing damage, and being out of breath. Staying in shape is easier than you think—a 30-minute power walks every day will suffice.

Don't Think Guns and Ammo Will Keep You Safe

Yes, you should have guns and plenty of ammo to defend yourself and your family, but you should try to avoid confrontation as much as possible. Learn to be stealthy and avoid drawing attention; guns will not keep you safe from those who have them.

Make a Plan for Getting Home

Many people fail to recognize that disasters do not wait for them. They can happen anywhere, so have a plan for returning home or a safe meeting place for you and your family.

Make No Assumptions

Some believe they will need to bug out, while others believe they will need to bug in. The thing is, you have no idea what will happen, so have a plan in place, as well as a backup plan. And another if necessary.

Examine Your Tools

Never assume that a tool will work when you need it; always test it. And don't keep a dozen of the same tool on hand—if it doesn't work, you might need a different one. Furthermore, the more tools you have, the more you carry.

Little Steps

Many DIY projects require significant time and education, and patience is essential. If you rush, you will become frustrated and tired. A lot of small steps go a long way.

The world will not end tomorrow. It might, but there's a good chance you'll get a heads-up. The issue is that some preppers get into the habit of thinking like this and panic, which leads to poor decisions.

Always Be Prepared, But Don't Forget to Enjoy Life on the Way

Don't lose yourself so much in your doomsday prepping that everything else passes you by, and remember—there is a chance that doomsday won't happen.

Important Documents

Keep a copy of important documents like copies of your prescriptions, birth certificates, and other necessary paperwork in a waterproof container. This will make it easier to replace these documents if they are lost or destroyed during an emergency or major disaster. I also have a copy of my will, insurance policy, and passport in my bug-out bag.

Ensure you keep essential family documents like passports, wills, and other legal papers in waterproof containers. It is also a g idea to keep extra copies of these items at home so they can be replaced if necessary. Family photos are also important because they can be used to help with identification in an emergency.

Keep a copy of your life insurance policy, retirement plan, and other essential papers in a waterproof container. In addition, keep photocopies of these documents at home as well.

Keep a copy of your birth certificate at home with photocopies available in an emergency or situation where ID is necessary for survival. In addition, have extra copies of this document at home so that they can be replaced or used in the event the original document is destroyed during an emergency.

Keep copies of your driver's license, passport, and other important documents with your medical records and prescription information in a waterproof container. I keep these at all times and copies of my health insurance card and prescriptions.

Make sure to keep a copy of your life insurance policy and other necessary paperwork at all times, primarily if you use it to protect property by ensuring that it is adequately insured. I keep these papers in an emergency kit or easily accessible for reference if needed.

Photocopies or digital images of important documents like prescriptions, passports, and social security cards should be kept in an easily accessible place as a reference more than anything else.

Record the important documents you have and keep copies of these in a waterproof container in a safe location. This way, even if you have a copy of the most important document, you can use it confidently just in case something goes wrong with the original.

These paper documents could matter more than any electronic documents you may have stored on a computer or electronic device like a tablet or smartphone because if they are lost or destroyed during an emergency, it will be impossible for anyone to access them from their location without your paperwork.

CHAPTER 3: WEAPON

This section is intended for preppers with little or no firearms experience. We'll give general tips on what to look for when stocking up on firearms and recommendations for prepper-approved options.

When it comes to weapons in a survival context, these are the items you will need to use if you find yourself in a situation where you need to defend yourself. You would also require weapons to be able to hunt and fish. Finally, you'll need tools to use as weapons, such as saws and axes. Let's take a closer look at the types of tools you'll require.

The first item on your list will be a firearm, which is a sophisticated weapon even in the best of circumstances and requires some investment and expertise. A firearm will be at the top of your list if you are already trained. It should be noted that ammo is classified as survival supplies. There is no one-size-fits-all approach to firearm ownership. When embarking on a survival mission, however, you'll want to choose a weapon that is light and efficient, as well as one that is most reliable. You must also ensure that you have enough ammo to protect yourself and your family, as well as to use for other tasks. If you intend to hunt with your weapon, make sure that it can take down the caliber of prey you desire. Certain weapons can be used for both self-defense and hunting. Remember that you may or may not be able to discharge firearms at will. Always be aware of the surroundings in which you find yourself.

Purchase a snake bore. A snake bore is a type of bore cleaner essential for anyone who owns a firearm. When you're out in the wilderness, proper weapon maintenance is critical. You'll need everything to work properly.

You could also create your weapons to use in combat. You can design and build these weapons as needed while in the wilderness, but you may lack the necessary materials and equipment. It's better to plan out what you'll need ahead of time. Homemade knives, stun guns, and flamethrowers are examples of customizable weapons.

You will also need a bow and arrow if you intend to go hunting. These weapons are ideal when stealth is required, and a firearm will not suffice. Their disadvantage is that they require some expertise to operate properly, and optimal conditions are required for their most effective use. Crossbows are also included in this category.

A tactical pen is another weapon you should carry with you. These are pressure-sensitive ink cartridges inside hardened metal pens. They do not kill but can be used as a last resort to strike an opponent. Furthermore, they are pens and can be used to make notes, maps, and a variety of other useful tasks.

Stun guns help deliver a burst of electricity that renders an opponent immobile for a few moments. They are only useful for self-defense and are not entirely reliable. However, they are ideal for situations involving imminent danger when they do work.

Mace spray is available in small pressurized containers. It can be fired at potential predators' and enemies' faces. It has a maximum range of 20 feet.

In addition to these weapons, you'll need spears, knives, machetes, saws, and other similar weapons to complete tasks while on the trail.

The first point to consider when considering what guns to purchase is this: ***there is no perfect solution.*** There is no ideal one-size-fits-all gun that will suit all your needs.

Due to this, many firearm experts recommend getting your hands on at least a few different types of guns that are good for different situations. Therefore, the type of firearms you need will depend on how you intend to use them. Do you want a firearm to shoot possible wild animal predators long-range, hunt in the wild, or as a short-range defense method if your home is raided?

Handgun

Are you looking for a small, lightweight gun that allows for concealed carry you can use for self-protection? Your best answer will be a handgun.

If you have a license to do so, this gun is the one that should be kept on you at all times, as it will act as your first line of defense against most threats.

Some general advice when looking for a good handgun is to make sure it is:

- Comfortable to carry
- Compact
- Reliable
- Simple to use
- It has ammunition, spare parts, and a holster that you can easily purchase a lot of

The key to a good handgun is finding one that is not too heavy but not too light - pocket handguns look cute but won't work as well. It will not be helpful if it's too heavy for you to carry day-to-day comfortably.

Some typical recommendations for handguns are:

- SIG Sauer P365
- SIG Sauer P320
- Glock 19
- Glock 43
- Smith and Wesson M&P

These five handguns are all highly rated as reliable by preppers, with the Glock brand being hailed as the most dependable and easy to use.

Like many things, the best type of handgun for you will come down to personal preference, so it's recommended that you take each gun for a test drive in a practice shooting range before you purchase anything.

Rifle

A rifle is a preferred solution for many if you're looking for a weapon for shooting or defense involving a long-range target. But experts also recommend a carbine, as it's more lightweight, so it will be easier to carry around.

A semi-automatic sporting rifle is an excellent choice for keeping things simple because it is suitable for self-defense and hunting larger-sized games. It's a good idea to outfit the gun with an optical sight and a sling to make it as easy to use as possible. For convenience, many preppers recommend purchasing a semi-automatic rifle.

Here are some good rifle recommendations:

- .22LR 10/22 AR-15 AK-47 from Rufer
- Lever-Action Repeating Rifle Henry .22

As with the handgun, the key is to get into the shooting range and try out a few different types to see what suits you best.

Pistol

Pistols are great for self-defense because they are simple to use and extremely effective. Finding a good pistol at a reasonable price is also reasonably simple.

When deciding on the best pistol for you, consider how cheap the gun and ammo are, how reliable the gun is, and how easy it is to transport. Accuracy is typically something to consider with other guns, but accuracy is less critical with pistols because they are shot at close range. If you want to buy a long-range hunting rifle, accuracy will be the most vital factor.

Some general pistol recommendations are:

- Kel-Tec P3AT
- Ruger Security 9
- Smith and Wesson 637 Airweight

Stabbing Weapons

As you might expect, a stabbing weapon can be used to stab someone physically. A kitchen knife, a letter opener, or a multi-tool would be the most accessible stabbing weapon. However, if you don't have any of those on hand, numerous alternatives can cause just as much harm. The only thing to remember is that stabbing someone with a car key or a corkscrew will require slightly more force than stabbing someone with a sharpened knife. So, if you want to harm someone physically, you must go for it.

If you're in danger, stab someone in the throat, ears, or nose to hinder them. If they're hurting you and you want the simplest solution, stabbing them in the eyes will do the trick but will almost certainly cause permanent damage (avoid this if you're just looking to scare someone off).

Here are some alternative stabbing weapons:

- Car keys/keys of any kind
- Screwdriver
- Fountain pen
- Sharpened lead pencil
- End of an umbrella (if the tip is metal)
- Tweezers

Beating Weapons

If you don't want to pierce someone's skin, the next best thing is to bludgeon them with a heavy object. In this case, we've labeled these weapons as "beating" because you'll be using them to beat someone. This weapon should be heavy enough to deliver a damaging blow to the assailant but not so heavy that you can't lift it properly. If you can't lift the item above your head, you won't be able to generate enough power to cause any damage to your swing. So, your chosen item will determine how much weight you can lift.

Another piece of advice for this type of weapon is to strike the person from behind, especially if they are larger and stronger than you. These weapons are most effective when the target is unaware of their presence.

Here are some excellent options for alternative beating weapons:

- Flashlight
- Dumbbell
- Vase
- Baseball bat
- Belt
- Chair
- Glass bottles
- Newspaper (read more about using newspapers below)

Alternative Weapon Ideas

Spray Weapons

One of the most commonly used and well-known defense weapons is mace (also known as pepper spray). Mace is an aerosol with an inflammatory ingredient called capsaicin. This ingredient causes pain and burning in the eyes, so the idea is to force the eyes closed and prevent vision. But if you don't have any mace, here are some excellent alternatives you can you that will just be sat around the house:

- Hairspray
- Perfume/cologne
- Spray bleach (any kind of cleaning product in spray form)
- Spray sun lotion
- Spray starch
- Powder fire extinguishers (only effective if sprayed in the face at proximity)
- DIY mace (see more info on how to make this below)

How to Make DIY Mace

You can develop a potent DIY mace by mixing cayenne pepper powder with 92% alcohol (rubbing alcohol) and vegetable oil. To make this mace, follow the instructions below:

1. Add 2 tbsp of cayenne pepper to a cup.
2. Pour the alcohol over the pepper until the powder is fully submerged. Stir well.

3. Add 1 tbsp of vegetable oil for each 2 tbsp cayenne pepper. Stir it well. If you don't have vegetable oil, baby oil would be a good substitute.
4. If you want to give your pepper spray a little more *zing*, you can add a little lemon juice or soap.
5. Once you're done adding things to the mixture, cover it in some plastic wrap and leave it to settle overnight.
6. After at least 12 hours, strain your liquid to remove all sediment. You need to strain it because the sediment can block the spray opening when you put it into a spray bottle.
7. Filter the solution by pouring it into another cup through material such as a cheesecloth or a coffee filter.

You can use a simple spray bottle with a manual mechanism to store this solution. If you use this bottle, take precautions to ensure that the solution will not leak out when it's not in use. But a lot of people prefer to use an aerosol spray. Here's how you can store your mace:

1. Get an empty aerosol can and drill a hole into the bottom to use an aerosol can. The hole should be around 9mm wide.
2. Transfer the mace solution into the empty can using a funnel or a syringe.
3. Use epoxy to patch up the open hole and leave a few minutes to set. Don't forget to wear gloves when doing this.
4. Put a tire valve into the hole before the epoxy has fully hardened. Add more epoxy around the valve to seal it. This tire valve will allow you a fast way to pressurize the can. Leave the epoxy for a few minutes to seal completely. Ensure the valve is in the hole deep enough to reach past the epoxy.
5. If you want to do so, decorate your can. This can be a good idea to make sure someone doesn't mistake it for something else, which could cause many issues.
6. The last step is to pressurize your can, using an air compressor. Fill the can with air and feel the pressure increase until you feel a difference in the can.

After you pressurize the can, don't forget to ***test it carefully***. The spray should stretch around 10 feet and works best when sprayed in short spurts.

How to Fashion a Weapon Out of a Newspaper

1. Get a newspaper and completely open it.
2. Roll it as tightly as possible from top to bottom.
3. Simply fold it in half once rolled. That's all!

To give your Millwall Brick more heft, stuff some coins in the middle or wrap it in packaging tape.

Of course, this weapon takes some time to prepare, so only use it if you have some time before the attackers arrive.

Anything with a bit of weight can be used this way; avoid large and difficult-to-pick-up items. Picking up a bicycle to throw at your opponent can cause you to lose your balance and not throw it as hard as you should. Remember to think realistically right now.

There are many ways you can defend yourself and your homestead. As mentioned many times, you shouldn't fall into just relying on your firearms to protect you. When planning your homesteading setup, don't forget to consider security parameters to ensure you and all your valuable resources stay protected.

CHAPTER 4: TRAPS

Turning your garden into a giant trap is not viable because of the time and effort it takes, especially if you have a large garden. Plus, any trip to your garden could be potentially lethal for you. Instead, you want to use traps strategically and use them to push the intruders towards an area you can easily defend. This is called funneling. This usually means forcing the intruders to reveal themselves and not letting them stay hidden. If an intruder wants to move from the garden gates to your front door, they will do so in the most efficient way; a straight line. In that case, you would want to have placed debris or anything that would make them deviate from that path and onto the path of the traps you have placed.

You need to be cautious about using traps to deter intruders because this puts you in an awkward position regarding the law. It can also be hazardous to you and genuine visitors, especially after dark, so steer clear of setting up random traps around your home. However, don't dismiss the area entirely.

Funneling is often used in hunting, and the idea is to push the prey into the right area to catch it. Although you aren't treating intruders as prey, a similar principle applies here. Instead, you are trying to push them into open spaces where they are more likely to be spotted and less likely to hang around.

To set up this arrangement, you must carefully survey your home's surrounding area and assess the different spaces. If you were trying to sneak around, where would you hide? What bushes, structures, and debris could provide shelter? What could you duck beneath?

These spaces you want to push intruders away from, forcing them to stay on the pathway or in the open. You can funnel an intruder into open spaces by making the other spaces challenging to pass through. For example, piling up boxes or old tools in hideaways or along the edges of the paths makes intruders far less likely to stray into these areas. They are also more likely to make a noise and alert you if they attempt it.

All these are designed to maim the intruder in some fashion, so please be careful when you employ them throughout your home.

A Not-So-Friendly Welcome Home Mat

The first thing you want to target is the intruder's mobility. Most intruders do not notice the carpet is frequently placed in front of the door and can be used as a defense.

You will need:

- A box of needle-like nails measuring 3 inches long
- A dark-colored carpet that is unassuming
- A piece of cardboard nearly the length and width of the carpet

Directions:

1. Insert the nails at least an inch apart into the cardboard.
2. Spread the cardboard out on the floor.
3. Place the carpet on top of the cardboard, and use the nails to remove the visible uplifting of the carpet.

You want the nails to be at least 3 inches long or longer because most common shoe soles are an inch to two inches thick, so they need to be longer to get into the foot. Even minor foot injuries cause excruciating pain and can sometimes render the person who stepped on the nail completely disabled. If the nail penetrates the Achilles tendon, the person may become paralyzed or walk with a limp.

All are tripped by clear duct tape. While clear duct tape is the cheapest and least visible option, you can easily replace it with another type of string or more secure material. The idea is to attach the duct tape to one side of the wall and then bring it to the other side of the wall to attach it there. Doing this two to three inches above the ground will capture the ankle of the foot rather than the front. Grabbing the front of the foot is less effective because the body will instinctively remove itself from the position if it detects anything abrasive against it.

Placing it where the ankle will travel means the foot is already in place and does not have the kinetic force to back out of the action to go upwards, resulting in the intruder tripping over the duct tape.

An Early Punch

What happens if an individual opens the door to an important room, perhaps a child's room or your own? This next trap is for landing the first punch on an unsuspecting intruder, which means you will need something heavy.

You will need:

- 2 Inter-connecting hooks
- 1 Board that is as long as the door is wide
- Something Heavy that can be attached to the board (optional)
- String
- Nail
- Hammer

Directions:

1. Hammer the nail in the door near the top of the door.
2. Tie the string to the nail.
3. Place the board with the heavy item towards the ceiling with the heavy item pressed against the ceiling.
4. Secure the hook to the wall and the other hook to the bottom of the board.
5. Ensure that there is enough pressure that the ceiling will hold on to the heavy item but that the string can pull it out of place.
6. Ensure the string is lax and not tight; otherwise, the heavy item will hit the door, not the perpetrator.

This will either damage the perpetrator or make enough noise that someone can wake up because of it. If this hits an intruder, they will likely be knocked out and have a mild to severe concussion, so if you put this in a child's room, be sure that while it can hit an intruder, it cannot hit the child.

A Shocking Turn

The following booby trap can be used for security, maiming, or as a prank on other family members. There are more lethal ways to make an electrifying doorknob, but if you just want to slow down an intruder rather than kill them, this is the best way. However, this method may still kill people, but it has a lower risk than other methods.

You will need:

- An RC battery of your choice, as long as it has wires
- Wire Stripper for Electrical Tape

Directions:

1. Strip the battery wires until you can access the copper wiring within them.
2. Attach the battery to the door with duct tape, but close enough to the doorknob that the wires can touch it.
3. Place the wires on the doorknob and tape them in place.

It will become quite hot when you place the wires on the doorknob. The only issue with this trap is that the feed will constantly run through the handle, eventually draining the battery and necessitating battery replacement.

You can make it much more deadly by plugging it into the wall, but it will not do much good if the power is out.

CHAPTER 5: SURVIVAL KIT

Water

- Plastic water storage containers
- Filtration system
- Bottles of bleach
- Rainwater collection system

Food Stockpile

- Freeze-dried meals/canned meats
- Cooking fuel source
- DIY food stockpile
- Daily multivitamins

Clothing and Warm Items

- Spare clothes
- Stocking cap/face shield
- Hand and toe warmers
- Footwear
- Rain poncho with hood
- Sewing/supplies
- Survival Gloves

Heat and Warmth

- Alternative energy and traditional heater
- Tact bivvy
- Woodstove

Smaller Energy Tools

- Biolite stove
- Light-weight rugged solar charger

Fire Starting Tools and Gear

- Stormproof matches
- Tinder
- Small magnifying glass/fresnel lens
- Ferro rod striker
- Electric lighter

First Aid and Medical Supplies

- Survival medical kit
- Neosporin (or similar salve)
- Sterile alcohol prep pads
- Hydrogen peroxide
- Personal medications
- Pain killers

- Vaseline
- Blood clotting sponge
- Super glue
- Antibiotics
- Wound gauze roll
- Surgical tape
- Tweezers and nail clippers
- Insect repellent
- Sun screen
- Band-aids/moleskin pads
- Tourniquet
- Cotton swabs

Personal Hygiene Items

- Soap
- Oral hygiene
- Female hygiene
- Hand sanitizer
- Razor blades
- Toilet paper

Essential Hand Tools

- Hatchets and axes
- Hand mill
- Survival knife
- Pliers
- Hammers
- Shovels
- Saws
- Hand pump

Illumination Tools

- Super bright LED headlamp
- Glow sticks
- Super bright LED tactical flashlight
- LED lantern

Communication Tools

- Ham radio setup
- Hand crank Am/FM/NOAA digital radio
- Two-way radio walkie talkies

Self Defense Items

- Survival firearms
- Window security film
- Motion trigger lights
- Ammunition
- Bow and arrows
- Armor concepts door armor
- Home defense items
- Camouflage

Misc. Survival Tools and Supplies

- Rechargeable batteries
- All forms of entertainment
- Corrective lenses
- Paper and pencils
- Gas mask and filters
- Electrical tape
- Duct tape
- Scissors
- Gold (not recommended)
- Vices

CHAPTER 6: FIRST AID

A well-stocked first-aid pack can mean the difference between life and death in an emergency. An injured person may have to wait hours or days for help in a survival situation, and with a severe injury, you may not receive any help at all. You want your first-aid package to help you treat accidents and illnesses effectively until professional medical help comes.

When you don't have access to medical services, you may take care of yourself and others with a sufficient quantity of medicines, bandages, & sterilizing tools. Don't rely on what you see in local stores regarding first aid kits.

Instruments for First Aid

Starting your survival first aid kit with the things you already have at home is a smart idea. These things are suggested for treating small cuts and scrapes that are common in everyday life. This also includes:

- Abrasions
- Burns
- Cuts
- Splinters
- Sprains
- Stings

These injuries may happen even after a disaster, so keeping the items that can treat them in your survival pack is a smart idea. However, you must supplement it with a few more injury-specific items and personal medications.

Don't forget to supplement your supply with some medication to relieve the symptoms of respiratory and gastrointestinal infections, including cough, fever, stomach pains, and diarrhea. If you have children, you should have medications in dosages that are appropriate for their age and current prescriptions. Make sure your kit has everything you'll need for an extended period since you may or may not have access to medicine stores.

The following are the items and utensils that should be included in your first-aid kit:

- Self-adhesive tape and bandages
- Anti-diarrhea and antacid drugs
- An antiseptic to clean hands and wounds.
- Antihistamines, both oral and topical
- Antibiotic cream or spray for minor scrapes and cuts
- Antiseptic lotion or spray for rashes and insect bites.
- Aspirin to relieve pain and prevent heart attacks.
- Bandages for wrapping sprains and splints and securing gauze to wounds
- Relief gel or relief cream
- Cough suppressant medications
- First-aid instructions
- Ibuprofen to treat pain, fever, and infection. repellant insect
- Knife
- A CPR mask
- Moleskin to treat minor burns and blisters.
- Instrument sterilization is simplified.
- Nasal decongestant for allergies and colds
- Non-adhesive sterile gauze pads can clean and cover wounds and burns.
- Prescription medications
- A phone card with at least 60 minutes of talk time, some spare change for pay phones, and a list of emergency contacts
- Other essential phone numbers, such as 911, poison control, etc.
- Resealable plastic bags
- Safety pins for bandaging and removing splints
- Ice packs and single-use gloves for infection treatment
- Sunscreen
- Scissors
- A tiny flashlight
- Corticosteroids applied topically to treat rashes
- Triangular sling and tourniquet bandages
- Tweezers to remove stingers, splinters, or ticks

You can get all of these items at any well-stocked drugstore, but it'll be up to you to put them together in a well-organized package. Remember to place the items in a resealable nylon bag with adequate visibility. You don't need to purchase a special case; a nice makeup bag will do as long as it is water-resistant. It's especially crucial to keep adhesives and sterilized items dry. Because this collection is far larger than a standard first-aid kit, labeling and categorizing everything is a smart idea. Each category of items may be divided into smaller bags, which can then be stuffed into a large backpack. This way, you can keep everything in one place and check to see if you need to restock anything regularly.

Make sure you know how to use all of the items in your kit properly, and teach your loved ones how to do the same in case you are the one who needs first aid. Keep the first-aid kit in a convenient location for anybody staying with you. It should be kept from heat and humidity since these variables reduce the medication's shelf life. This is why you should never store your medication in the bathroom. It's excessively humid, which might make the medication ineffective. If you're moving, take your gear with you everywhere, but keep it out of direct sunlight and water.

Keeping Your First-Aid Kit Updated

Examine your first-aid kit at least twice yearly to ensure everything is current and in working order. You can also use this time to sanitize the bag that holds your equipment and any non-packaged utensils. Take everything out of the bag and spritz it with antiseptic. While you wait for the bag to dry, spray the tweezers, scissors, and anything else that can withstand moisture. Then go through the rest of your belongings to see what you can get rid of or replace. Another reason to label items is to make it easier to track them. Make a labeled checklist to ensure you don't forget to replenish any essential items in your kit. Examine individual package seals, mainly if the item contains adhesives or medicines. They should not be used on or near an open wound if any of them appear suspicious (have holes or moisture). You should get rid of them and purchase new ones.

Most of your items should last for years if you keep them in a watertight, puncture-resistant, and drop-resistant bag and keep your kit from being tampered with. Gauze, bandages, and metal utensils have an almost infinite shelf life. Even those that aren't typically used for a long period after their expiration date. Most over-the-counter medications are the same way. Most drugs have an expiration date from 12 to 60 months after they were manufactured, but this does not preclude them from being used after that date.

On the other hand, the expiration date takes storage and handling into account. For example, if a pharmacist removes a medication from its original packaging and places it in a different container, the drug's potency, lifespan, and safety may be compromised. For stress-free handling, it is recommended that the medication in your first aid kit be kept in a sealed manufacturer's container.

When kept in an unopened container, most over-the-counter medications in tablet or capsule form retain their potency for 3-5 years after expiration. Liquid medications are different because they contain additional ingredients that may become unstable after expiration. You should thoroughly inspect any liquids in your pack, whether they are medications, disinfectants, or something else. If they're foggy, discolored, too thick or liquid, or smell bad, it's time to replace them.

The two most notable exceptions to the use beyond the expiration date rule are Pi-Pens and antibiotics. Pi-Pens contain epinephrine, a substance that rapidly degrades after its expiration date. Similarly, even if they are unopened and stored in a cold, dark, and dry environment, most antibiotics degrade quickly after expiration. Regardless of their expiration date, antibiotics should only be used for a few weeks or months. Antibiotics, whether tablet or capsule, should be kept unopened in your first-aid kit. Spray antibiotics may be used, but they must be replaced after six months. They would be too dangerous to use on an open wound otherwise.

In terms of specific dates, here are some guidelines for how long you should keep medications in your first aid kit:

- **Tylenol:** This should be used within five years of opening. The same holds for its unopened form, as it loses potency after five years.
- **Aspirin:** This is most effective when taken within 4-5 years of surgery. Its pain-relieving properties may fade significantly, but its blood-thinning properties deteriorate much faster.
- **Antibiotics:** Most antibiotics can be stored for up to a year if not used. Prescription antibiotics should be taken as soon as possible, and generic antibiotics (primarily topical) should be taken within 6-12 months.
- **Cough Syrup:** Use within 24-36 months of the expiration date if unopened. When you open it, the liquid is contaminated and begins to degrade, so use it within a few weeks.
- **Nasal Sprays:** Nasal decongestants degrade quickly because they contain preservatives. It's best to use them within a few weeks of opening, or at the very least before they expire.
- **Prescription Medication:** Because of the medication's potency, manufacturers limit its use to one year after prescription. They usually have an expiration date of less than a year after they were prescribed, after which they are no longer safe to use.

Note: While not advisable, most medicine can be used for up to 5 years after opening, regardless of the expiration date or if it has been dormant for over a decade.

You Can Grow Medical Herbs

Another approach to being self-reliant in an emergency is to grow your own culinary and medicinal herbs. Many plants have regenerative and healing properties. Most likely, you already have some on your spice rack. However, if something unexpected happens, such as a natural disaster, you may not be able to purchase them in a store. Growing them is a great way to ensure access whenever you need them. The recent coronavirus pandemic has brought the importance of high immunity to light.

Many herbs may assist you with this, as well as much more. Spices such as pepper, cinnamon, cayenne, and cloves, as well as herbs such as oregano, garlic, basil, fennel, and sage, should be included in your daily diet. These herbs may be cultivated in pots and gardens.

If you live in an apartment and don't have enough space to grow your herbs, dried onions may be stored. If desired, they may be stored for up to a year. They will keep their healing properties in unopened containers for roughly 12-18 months.

The following is a list of essential spices having healing properties:

- **Black Pepper:** It has a high energy level, which warms the body and improves circulation, but it can also be used to stop blood flow from wounds.
- **Cayenne Pepper:** It stimulates the cardiovascular system, increasing blood flow, accelerating digestion, and even stopping minor bleeding. Cayenne may keep the body warm throughout winter and boost immunity to colds and viruses.
- **Cloves:** Because of their analgesic and antibacterial properties, clove oil may help treat tooth and gum infections. Cloves' antibacterial properties make them ideal for including in a topical ointment to treat burns and skin irritations. Cloves may be reduced more efficiently in teas.
- **Cinnamon:** In small daily doses, cinnamon improves digestion, relieves stomach cramps, and stimulates circulation throughout the body.
- **Ginger:** This spice relieves nausea, prevents urinary retention, and stops diarrhea. It may also be used as a nasal decongestant or to soothe a sore throat.

Here are a few medicinal herbs that you can grow:

- **Bay Leaves:** These are excellent digestive aids, especially when made into tea. Bay leaves will have a less potent effect when added to your meals. They keep stomach acids at bay when consumed regularly.
- **Basil:** It is another well-known sleep aid since it reduces anxiety and tension. Its calming perfume can elevate one's spirits and alleviate mental problems.
- **Garlic:** Garlic is a strong antibiotic that can help you fight colds and flu by boosting your immunity and preventing infection.
- **Oregano:** A rich source of antioxidants and potent immune boosters that may help you fight infections. Oregano may also help to relieve coughs, settle the stomach, relax the mind, and promote restful sleep when used in tea.
- **Sage:** Sage is recommended for improving digestion and calming cougars, particularly in the winter. It may also be used as a natural antibiotic source and can be taken orally or made into an ointment.

Your garden might also include other medicinal herbs with potent healing properties. Many medicinal herbs with potent regenerative properties, such as peppermint, thyme, rosemary, and fennel, should not be overlooked. Growing and stocking up on healing herbs might come in handy in an emergency. Not to mention the money you could save by substituting natural medicines for costly supplements.

Survival Guide for Medical Emergencies

Keep Calm

Panic can be just as harmful to our health as the conditions that brought it on. Given the recent increase in medical emergencies and the ever-increasing complexity of healthcare, having a plan has never been more critical.

Panicking will not solve your problems and will only make them worse. It will not help you; it will only make you weaker. As hard as it may be, pull yourself together and remain calm.

Utilize Your Assets

Please seek assistance! Determine your objectives by locating someone who can interact with doctors or nurses. Call an ambulance (or dial 911) if no one is present. Maintain adequate oxygen levels in your body by breathing deeply.

Avoid Squeezing the Needle

The ER doctor knows precisely what they're doing but refuses to place an IV if you have a vein. You can cause many problems by struggling against it and possibly shattering it, so try to take deep breaths and relax.

Remind Yourself to Breathe

While this may seem obvious, people occasionally hyperventilate and pass out.

Remember your ABCs:

- Any minor injuries (cuts or bruises) must be washed and air dried.
- Cover them with a clean cloth and gently pat them to promote clotting.
- Examine for signs of infection.
- Apply pressure to severe lacerations to reduce blood flow and stop the bleeding.

- Lift any nearby objects off the ground and place them behind the incision to help limit blood flow until medical help arrives. Always let them understand where you are and follow up with them later to see how they are doing. If somebody is willing to assist, inquire if they are being provided instructions. Be open and honest regarding your physical health and any medical concerns so that they can assess your needs and provide appropriate care.

CHAPTER 7: TOOLS

Although tools may not be as essential as food or water, we should consider them and gather them over the years. We will not mention every single tool in this chapter, which would be redundant and require a lengthy list, but we will talk about the common ones that might help you in a survival situation.

One last note regarding tools is their maintenance. You must have the means to fix or maintain your tools, mainly because you can't just go to the shop and grab a new one. Ensure you have a few extra handles for axes, hammers, whetstones, and files to sharpen blades. Also, maintaining some of the tools we will discuss may not be as easy as sharpening a knife; an ax, for instance, requires a little more technique. Ideally, you would have already learned how to appropriately maintain your different tools before disaster strikes.

Main Repairs and Basic Tools

If you need repairs done in your home, you won't be able to hire a handyperson. You must complete the task yourself. Tools will vary depending on what you want to fix, but basic tools can usually be adapted to most situations.

Hammers, for example, are one of those tools that are always useful and come in various sizes. Make certain that the hammer is high quality and that the connection between the handle and the head appears solid. Check that it fits comfortably in your hand. It is a good idea to buy at least two hammers to have an extra in case one breaks or goes missing and work on a project with two people.

Adjustable wrenches are also essential; having at least a couple of them on hand will be beneficial.

When it comes to screwdrivers, you should have a variety on hand. Many jobs will be impossible to complete without them.

Pliers are another vital tool. They come in wide varieties, but a ten-inch plus two or three smaller ones are sufficient. Below is an essential list of the tools you will need:

- Hammers
- Screwdrivers
- Wrench sets
- Pliers (at least 2 or 3)
- Duct tape
- Hand saws
- Tape measure
- Flashlight
- If you still have access to power and electricity, a cordless drill will also be helpful.

Demolition Tools

When you think of tools, you think of building something. However, sometimes you need them to take things apart. Getting rid of debris or fallen trees will require a variety of tools, including a framing hammer. The difference between a framing hammer and a regular hammer is that the handle is usually longer, and it is easier to maneuver the straight claw at the back of the head. Having a couple of pry bars of different sizes is also essential, especially if you need to open or destroy something in tight spaces. A ratcheting device with a handle can be extremely useful when you need to move heavy things, and these are usually called come-along wrenches. You might already have them in your basic tool kit.

Cleaning Supplies

Cleaning supplies may not be the first thing that comes to mind when making a list of all the items you'll need in an emergency, but they're pretty important.

Dirt can quickly accumulate in your shelter and degrade your quality of life. Cloths or rags and an all-purpose cleaner should be the first items in your cleaning kit. You are not looking for gleaming floors and sparkling windows, but hygiene is essential and difficult to maintain in an emergency.

If you have carpets in your home, they may be difficult to clean unless you have a carpet sweeper, which cannot be electric. If you have rugs, you can simply beat them outside.

Apart from that, all you need is a dustpan and a broom to keep things tidy. Here's a useful list of cleaning items to add to your kit:

- Cloths or rags
- All-purpose cleaner
- Bleach/vinegar
- Dustpan/broom
- Carpet sweeper (if you have one)

Lighting Tools

Candles and oil lamps can light your home and help you guide yourself at night or if you need them while dealing with an issue. However, as well as being dangerous, they are fairly inefficient compared to other lighting solutions. The best thing you can do is purchase a solar-powered light. They may be slightly more expensive but will provide a safer, more reliable light source.

Alternatively, glow-in-the-dark lights can also help you; however, these lights are not as strong as solar-powered lights but will do well if you intend to mark a path or create more ambiance lighting.

If you have a way to charge batteries, you can get flashlights. Nowadays, you can buy ones that have LED light technology that doesn't consume as much energy, allowing for more hours of light.

Firewood Tools

You may need to build a fire in a fireplace or outside in a fire pit, so you will need some specific supplies. First, you will need a lot of wood, hand saws, and other cutting tools to enable you to cut the wood down to an appropriate size. A bow saw can be helpful with cutting the thicker branches. For the thick logs, you will need at least one good axe. Gardening shears and loppers can come in handy to cut smaller branches, although they are not necessary. The more variety of firewood tools you have, the better because how you cut wood depends on the type of wood and the thickness of the logs and branches you find. You can get the job done quicker and more efficiently if you have the essential tools.

Gear for Protection

When using and carrying tools, particularly sharp tools, the risk of injury is relatively high when you consider that the tools may not be as well maintained as they should be, as well as a potential lack of light or anything related to a disaster, the chances of getting hurt increase.

Accidents happen even when these conditions are met, so we should include protective gear in our survival kits. Safety goggles or glasses, as well as thick gloves, are essential. If something flies into your eye, it will be difficult to locate an eye doctor. The gloves will shield you from any cuts or splinters that may become infected.

If, by any chance, you will be working with sawdust, smoke, or even fumes, you will need to pack some face masks. Ideally, you would be looking at N95 types of masks. Below is a list of helpful protection gear.

- Thick gloves
- Dust mask
- Safety goggles
- Steel-toe boots
- Ear protection (if necessary)

Communication Tools

In a disaster-stricken world, having access to information is extremely valuable. Unable to share or receive information can isolate you, which, aside from being extremely stressful, can be detrimental to long-term survival.

Communication devices, of course, require power, which can be a problem. Because these devices are typically battery-powered, having a supply on hand is critical. Let's take a look at the different communication options available to you.

Two-Way Radio

Two-way radios are similar to the walkie-talkies you used to play with as a kid, and while they have improved significantly since then, they still have drawbacks. For example, their range is limited in comparison to other modes of communication, and any physical obstruction between the two points of communication can cause connection problems.

Two kinds of two-way radios exist: General Mobile Radio Service (GMRS) and Family Radio Service (FRS). These are the various frequencies that radios can operate on. To use GMRS, you must have a license; however, to broadcast on the FRS channels, you do not. Some devices enable you to broadcast on both of these frequencies.

Amateur Radio

An amateur radio, also known as a ham radio, is one of the most useful tools for long-distance communication. You will need a license, but you should strongly consider getting one because amateur radio operators are excellent at sharing information, particularly during times of crisis. There are ham operators in every state and county; you can contact some of them to help you get started. Furthermore, by becoming acquainted with the local ham operator community, you can easily establish communications with them in a crisis.

Shortwave Radio

These shortwaves can travel across the entire world and are great ways to understand what is happening in other countries and to have an unbiased vision of what is happening in your own country. Having a shortwave receiver can be helpful in an emergency, especially a long-term one.

Health Tools

Living off-grid allows us to be more in tune with the natural world and its rhythms and patterns. Unfortunately, this may also imply that we are exposed to more germs. The following items should be included in your first aid box, in addition to the usual supply of plasters and sterile dressings:

- **Antiseptics:** These work by slowing the rate at which germs grow or infect the area where they are applied. For example, if you plan to do some woodworking, you should apply antiseptic to your hands to reduce the risk of illness if your skin becomes damaged. When used as directed, bar soap dissolves viral membranes and cleanses the hands of harmful germs. Hands should be washed with soap regularly.
- **Tweezers:** They're great for removing makeup and facial hair, as well as splinters and ingrown hairs. A straightforward yet fully functional, multifunctional health tool. Being in good health is important for more than just illness prevention. Off-grid dwellers almost always have to spend significant time working with their hands. If performed without the proper equipment, this work may be harmful to the body over time.
- **Safety Glasses:** Never leave your eyes to change what they see. The most important thing you can do is get into the habit of wearing safety glasses whenever possible.
- **Earmuffs:** The sound of hammering, sawing, and using power tools generally may not appear loud at first. However, cumulative noise pollution may harm your hearing over time. Earmuffs, like safety glasses, should be worn daily.
- **Fire Extinguisher:** You will be disadvantaged if a fire breaks out unexpectedly while living off the grid. In such a case, you'll need to extinguish the fire as soon as possible. Remember that you must choose the appropriate fire extinguisher for the fire most likely to develop.

Everyday Tools

Your off-grid existence may be made or broken by your daily equipment. It is essential to consider them and to do so thoroughly. For example, although wearing walking boots may appear unimportant, the danger of damage is greatly increased.

- **Chainsaws:** For obvious reasons, these motorized beasts are excellent for clearing brush and trees and chopping firewood.
- **Work Gloves:** It is critical to obtain high-quality gloves, preferably several pairs. Choose a long-lasting, well-insulated, and comfortable brand, and you will save your hands from the agony of blisters and pains for many years.
- **Walking Shoes:** A good pair of hiking boots have an average lifespan of ten years. The best ones have steel toes, are insulated, and are chemical and cold-weather resistant. If you're doing a lot of physical labor, like chopping and transporting wood, you should consider wearing steel toes to keep your feet from being crushed by a board.
- **Bicycles:** These are so cleverly designed that our forefathers and mothers will almost certainly be riding them thousands of years from now. They are easy to repair when they break down, are eco-friendly, and never run out of gas. For those who need to get somewhere quickly, a bicycle is an excellent mode of transportation.
- **Solar Energy:** The Sun provides limitless, renewable, and cost-free energy. Do you think it's reasonable? Even briefcase-sized solar panels can now be purchased to charge your batteries, power your phone, and heat water for a quick shower in four hours or less.

- **A Knife or Multipurpose Tools:** Examples are a Swiss army knife or Leatherman tool. These are essential for making tasks easier when the worst happens. A sharp tool that allows you to quickly complete tasks like chopping wood, setting traps, or opening food cans can make a huge difference. A knife or multirole is also helpful for self-defense, so keep one on hand at all times.

In any situation, hand protection is essential for comfort and safety. Gloves protect your hands from cuts, scrapes, abrasions, and the elements. Make sure you have a good pair of waterproof gloves if you need them for the weather conditions you're anticipating or even for dirty tasks like gathering firewood or cleaning fish and game.

In an emergency, a quality first-aid kit is critical for your health and your family's health. Bandages, gauze, and antibiotic ointment should be included. As well as other equipment to keep you healthy and safe. Ensure you have enough medicine if you or another family member sustains an injury.

Medicine is essential regardless of the situation you are preparing for. Stock up on aspirin, ibuprofen, and antacids for any aches and pains you may experience. Take any medication only when necessary to ensure that it lasts as long as possible.

Staying informed about emergencies or learning about local weather conditions requires a radio to pick up AM, FM, and shortwave bands. You could even pick up a shortwave radio in an emergency and listen in on other countries. Many shortwave radios can be used as flashlights or power sources.

Flashlights are essential in any situation, from navigating the dark to finding your belongings during an emergency evacuation. Make sure you have flashlights in every room of your home and that they all work when you need them the most.

When the power goes out, portable power is essential for keeping electronics charged. Car chargers are crucial for keeping your cell phone or other portable devices charged in an emergency. You can also use a solar-powered charger to keep your batteries and devices charged while traveling, ensuring that you always have access to information from radio stations or electronic devices such as your GPS.

A compass is necessary for navigation. Because the earth's magnetic field points north, it can be used to determine which way to go if you get lost or need to navigate around obstacles during an emergency.

Headlamps are helpful in inclement weather and can also be used to illuminate rooms, paths, and other areas when it is dark outside.

Waterproof bags are essential for keeping your belongings dry, particularly if you must evacuate your home. They can also be used to keep electronics dry when traveling and need to protect them from water.

A watch or wristwatch is vital for helping you keep track of the time, especially during emergencies when it may be challenging to know what time it is. It will also help you keep up with the past and understand how many days have passed since the disaster occurred or after it was announced. In addition, wrist watches can be used as tools for survival in an emergency.

CHAPTER 8: FOOD AND WATER

Water

In a Survival Situation, How Do You Store Water?

You can go for a few days without food in an emergency, but your body requires water to function properly. If you don't have access to safe drinking water, you may become dehydrated and suffer from various medical issues, making it difficult to defend yourself against looters. Keeping several gallons of safe drinking water in your pantry or basement can ensure you have enough for everyone in your home during a disaster.

To keep drinking water fresher for longer, only store it in food-grade plastic containers with sealed lids. For best results, clean your containers with dish soap and thoroughly rinse them before refilling them. If you don't have enough clean containers for your entire water supply, you can store them in many gallons before moving them into buckets.

Purchase commercially packaged drinking water rather than tap water to ensure consistent quality and safety. If you're concerned about tap water's safety, you should purchase a reverse osmosis filter.

Keep a manual can opener and other equipment with your food storage containers to make it easier for you and many others in your household to enjoy the contents of your pantry.

As an added precaution, keep multiple water purification pills on hand so you can always mix safe drinking water with contaminated or suspicious water sources if necessary. These pills can also clean the plastic container that holds your drinking water before refilling it.

Even if you grow your fruits and vegetables, know how to hunt in a survival situation, and have a sufficient water supply in your pantry or basement. You should still have enough food to avoid going outside during a crisis.

Following the suggestions presented here should have no trouble keeping yourself and your family completely self-sufficient. Keep protein, carbohydrates, fiber, antioxidants, fat, vitamins, minerals, and cholesterol-boosting foods on hand. Foods with a long expiration date, such as dried fruit or canned goods, should be kept near the bottom of your storage shelves so you can use the freshest ingredients first.

As with any type of emergency, gather as much information as possible before a disaster occurs.

The amount of water you need to store depends on the individual. There are a lot of factors that will determine how much water you should have stored. Each person has a different weight and level of activity, which impacts how much they drink daily. People who live in warm climates drink more than those who live in colder temperatures. Also, the more people you have in your household, the more water you will need to store.

How to Purify Water?

To cleanse the water you collect in the wilderness, you may employ a few methods using only a few resources. Boiling is one of the safest and simplest methods. Of course, you'll need the appropriate equipment to heat the water. In the best-case scenario, you'll have a portable stove and a heat-resistant metal container. It is a good rule of thumb to allow your water to boil for at least 5 minutes and then to cool entirely before drinking it.

Another common choice is purification tablets. Simply drop a couple of tables into the water and wait about 20 minutes before serving. Iodin or chlorine may be found in tablets. While this method is simple and inexpensive, it does not provide the best results. You may use a flavored powder mix to cover up the unusual taste of water.

Another option is to use purification pumps to filter your water. Numerous brands specialize in camping equipment that you may find at stores that specialize in camping equipment. These pumps will come in handy if you come across any polluted water in the woods. The filter purifies the water, making it safe to drink. The system includes charcoal particles that absorb dirt and debris while eliminating pollutants. You may also get a more advanced water bottle with filtration for easier use.

There are other methods to filter water if you don't have access to these technologies. First, remove any visible debris, such as sticks, dirt, leaves, or visible live creatures. Examine your surroundings for filtering materials such as pebbles, sand, charcoal, and a piece of fabric from your clothes. These items may be used to make your water filter. Allow time for visible debris to float to the surface to remove when you first collect water.

Place your towel on top of a container, then add the pebbles you discovered before pouring the water on top of them. The pebbles act as a filtration system, catching any large particles. Then, to collect finer debris, repeat the process using sand as the filtering material. Crushed charcoal is better, but you won't always have access to it outdoors. The best way to filter foreign materials and improve water taste is to use charcoal. You may make charcoal by lighting a campfire and covering it with ash and earth until it cools down. You may then smash it and use it as a filter, but be sure to run the water through it many times to ensure proper purification.

If possible, make a multi-layer filter by cutting fabric into pieces and layering pebbles in the first layer, sand in the second layer, and charcoal in the third layer. You'll notice the water becoming clearer as you repeat the process. If you don't have one, bamboo shoots may be used to make one. Any hollowed bark may be used as a container. Remember that you should only use these strategies in extreme cases if you must remain dehydrated. There is a chance of becoming sick no matter how careful you are while filtering your water, so only use it in an emergency.

Food

Best Foods for a Bug-Out Bag

You might be forced to leave your home and 'bug out' in the wilderness. If you find yourself in this situation, you do not want to carry a backpack full of heavy canned goods.

In situations like these, you must prioritize calorie intake over everything else. Consider the quantity and type of food you bring. The most important thing you'll need is water. After all, you can only go three days without water, but you can go thirty days without food. Bring a water filter and a water collection device if you encounter water in the wilderness.

However, you should ensure you have enough food for the duration of your "bug out." That means two meals per day plus snacks for each person, plus an extra day or two in case things don't go as planned. Keeping your bag as light as possible necessitates careful food selection, and freeze-dried and dehydrated foods are some of the best options. These are typically light in weight but high in nutrition and calories.

Consider the following foods:

- **Dry Pasta:** This requires only boiling water and a pinch of salt and weighs very little.
- **Dehydrated Food:** Any food that only requires water will work well, but keep in mind how much extra water you will need to carry.
- **Peanut Butter:** Peanut butter is high in protein, and a little goes a long way; jars are too heavy, so opt for single-serve packets.
- **Pouches of Meat, such as Chicken, Tuna, and Spam:** These are high in protein and easy to transport.
- **Rice:** While small bags of rice aren't particularly heavy, buying boil-in-the-bag rice is a better option; simply add water and a pinch of salt, boil it up, and top with pouched meat for a nutritious filling meal.
- **Dried Fruit and Nuts:** These are great for snacking but won't last long in hot weather.
- **Instant Coffee:** In some stores, single-serve sachets with creamer and sugar are available; simply add hot water for a tasty alternative to water.

These items require a little hot water to make a filling meal. They also take up little space, weigh little, and come in various flavors.

Don't forget that "bugging out" means getting from one point to the next as quickly as possible. That means choosing foods that require the minimum preparation and cooking so you don't need to carry heavy cooking equipment. Choose foods that require the minimum prep, preferably those you can eat raw or just add hot water to.

Best Foods to Stockpile

Providing your body with the necessary fuel during a disaster is vastly different from an everyday diet. You'll be spending more energy than usual, so you'll need to eat high-energy, high-protein foods. If the emergency is related to a disease such as the COVID-19 pandemic, you'll need to eat nutritious foods to maintain good health. Since you'll only be able to keep a limited food supply, it is best to have a small supply of high-end foods.

What to Keep on Hand

The following foods are non-perishable or close enough with lengthy expiration dates, so you can keep them on hand for long periods, even if it's not disaster season. Remember to keep a list of everything in your food stockpile and check the expiration dates every six to twelve months to keep things fresh.

- **Peanut Butter**

This is a high-energy food that also contains healthy fats and protein. You won't need to refrigerate the peanut butter once it's opened unless the jar says otherwise. Peanut butter that is low in sodium and gluten-free is the best option because it can meet various needs while not increasing thirst.

- **Crackers with Whole-Wheat Flour**

This is an excellent substitute for bread, which can mold and become stale. If you need to make sandwiches, crackers are a great substitute. Whole-wheat crackers, on the other hand, have a shorter shelf life than plain crackers due to their higher fat content. When you're hungry, however, you need more fiber. You can keep the crackers fresher for longer by vacuum packing them.

- **Trail Mixes and Nuts**

These are essential high-energy foods. They are nutritious and can also be beneficial for snacking during or after an emergency. If possible, buy them in vacuum-packed containers to keep the nuts from oxidizing and losing their freshness.

- **Cereal**

Choose multigrain cereals with individual packaging to avoid them going stale once opened.

- **Granola and Energy Bars**

These are both filling and nutritious. They typically keep fresh for at least six months when used as a portable snack. They are also a good source of carbohydrates, which provide you with more energy without requiring you to eat a lot of food. You can also get them in a variety of flavors to please everyone.

- **Fruits Dried**

This option can provide potassium and dietary fiber when fresh fruit is unavailable. This provides both calories and nutrients.

- **Meat or Fish in a Can**

These can often be stored in the pantry for two years and provide an essential source of protein after a disaster. The vacuum-packed pouches have a shorter shelf life, but they can still last up to six months. However, the pouches may take up less space and do not require a can opener.

- **Vegetables in Cans**

If you cannot obtain fresh vegetables during or after an emergency, canned vegetables will still provide you with the essential nutrients you require. Keep a variety of vegetables on hand to ensure a variety of healthy vitamins and minerals.

- **Soups and Chili in Cans**

These can often be eaten straight from the can and provide a variety of nutrients. To avoid increasing your thirst after a disaster, choose a low-sodium option.

- **Pasta Sauce and Dry Pasta**

These are carbohydrate-heavy and gluten-filled, but they are a filling option. Furthermore, dry pasta and jarred sauce can be stored for months. If you or your family has dietary restrictions, consider gluten-free pasta or pasta made from a different material.

- **Water in Bottles**

You should try keeping at least three days' worth of water. This equates to at least one gallon per person per day. A typical active person consumes at least a half-gallon of water per day. You'll also need at least another half-gallon per person daily for food and washing. You can also buy a case of water with added essential minerals and electrolytes to help with hydration and improve the taste.

- **Sports Drinks**

Sports drinks contain electrolytes and carbohydrates, which can help you rehydrate and replenish yourself when water is scarce. Be careful not to add too many additives, such as sugar or artificial sweeteners.

- **Milk Powder**

Except for powdered milk, nearly all dairy products must be refrigerated. This is an excellent calcium and vitamin D substitute if you don't have access to fresh milk.

- **Salt, Pepper, and Sugar**

If you have a propane or charcoal stove to prepare your food after a disaster, you will most likely be cooking it. If you keep a basic supply of seasonings and sweeteners, you can improve the flavor of fresh and packaged foods.

- **Multivitamins**

Supplements are important because they can replace nutrients you usually consume through your diet but may be in short supply after a disaster. Vitamins don't need to be boring so if needed, consider purchasing fruity gummies or other vitamin types. Choose a vitamin that has a whole day's worth of vitamins and, if possible, even omega 3s and folate, so you have complete coverage.

Food Production

Keep in mind that we're talking about long-term survival preparation. You may have to save those seeds and sow them across many seasons. Make a list of the veggies you and your family consume daily to begin starting. Add any vegetables you haven't tried yet but would be willing to try to the list. Then conduct your research, determine which garden crops thrive in your location, and stock up on seed packs. Also, don't wait till a collapse to get your hands dirty. Begin with modest garden beds or perhaps a few container gardens right now. You'll almost certainly make errors, and it's better to learn from them now than later when it counts most.

Raising food animals is another something to think about. Rabbits, chickens, and even goats will thrive in a limited space. However, unlike gardening, this isn't something you can start doing at any time. You won't be able to stroll to the feed store and pick up a few chicks to raise for Sunday meals after the grid goes down. On the other hand, a half-dozen hens will keep you in eggs and fresh meat for a long time if you start now.

Foraging for Edibles in the Wild

Outside the extreme northern and southern reaches of the earth, wild edibles can be found almost anywhere. Learning what foods can be foraged in your area, on the other hand, takes time and effort. Once you've mastered the art of identifying plants, experiment with incorporating them into your regular meals on occasion. This will assist you in determining which ones are compatible with your palate and digestive system.

Trapping, Hunting, and Fishing

These pastimes are frequently the foundation of a person's long-term survival strategy. Some survivalists believe hiking a few times per week will keep their pantry stocked. This could work for people who live in the middle of nowhere, off the beaten path. The competition will be fierce for those living in cities, suburbs, or even small villages. Forests will be quickly depleted, and small lakes will be fished out. We're not saying you should abandon all efforts to supplement your diet with wild game. What we mean is that this should not be your primary strategy.

Trapping

This is the least energy-intensive of the three options for obtaining wild meat. Traps will work for you 24 hours a day, seven days a week, but you must check them regularly. If you take this route, we recommend checking all traps at least once daily. While you don't want to spend hours going over your trap path, possibly disturbing the wildlife you're trying to catch, you also don't want another predator (on two or four legs) to discover your catch before you do.

Fishing

On a calm day, a few things are more relaxing than lying on the beach with a line in the water. The goal here, however, is not leisure; it is to fill stomachs. Increase your chances of success by using trotlines and automated fishing reels. Trotlines are a type of fishing where multiple lines are in the water at the same time. They are usually found in rivers or streams rather than lakes or ponds. A rope or cable is stretched straight across the river from one bank to the other. At regular intervals along the journey, smaller lines known as snoods drop into the water. At the end of each snood is a baited hook. Add weight to each snood if you're fishing in fast-moving rivers or streams to keep the bait from rising to the surface. The snoods must not come into contact with one another. This can be avoided by separating them based on their length.

Hunting

Those of you who go fishing or spend a lot of time outside may have noticed that the tactics we've discussed thus far, such as trotlines and snares, aren't always permitted in today's world, at least not in most places. We do not recommend that anyone risk provoking the wrath of their local government. However, if the type of long-term tragedy we're discussing occurs, such regulations will likely become obsolete. In reality, by removing certain current constraints, you may receive helpful recommendations and suggestions to improve your chances of success.

Remember that you may not want to focus all of your hunting efforts on large games such as deer. Sure, a single shot may grab a large amount of flesh, but you must have a technique to preserve that meat, or it will go to waste. Our advice is to be ready to hunt everything you come across, from squirrels to deer.

Look for Edible Flowers, Nuts, Fruits, and Berries

Most people stuck in a forest with a survival situation often start their food search by looking for small animals. Protein is important for survival, but plants are prevalent and have more nutrition to help you sustain yourself in those critical times. You need to look for the flora or edible flowers first. The barks of trees and grasses are highly edible, but the first approach should always be to look for flowers because recognizing their edibility is quite prominent.

If you are an adventurer or explorer, it is evident that you know some basic wild nuts, flowers, and plants. The knowledgeable resources are the easiest to access at any time. All the adventurers should get a handbook of edible plants and flowers they will find in the wild. It is for their safety and research purposes to have access to the knowledge on which plants they can eat. The nuts, berries, fruits, and other edibles can give you the nutrition you need until you find other potent satiations.

You will find different berries in the wild, but you cannot just pluck all of them and eat them. If you do not know which berries you should eat, you should at least know which ones to avoid! Some of the berries of plants you need to avoid are holly, Yew, Dogwood, and Pokeweed. You can count on eating gooseberries, mulberries, muscadine, elderberries, and others.

Methods of Preserving and Keeping Food

Drying/Dehydration

This technique is precisely what it sounds like. It will prevent the food from deteriorating if it is dried and removed from the environment. It will also keep it edible for far longer than it would usually be if it were eaten while it was still fresh. If you don't have a smoker, you may use a store-bought one; if you don't want to smoke your food at home, you can use an oven on a low heat setting or a dehydrator. Certain fruits and vegetables, such as different peppers, bananas, berries, apples, and so on, are particularly well suited to this procedure. It is also a fantastic technique for making jerky out of whatever cut of meat you want, and it will help you get more use out of your food supply over time.

Root Cellars/Cold Storage

Ideally, this should be a cold and dry environment. There are several options for storage, including an unheated cellar or pantry, a hole excavated into the earth, or any other location where you can guarantee that the food remains cold and dry to ensure that it stays fresh for a longer period. One should only use this technique for root vegetables, but it also works well with other foods such as dry maize, beans, onions, and potatoes.

Canning/Preserving

This is a popular technique, and people use it to produce and preserve a broad range of goods, ranging from jams and jellies to salsa and preserved fruits, among many others. There are many methods for canning foods, each of which requires its own set of materials and is best suited for various foods. High-acid foods should be canned in a water bath or steam can, whereas low-acid foods should be canned using a pressure canner.

Pickling

The technique we're discussing is vinegar pickling since it is the most popular and easiest. To put it another way, it's just soaking your food in vinegar to preserve it. That's all there is to it. During this process, however, you may include spices, sugar, herbs, and other ingredients to make your unique mix. Cucumbers of various sizes, especially tiny ones, are the most popular pickled food, but people also pickle carrots, eggs, beets, and even meats. Due to the strong acidity produced by the vinegar, bacteria cannot develop, and your food will remain safe to consume for an extended period.

Pasteurization

The hygiene of your milking process is critical. Pasteurization isn't necessary for raw milk to be safe and nutritious; nevertheless, you'll need to be meticulous about barn cleanliness if you want this to happen. You may simply pasteurize your milk on the stovetop if you so choose. For 35 minutes, heat your milk to 140 degrees Fahrenheit in a stainless steel boiler. The milk will be ready after 35 minutes, so place it in an ice bath and let it sit there for the remainder of the time. Stir the milk continuously until it reaches a temperature of 40 degrees Fahrenheit (4.4 degrees Celsius).

Freezing

It's a very straightforward process. You can freeze nearly anything, but certain things will work better if you do a little prep work ahead of time. Most veggies may be blanched before frozen, which is a good option. As a result, they will remain fresher in appearance and taste. Blanching most vegetables requires three minutes of boiling, followed by an instant cold bath. When it comes to frozen foods, most meats and fruits may be left as is, but for long-term preservation, you may wish to freeze them in smaller quantities on cookie sheets first. The amount of freezer space you have and your ability to purchase more freezer units are factors to consider, but even a modest chest freezer may offer enough capacity to store various delectable foods.

Fermentation

Because it is a safe food preservation technique, fermentation has been around since the dawn. Chopped vegetables in salty brine, stored in jars or porcelain crocks, can keep for a month or more. Jars that are kept at a lower temperature will survive even longer. Fermented foods have the additional benefit of being a great source of probiotics, which will aid in the development of excellent gut health and provide a welcome boost to the immunity of those who consume them. You can lacto-ferment just about any vegetable.

Salting

Salt curing meat is a fantastic method to preserve meat for a lengthy period without electricity. Settlements and ship crews used this method to preserve slaughtered meats throughout the year in the olden days. It is still practiced today. You may keep raw meat at room temperature for months by coating it with salt, draining it, and hanging it to age for approximately two weeks.

CONCLUSION

Thank you for reading this book. Off-grid living isn't for everyone, but prepping is. In this day and age, being prepared is critical. After all, we live in a time when things have been so good for so long that the wheel has finally turned.

Disasters happen to everyone. Some are significant, affecting millions, if not billions, of people worldwide. Some are smaller, affecting only a single city, neighborhood, or household. Like everyone else, you will likely go through at least one of these. The only difference between you and others is that you can plan ahead of time.

Being ready is more than just a state of mind. It is being prepared to deal with whatever comes your way. A good prepper is ready in the event of a car breakdown, a pandemic, a blizzard, or the breakdown of law and order.

A good prepper knows that if a blizzard forces them to stay inside their homes for a week, they will have enough food, water, toilet paper, and energy sources to cook and heat their homes.

Natural disasters can devastate infrastructure, and human life is impacted in various ways. Worse, most people who are affected by disasters are unprepared. In other cases, they are unsure how to respond effectively in an emergency. The good news is that you can access this comprehensive beginner's risk preparation and management guide. We created this helpful workbook with people like you in mind.

When disasters strike unexpectedly, most people panic and become confused; as a result, some may unnecessarily lose their lives over something that could have been avoided. When you read this survival workbook, you will realize that saving your life and the lives of your loved ones is not that difficult.

You can be there to see what happens next if you plan ahead of time. I told you we survivalists and preppers are optimists!

A good prepper keeps a bug-out bag in their car, a family member's house, and another location away from home. They can survive in the wild for several days with this, regardless of the conditions. Good luck.

THE PREPPER'S SURVIVAL MEDICINE BIBLE

5 in 1

The Most Complete Guide to the U.S. Army Procedures for Emergency Preparedness

Tyler Gordon

INTRODUCTION

Preppers are people who plan for the worst-case scenario. Preparing for the worst allows you to deal with any problems more confidently. If you are prepared, you will know what you are putting into your body and can avoid things that may harm you. This can help protect your current health as well as your long-term health.

As a prepper, you know that growing and producing your own medicine is just as important as being able to source food. When leaving your home is dangerous, or western medicine is completely unavailable, you must have a backup plan or medicines on hand. Treating minor ailments such as a toothache may imply, at best, avoiding a painful period in which you are unable to eat, lose weight, or feel happy due to constant pain. In the worst-case scenario, you may become toxic or even die from a severe infection.

If you're a prepper, you understand the value of planning ahead of time and having backup systems for critical systems. You understand the importance of gardening, preserving food, and storing seeds for the following year.

On the other hand, the medical aspect of prepping is frequently overlooked. What if you become ill or injured and no expert medical help is available? Could you meet the healthcare needs of yourself and your loved ones if our health-care system became overburdened or cut off after resupply?

Preppers frequently begin with a well-stocked first-aid kit, then supplement with non-prescription drugs in bulk, such as pain relievers, antibiotic ointments, and cough syrups. Many people even go so far as to use fish antibiotics.

While I keep all these materials on hand, there are disadvantages to using only conventional biomedical supplies. Supplies will eventually run out or outlive their shelf life, and there will be no way to replenish them. There is no treatment strategy for chronic disease or severe pain; the only options are over-the-counter medications. Antibiotics, whether fish or otherwise, steady decline in the fight against drug-resistant bacteria. As part of their well-planned survival strategy, preppers require a continuous supply of effective medications that they can make and duplicate.

Preppers also require a method to diagnose disease and injury without laboratories and diagnostics. One method is to incorporate natural remedies into an emergency preparedness strategy.

While there are numerous reasons to choose natural remedies, prepper concerns make natural medicine especially valuable.

Simply put, the main reason to use natural medicine is its work. It is used worldwide because it works and has done so for millennia. Thousands of studies demonstrating the utility of medications and alternative medicines are free to review at www.PubMed.gov.

Understanding what herbs you already have in your kitchen and what they can do to optimize and assist your health and ailments. Understanding what herbs and spices are available to treat other more severe conditions, how to use them, and even grow them could be a future survival decision.

This book is aimed at the beginning or low-level preppers who want to learn the fundamentals and what is easily accessible because it can be overwhelming at first.

There is something for everyone, from discovering that a simple cup of tea can help your immune system to the more complicated system of companion planting herbs to maximize the life and health of the plants.

For example, to relieve irritable bowel syndrome cut an aloe vera leaf and rub it on sunburn. You can also flavor your coffee with spice powder. Even if the worst-case scenario does not occur, knowing how to treat simple health issues may allow you to save money. Begin your self-sustaining journey into natural herbalism with this gentle overview of a preppers herb and spice medicine cabinet.

BOOK 1: THE PREPPER'S HOME PHARMACY

Your list of home remedies is about to become a lot more interesting. Even though these natural herbs have been used for hundreds of years, doctors and scientists now recommend that they be used for healing. Traditional healing methods can easily replace these natural medical resources. To name a few, some plants can heal and reduce cholesterol, high blood pressure, and arthritis pain. Some of the best healing herbs can even treat cancer cells and help alcoholics quit drinking.

Herbs, other natural remedies, and natural medical resources are just as effective as conventional treatments. They can be even more effective and have no adverse side effects. Here are some of the most effective natural medical resources. These super healers and your favorite recipes can be added to your herbal medicine or natural medicine cabinet. Some of them can benefit your body if you include them in your daily routine.

CHAPTER 1: THE PROCESS OF MAKING HERBAL MEDICINES AT HOME

The best time to collect herbs is when they are at their height in terms of flavor and scent. The ideal time to collect a plant component depends on what you are harvesting and how you want to use it. A herb may be harvested as long as enough foliage is on the plant to sustain it. Annual herbs can be pruned to 60% to 70% of their original size without harming their growth. Trimming one-third of perennial herbs at a time is required. To make precise cuts, use a sharpened knife or pruners.

Harvesting is best done early in the morning when the crops have dried out but before it becomes too hot. Take your herbs before they begin to flower to get the most out of them. Remove the blossoms from the plant as soon as they appear to continue harvesting leaves.

Ensure the plants have not been sprayed with pesticides before collecting herb leaves. Certain pesticides and fungicides have been banned from being used on plants meant for human food, including herbs.

The world is taking chances on pharmaceutical medications and is ready to surrender completely to what chemical formulations offer. Indeed, conventional or pharmaceutical medications work well upon critical symptoms. Still, they should not be your immediate approach when the symptoms are mild or you intend to take preventative measures for specific conditions.

Herbal remedies or solutions should be used to strengthen your bodily functions and give them the ability to fight viruses and bacteria that infiltrate your body and weaken you. People who use chemically formulated medications for such preventative measures eventually develop a dependency. You might get the impression that your body's ability to fight diseases is directly proportional to the number of pills you take.

Ingredients

Some other supplies are difficult to replicate at home. You must acquire the necessary supplies and not wait until the last minute to create a stock of needed medicine. For example, if you want to make capsules at home, you'll need to buy them. When properly stored, they last a long time. Furthermore, they are inexpensive, allowing you to stock up on several years' worth of capsules. Even if manufacturing or distribution services are disrupted, you will have the necessary ingredients to make the required medicine.

Herbs

If you have harvested fresh herbs, ensure you preserve them right away. There are two ways to preserve herbs: maceration and drying. To macerate herbs, you need to steep them in a solvent or a menstruum such as vinegar, alcohol, or honey. On the other hand, when it comes to drying, simply leave the herbs out in the sun and let them dry naturally. You can also dehydrate them using a dehydrator or an oven. Ideally, dried herbs are your best bet.

When drying herbs, make sure they are appropriately stored. Mold could form if this is not done. If you notice any mold, throw out the herbs and start over. Consider the health conditions or problems you want to treat before growing, purchasing, or storing herbs. The type of herbs you require will also vary depending on their occurrence.

Alcohol

Alcohol has many applications, from dulling pain to disinfecting wounds and extracting therapeutic compounds from natural ingredients. Distilled grain alcohol is the best choice for making tinctures. Alcohol aids in the rapid absorption of herbal remedies into the bloodstream, which is critical in an emergency. It aids in extracting alkaloids, balsams, resins, and other active compounds from non-water-soluble plant materials. It also extends the shelf life of herbal medications. There are various types of alcohol, and the strength of each varies. Grain alcohol, vodka, brandy, and wine are the most common types of alcohol to stock up on.

Vinegar

Humans have used vinegar since the olden days. Leftover wine makes vinegar, typically made from apple cores and peels. Vinegar can be used as an alcohol substitute when making tinctures, and such tinctures are known as acetum. Herbal vinegar can be used to rinse laundry, wash hair, and even as medicine. Apple cider vinegar is the most common type used in natural medicine. Because it contains acetic acid, it can also be used to clean surfaces. To be effective as a disinfectant, the vinegar must contain at least 5% acetic acid. You can buy apple cider vinegar or make it yourself.

Bentonite Clay

This beneficial ingredient aids in the removal of toxins from the skin and gut. It works through a process similar to absorption known as adsorption. The molecules, ions, and atoms in the body or face stick to the surface of the clay rather than being drawn out by it during adsorption. The adsorption level is proportional to the available surface space. There are two types of bentonite clay, and they are calcium and sodium bentonite. Calcium bentonite is preferable for demineralization, whereas sodium bentonite aids in toxin leaching.

Kaolin Clay

Kaolin clay is popularly known as China clear and is commonly used in facial masks. Kaolin clay is a critical ingredient in Quick bandages used to stop bleeding in case of emergencies. A simple DIY version of a quick clot bandage is to pour kaolin clay directly on the wound. Another wonderful thing about this product is it doesn't have any shelf-life expiry.

Activated Charcoal

Activated charcoal, like bentonite and kaolin clays, leaches out toxins. The tiny pores on its surface enhance its ability to draw out more toxins. This is different from regular charcoal. The term activated charcoal refers to the fact that this charcoal was explicitly created to draw or pull toxins out. By sucking out toxins from stings and bites, activated charcoal can treat intestinal infections and ingested poisons. Activated charcoal is said to be capable of absorbing up to 4000 different types of poisons. Activated charcoal capsules should be in your first aid kit.

Salts

Epsom salts are required whether you make salt scrubs or bath salts. Epsom salts have a high mineral concentration and give your body its daily magnesium dose. Bath salts can be infused with herbs, oils, and even essential oils, which are released when the salts are mixed with warm water. Bath salts can be customized to reduce pain, soothe nerves, relieve flu symptoms, and promote general relaxation. Epsom salt and regular table salt are not the same things. So, if a recipe calls for Epsom salts, don't try to make it with table salt.

Basic Equipment

You will need basic equipment to make natural medicine at home. Consider the items on this list to be a one-time investment. You may also already have some of the necessary equipment.

Containers

You will need to store the medicine once you have learned how to make it. As a result, you will require various types of containers. The best option is to use glassware. Glassware is not only reusable but also the safest option because none of the ingredients listed above can interact with it. It does not leach into your herbal formulas and is not harmful. To store tinctures, use Mason jars or opaque and dark-colored bottles with a rubber bulb and flint jars to store salves, lotions, balms, and creams.

Capsules and Capsule Machine

The most convenient way to consume dried herbs, powdered mushrooms, or even activated charcoal is in medicine capsules. This makes natural remedies easier to take and effectively masks their unpleasant taste. Natural medicine capsules are an easy and affordable way to make and store natural medicine. Simply take the capsule apart, fill it with powder, and put it back together.

For example, bladderwrack is a nutritious seaweed with an unpleasant taste and odor. It contains a lot of iodine, but the odor and flavor make it challenging to consume. You can consume it without worrying about the taste by converting it into a capsule. Consider purchasing a small capsule machine in addition to the capsule shells. This straightforward device allows you to fill multiple capsules simultaneously and achieve more consistent results. Select a machine based on the size of the capsules you intend to produce. A capsule machine can be purchased for under $20.

Pestle and Mortar

A coffee grinder, mortar, and pestle can be used to grind the desired ingredients into powders. Powdering dried herbs or other ingredients will take longer if you use a mortar and pestle, but this is a simple and inexpensive instrument and a traditional herbal tool. You can also do this with a coffee grinder. It will only take a few seconds to powder the ingredient, but the results will not be as fine as with a mortar and pestle.

Scale

It is best to measure the ingredients you use for the best results. Whether you're making a lotion or a salve, it's always a good idea to measure. A scale will come in handy here. A small scale helps measure specific amounts of fats, beeswax, or other similar substances. Choose a non-electronic scale that runs on batteries, if possible. Don't forget to keep a supply of batteries on hand as well.

Blender

In addition to the mortar and pestle, a blender is required. Any liquid can be emulsified with the help of a blender. Combining a soluble liquid with a non-soluble liquid is known as emulsification. This is the method by which the lotion is created. The ingredients for a lotion can be whisked by hand, but it takes a lot of elbow grease. To make this process easier, invest in an inversion blender.

Funnel

A wide-mouth funnel can be used to fill any bottles or containers, such as mason jars. This reduces the likelihood of spills and makes cleaning easier.

Strainer

If you have any filters at home, you can use them to make natural remedies and medicine. A traditional tea ball mesh strainer or one that resembles a basket that sits on the cup's rim will also suffice. On the other hand, Muslin and cheesecloth can be used as natural strainers.

Labels

Labeling everything is one of the most critical steps in making herbal remedies or medicine at home. Label the ingredients, the recipes that call for them, and the date they were prepared. As a result, always label your herbal concoctions.

Miscellaneous Items

Apart from all the ingredients, items, and equipment mentioned until now, you will also need basic kitchen essentials such as mixing bowls, spoons, double boilers, measuring spoons and cups, and multiple rubber or silicone spatulas.

Forms of Herbal Medicine

Here are some of the forms of herbal medicines that you should count on making at home and prepare yourselves with good health for any upcoming emergencies:

Tinctures

Tinctures are favorite among other forms of herbal preparations or consumptions. Tinctures are the concentrated form of herbs best used in teas and other medicines. They have a long shelf life, so that you can use them for your survival scenarios. Making tinctures is relatively simple, and they are prevalent among residents for use in their homes.

But remember that the tinctures are incredibly concentrated, so you must know the dosage you intend to administer. If you have any doubts, you can consult with your herbalist and get a dosage schedule. Don't worry; they won't force you to buy their tinctures! Natural medicine experts are relatively open about growing herbs and creating medicinal solutions.

The tincture recipe requires you to make arrangements for alcohol. You can use 80-proof vodka instead! It is okay to purchase the cheapest available in the store. If you are not a drinker and are concerned about what to do with the leftover vodka, you can substitute high-quality apple cider vinegar or glycerin.

Get a pint jar with a tight-fitting lid and plan out the herbs you'll use to make a tincture. Fill the jar with herbs until it is about two-thirds or three-quarters full. If you're using the bark, berries, or roots, pour enough alcohol into the jar to cover the plant material completely. Allow it to sit for 6 to 8 weeks in a dry or cool place. After the period has passed, simply strain the herbs and transfer the filtered solution to amber glass bottles. Your tincture is now complete! You can do the same thing with any herb you grow in your garden or buy in the store.

Capsules

People prefer to drink tea from a capsule rather than a tincture solution. As a result, the herbs can be blended and formed into capsules more effectively. The process is a little complicated, but you can easily prepare herbal capsules with the right equipment and technique.

To make the herbal capsules, you will need gelatin capsules of regular or desirable size. The capsule-making machine will then be required. For your convenience, some machines are sold in conjunction with gelatin capsules. Finally, gather your favorite herbs.

Fill the capsules to the maximum capacity permitted by the capsule machine. It is entirely up to you whether to fill it or leave some space. Make enough for a month to use the capsules as a preventative measure. Make them according to the dosage cycle if it is for a medical condition.

You can also make extra for a long-term plan or an emergency. Fill your mason jars to the brim with capsules. Seal the lids, then add some 100cc oxygen absorber to keep them fresh until you need them again.

The most popular herbal option is Valerian root capsules. You can get up to 1000mg of medicinal content per capsule by filling #00 size capsules with herbs.

Creams for the Skin

There are numerous topical creams and medications available. Balms and salves are great examples of this kind of product. Typically, these herbal topical solutions treat scrapes, cuts, achy muscles, and abrasions. These solutions are made with herbs, oils, and beeswax. They are applied to the skin rather than taken orally.

Herbal salves treat scrapes, abrasions, rashes, cuts, and other skin problems/irritations. Lemon balm, calendula, tea tree, plantain, and other wound-healing herbs may be preferred.

Balms: Balms are well-known for relieving achy muscles, strains, and sprains. Herbs like arnica, comfrey, and others are commonly used to make balm. Muscle pains can sometimes be unbearable at times. As a result, relying on over-the-counter pain relievers or balms should not be the only option. Herbal balms are now taking over as your go-to sprain and strain treatment.

You will need the following ingredients to make a herbal salve or balm:

- 1 to 12 cup herbal oil (infused). You can make your herbal-infused oil at home by combining your favorite herbs.
- 1 ounce of beeswax
- 12-24 drops essential oils to enhance the aroma and medicinal properties

The following is a recipe for a herbal salve:

You'll need the infused oil first. Heat the herbal oil in a double boiler. It is best to heat the oil in a metal bowl. You must melt the beeswax after adding it. Before adding it to your oil, you must first break it up. Stir in the beeswax until it is melted. Turn off the heat for 1 minute. To stir the mixture, add the essential oils to the pot. Pour your hot balm or salve into small tins or jars with care. Amber jars are preferred for protecting and extending the shelf life of the solution. Allow the solution to sit uncovered for a few minutes until the medicine hardens. Put a lid on it and store it in a cool, dry place for a few months. Finally, the balm or salve is complete!

Teas

Teas are one of the simplest and most convenient ways to medicate oneself with herbs. People are familiar with this type of herbal consumption because they have been using teas for a long time for various reasons. Herbal teas work and are simple to make!

The tea is also known as a herbal infusion. It is made through the steeping process of herbs in hot water. This method requires little time to extract the herbal goodness from the fresh or dried plant. You must enjoy it as soon as you begin the making process. The herbal preparation requires you only to use the plant's aerial parts, such as leaves or flowers.

1. Combine 4 to 6 tbsp. of a quart jar of dried herbs to make an infusion or herbal tea.
2. Fill the jar halfway with boiling water and add the dried herbs.
3. Allow the herb to steep for 30 to 45 minutes in the water. The herb used to make the tea determines the steeping time.
4. When the time for waiting or steeping is up, strain the herb and drink the infusion.

The herbal tea will be called a decoction if you use non-aerial parts of the plant, such as bark, roots, and twigs. The herbal solution results from slowly simmering the herbal root on low heat.

1. You'll need 4 to 6 tbsp. 1 quart water and 1 cup of dried herbs in a saucepan.
2. You must bring the solution to a slow boil.
3. Cook for 25 to 45 minutes over medium heat. To reap the health benefits of the herbs, simply strain them and drink the herbal tea.

Infusions

Infusions are made from the plant's delicate parts, such as the leaves and flowers. To make an infusion, the plant parts are steeped in water. To make an infusion, heat water just below boiling, then steep the herbs in it for up to 15 minutes. Put a lid on the container to keep the essential oils in the herbs from evaporating as steam. Infusions typically require a teaspoon of herb per cup of water. If you want it to be stronger, use one tablespoon of the desired herb per cup of water. You can steep it for as little as 15 minutes or overnight.

Alternatively, a French press can also be used for infusion. Place the plant material in the carafe and pour hot water. Place the lid with the plunger on top to prevent evaporation. Once the time is up, press down on the plunger, and the infusion is ready. For single servings, a mesh strainer can be used too.

Sometimes, cold infusions are preferable, especially if you want to extract mucilage from demulcent herbs such as marshmallow root. Any herb that helps reduce inflammation is known as a demulcent herb. The sticky, gooey, and slimy texture of demulcent is due to the mucilage present in it. It lubricates the mucus membranes upon consumption and reduces inflammation.

Decoctions

Decoctions are made from tough plant parts such as roots, seeds, bark, stems, and even dehydrated fruits. In contrast to an infusion, where evaporation is avoided, evaporation is required to make a decoction. A decoction requires two cups of water for every ounce of plant material. Bring the water and plant material mixture to a boil, then reduce to a gentle simmer for another 20 minutes. The decoction is ready when the liquid has been reduced by half. To make a thicker decoction, boil the liquid for a longer period. This produces a double decoction, which is commonly used to make syrup.

The herb ratio is critical when making tisanes, whether infusions or decoctions. You can use a single herb or a combination of herbs. The standard formula uses approximately 70% of the herb that treats the primary health problem, 25% of the herb that supports the primary herb, and the remaining 5-10% of the herbs used to strengthen the tonic or increase its anti-inflammatory properties.

Syrups

You get herbal syrup when single or double decoctions are combined with honey, molasses, glycerin, or even simple syrup. Simple syrup is a solution of sugar in water. Simple syrups are used as sweeteners, particularly in herbal remedies for children, but they have no nutritional or medicinal value. Syrup has a shorter shelf life than acetum, glycerite, or tincture, but honey may extend its shelf life. However, syrup usually spoils within a month. You can extend its shelf life even further by using a double decoction to reduce the total water content in the syrup. Cold infusions can also be used to make syrup. Elderberry syrup, for example, is an age-old remedy for colds, particularly during flu season.

Elixirs

An elixir is created when herbs are macerated in brandy or honey. The combination of these ingredients has a long shelf life. Herbal remedies made with vodka or alcohol-extracted herbs taste much better than elixirs. Aside from that, they work faster than syrups. You can drink an elixir-like syrup, but it is not the same.

Instead of making a decoction, you will macerate herbs to make elixirs. Elixirs contain no water and take 2-6 weeks to complete. On the other hand, Syrups can be made in under an hour. When compared to an elixir, the syrup has less alcohol content. Elixirs can be used to treat a violent cough caused by a condition such as bronchitis. Its alcohol content temporarily relieves coughing while numbing a sore throat. However, you must be mindful of the total alcohol consumed, as excessive consumption can suppress the immune response. If you don't want to drink alcohol, try an oxymel instead of an elixir.

Powders

If you don't mind a little elbow grease and are patient, the traditional method of powdering herbs is to use a mortar and pestle. If this seems too much work, you can use a coffee grinder to powder the herbs. It is more convenient to grind the herbs into a fine powder. You will have a slightly coarse powder regardless of the tools or equipment. Pass this through a fine sieve to obtain a smooth and fine powder. Fine powders, such as baking flour, can only be produced by a flour mill.

When the herbs are powdered and stored, they begin to degrade. Powder the herbs just before using them. Capsules can be made from herb powders. On the other hand, certain powders, such as wound or dusting powder, can be stored and used topically later. Tinctures can also be made from powders, but straining the mixture is difficult. Encapsulation is also a more effective method of consuming powders, especially if the herbs are bitter or have an unpleasant taste. Keep the capsule casings in a cool, dry, and dark place away from direct sunlight after filling them with your preferred herb mixture.

Pastilles

Pastilles are lozenges that are incredibly easy to make. Pastilles are created by combining powdered herbs and liquid. Allow the pastilles to dry for a few weeks after mixing the two ingredients like an electuary. The powder-to-liquid ratio will vary depending on the recipe. When making pastilles, you must pay close attention to the texture. When combined, the ingredients should form a paste that can be shaped into pastilles.

The best way to accomplish this is to incorporate powdered mucilaginous herbs such as slippery elm or marshmallow root. Depending on the purpose of the pastilles, the herb combination will vary. Similarly, there are several options for the pastilles' liquid portion. You can make decoctions, cold infusions, tisanes, or even infused honey to combine with the dried herbs.

Poultice

A poultice is a moistened herb applied topically to a specific area or injury to promote healing and pain relief. Warm the poultice slightly before applying it to the lower back or tight muscles. It can also treat inflammation or sprains when applied to cold. Making a poultice is simple. Begin by heating some water with the necessary herbal powders until a paste forms. The infused water will clump together. Depending on the application, you can use it immediately or let it cool.

Oils With Infusions

The infused oil is any liquid fat infused with one or more herbs. This procedure is similar to the previous section's infusion. Allow the herb to macerate in the oil for a few minutes. Once macerated, the infusion is ready. You can make cold or warm infusions at home. Let us examine both processes.

Fill a jar halfway with your chosen dried herbs, then top with oil. Simply leave the herbs in the oil until they have macerated completely. Allow fresh herbs to wilt slightly to ensure the water content has evaporated. Because water can quickly ruin an infusion, dried herbs are always preferable. Remove any air bubbles by running a knife or other flat utensil along the jar's side. You can always add more if the oil content falls below a certain level. Allow this to macerate in a cool, dark place away from direct sunlight for 2-6 weeks. Meanwhile, gently shake the jar daily to ensure the contents are in good condition. This is how cold infusions are made.

The infusion of herbs into oil can be sped up by heating it gently. One of the reasons why warm infusion is so effective is because of this. A warm infusion aims to gradually warm the oil without cooking it. Fill a slow cooker halfway with plant material, cover with oil, and set the temperature to warm. In a slow cooker, you can only use the warm setting. If you set it too high, the herbs will become fried in the oil, losing their medicinal properties. Instead of a slow cooker, a double boiler can be used to heat the oil infusion indirectly.

Making the infusion, once again, will take up to two weeks. Allow the herbs to soak in the warm oil for up to two hours before macerating for two weeks. Olive oil and coconut oil are ideal for infusion. You can also use grapeseed oil, mainly if the infused oil is applied topically.

CHAPTER 2: THE MOST IMPORTANT MEDICAL HERBS FOR YOUR HOME PHARMACY

Find new ways to incorporate these unusual plants into your daily routine, and you'll be glad you did. The following are some of the essential, naturally occurring medicines that a prepper can use for a variety of injuries and illnesses:

Blackberry

Blackberries are popular not only for their undeniable sweetness but also for their nutritional and medicinal properties. These berries have been known to prevent and cure diarrhea, which can be a major inconvenience when trying to survive in harsh living conditions. When these berries are almost ripe, they are pink, but as soon as they are ripe enough to eat, they turn black.

Besides being useful in treating diarrhea, blackberry leaves can also be used to make homemade mouthwash due to their acidic nature. Because the procedures are the same, the process is simple if you know how to make tea. The fresh blackberry leaves must be immersed in boiling water and steeped for five to ten minutes to release their astringent properties.

Once your mouthwash is ready, you can confidently treat oral-related issues quickly and cheaply while you are still alive. The good news is that this homemade toothpaste lasts a long time and is highly effective at cleaning your teeth.

Cinnamon

A recent study on type 2 diabetics found that taking cinnamon extract daily reduced blood sugar levels by 10%. It reduces cardiovascular risks and cholesterol by about 13%. 1 g cinnamon extract capsules help control blood sugar, while 1 to 6 g capsules lower cholesterol. However, consuming a large amount of the current spice harms your health. As a result, it is preferable to use a water-soluble extract.

Rosemary

HCAs, or heterocyclic amines, are known carcinogens in various cancers. When meat is grilled, fried, or roasted at high temperatures, amines are produced. HCA levels in the body are reduced by rosemary extract, a common powder mixed into cooked meat. Rosemary extract prevents carcinogens from binding to DNA and entering the body. It's the first stage of cancer development, and rosemary extracts can help prevent it. As a result, ingesting rosemary extract kills carcinogens before they can form tumors. Although this study was conducted on animals, the extract appears to have anti-cancer properties. To help reduce HCAs in the body, add rosemary extract to any spice blend. It will also enhance the dish's flavor, making it more flavorful. Combine the herb with oregano, parsley, thyme, and onions for a perfect blend.

Ginger

Ginger can help with motion sickness, pregnancy, and chemotherapy, to name a few. Our mothers and grandmothers frequently mention this old home remedy. They are correct because it is effective! Ginger is a powerful antioxidant that inhibits the effects of serotonin in the body. When you feel sick, your stomach and body produce this chemical, which inhibits the production of free radicals, another cause of stomach pain.

Garlic

Garlic consumption has been shown to cure colorectal and ovarian cancer. There has also been a decrease in the number and size of precancerous growths. Garlic benefits include not only cancer prevention but also blood pressure reduction. Garlic has about 70 active phytochemicals, including allicin, which has been shown to lower blood pressure by 30 points. Garlic in your diet helps to prevent arterial blockages and strokes. The best cancer and cardiovascular benefits come from fresh, crushed garlic. To reap the full benefits, however, at least five cloves of crushed garlic should be consumed.

Holy Basil

Several animal studies back up holy basil, a type used in pesto. Holy basil effectively reduces stress in the body by increasing norepinephrine and adrenaline while decreasing serotonin. The herb is also used to treat headaches and indigestion. Holy basil tea leaves are an excellent natural resource that outperforms traditional pain relief methods.

Aloe Vera

Aloe vera has traditionally been used to treat skin conditions, constipation, infections, worm infestations, and colic. It's widely used in Chinese medicine to treat fungal infections. Nowadays, various cosmetic products use this herb to soften the skin. Surprisingly, there are over 78 active ingredients in Aloe Vera. Furthermore, studies have shown that the herb has antiviral, anti-inflammatory, and antifungal properties. It boosts the immune system and contains no known allergens.

Feverfew

This well-known herb has been used to treat headaches, toothaches, stomachaches, infertility, menstrual problems, and labor during childbirth. Parthenolide, a biochemical found in the herb, is responsible for the healing effect. It prevents blood vessel dilation during migraines. The herb also prevents blood clots and dizziness, alleviates allergies, and alleviates arthritis pain.

St. John's Wort

St. John's wort treats physical symptoms and mild to moderate anxiety and depression. Best of all, it works just as well as any other medication and has no side effects.

Saw Palmetto

Saw palmetto is a supplement used to treat prostate cancer in men. It also contributes to several men's health issues, such as hair loss, low libido, and prostate enlargement. It is also said to help with relaxation, respiratory conditions, and immune system strength.

Burdock

Numerous cases leave your blood infected while fighting or living in poor conditions. When exposed to tetanus, venom, or infected food, survivors must find a way to cleanse their blood regularly. If not treated promptly, blood poisoning can result in long-term complications or, in the worst-case scenario, death.

The burdock plant has proven to be invaluable in terms of blood purification, as well as an excellent liver tonic. Its leaves and roots can be processed for blood purification, and it can also be used to clean the body in general. You are exposed to various agents that will contaminate your body in the wild. Therefore, eliminating these toxins is advisable if you want to perform optimally.

Aside from purification, the burdock root-alcohol tincture can be used to effectively eliminate eczema and other skin-related disorders without causing any side effects. If you don't like bitter herbs, you can eat the fresh leaves immediately or boil them to remove the bitterness. Just remember to drain the water after you've finished boiling it.

Willow

Willow trees thrive in moist areas, so survivors should watch them because they have some powerful medicinal properties they may want to use while out in the wild. For centuries, the bark and branches of the willow tree have been used to treat various ailments.

If you take the boiled willow with the remedy and the symptoms do not go away immediately, try sipping it once every two hours until you are cured.

Boil its green leaves for about ten minutes or until an astringent is formed. After that, soak a cloth or a ball of cotton in it and gently press it against ulcers, boils, carbuncles, or abscesses. You can also boil the willow tree back and drink it. For centuries, this has been used to treat inflammation and as a pain reliever.

A sip of the acidic willow solution can also serve as an effective anti-diarrhea drink, allowing you to stay healthy while surviving in the wilderness or during a difficult period. If possible, plant a willow tree in your garden for its nutritional and medicinal value; you will not be disappointed.

If you have a stomach for bitterness, you can chew these herbs, which will relieve your fever if you have one. Make it a habit to keep some willow bark in your medicine cabinet because it will give you a fighting chance when you think you aren't fighting an infection.

Plantain

As small and insignificant as it may appear, plantain can save your life in the wild due to its medicinal properties. Small, green weeds that grow in lawns can be identified with their plausible, parallel veins. As a well-trained survivalist, you will never be without these useful herbs. If you ever have the opportunity for easy access, you should make a point of planting plantain in your garden.

A plantain tincture should be taken three times daily to achieve the desired results. A plantain tincture can help deal with venomous bites and stings, but it should only be used as a supplement, not as a replacement for a snakebite kit (since snake venom is too potent). However, this simple tincture can be used to combat bee, scorpion, and wasp venom. It can also treat other insects that bite or sting, causing pain and discomfort.

Plantain paste is simple to make because all you need to do is crush it, and the dough will form gradually. Always keep the dough over the stung or bit area until you feel immediate relief. If not, apply more plantain paste to the sensitive area, which should alleviate the discomfort.

Dandelion

To survive in the wild, you may not have the luxury of choosing what you eat. As a result, you may experience indigestion, but you can alleviate this by making a tincture of dandelion and consuming it three times per day for the best results. Because dandelion is highly soluble in alcohol, many experts recommend an alcohol-based tincture. This increases the overall effectiveness of the tincture.

Numerous reports have been of people losing their appetite while out in the wilderness due to infection or other factors. Because of its mild diuretic properties, dandelion can be used to treat this condition and boost your appetite.

You must prepare dandelion tincture before using it as an appetite stimulant. This will require 1-2 tablespoons of dandelion leaves added to a cup of boiling water, then allowed to settle for a few minutes before drinking as a decoction. To achieve the desired results, drink it three times per day.

Echinacea

For a long time, Echinacea has been used effectively to treat fungi and yeast infections, which are known to thrive greatly in the wilderness. It is, therefore, critical for a survivalist to understand how to identify, prepare, and use Echinacea because it will significantly improve their overall survival chances. At the same time, out in the wilderness, where conditions are moist. Apart from assisting in the fight against fungi and yeast infections, you should also ensure that your overall immunity has been boosted.

As a serious prepper, you must have Echinacea on hand because it helps prevent recurring ailments like the common cold, which can be inconvenient.

You can make tea from the dried leaf or use it to ensure that you can easily survive whatever harsh realities you face.

You should also consume Echinacea roots and leaves to strengthen your immune system and live healthier lives. According to studies, Echinacea is highly effective in treating vaginal yeast and reducing adults' common cold.

It has yet to exhibit any side effects, as with conventional, artificial medications, which is always a good sign. When combined with creams, echinacea products have also improved skin conditions, which is always a good sign.

Yarrow

Yarrow is known for several medicinal qualities that a true survivalist should always pay attention to, in addition to its undeniable aesthetic appeal. Yarrow has been shown to sterilize cuts, wounds, and bruises and speed up the healing process, especially when applied early.

Aside from its medicinal properties, Yarrow can also be used as a poultice, particularly when the bleeding does not appear to stop. When applied to the wound, it absorbs all the blood and forms a thick barrier, preventing blood from spitting out and infectious microorganisms from entering the bloodstream.

Aside from the leaves, the Yarrow flowers have pretty impressive healing properties. Yarrow can also be dried and mixed with comfrey water or plantain (or both) and applied to wounds to speed up healing and eliminate mild poisons and venom. Yarrow can be grown in a home garden and used for the abovementioned purposes.

Comfrey

Comfrey is another naturally occurring medication every survivalist should watch for while in the wilderness. It has long been a topical treatment for arthritis, sprains, burns, and bruises, especially when young, tender leaves and roots are used.

Comfrey roots are considered unsafe for internal use due to an alkaloid element called Pyrrolizidine, which can cause extensive liver damage. Preparing the comfrey leaves and roots is a relatively simple process that should not take a survivalist long to master.

However, you can use it solely for the external applications mentioned above and benefit from its rapid healing properties. If you can successfully remove the alkaloid element, you can drink comfrey tea without worrying about liver damage. However, taking chances in the wild or under duress is not good.

Birch

In the face of danger, many things can end up causing you much pain. These causes are stings, bites, fists, kicks, bullet wounds, concoctions, fever, or fractures. In short, there are numerous causes of pain, and to think clearly, you must find a way to alleviate the pain. There are multiple pain relievers available over the counter that you can keep in your medical bag.

However, birch bark should be considered if you are looking for an effective, natural analgesic (pain reliever) that you will enjoy taking because of its sweetness. You may also be interested in learning more about birch leaves if you are in a situation where you do not have access to over-the-counter medications and require pain relievers.

Apart from being simple to prepare, it is also simple to obtain in the wild; however, you must ensure that you have it on hand. When consuming birch, exercise caution because too much of it can cause nausea, tinnitus (also known as ringing ears), and stomach upsets. Once you start experiencing the above-mentioned symptoms, you must discontinue its use.

Jewelweed

Impatiens Capensis, also known as jewelweed, is well-known for its ability to eliminate plant toxins as quickly as possible. Plant toxins in the context include, among others, oak, sumac, and ivy poison. This means that if you come into contact with these toxins, your first response should be to gather some jewelweed and make a mush of it before applying it to the affected area of your body.

This must be done as soon as possible if you are to be successful in combating the poison's effects. A survivalist may be unaware that they have come into contact with poisonous plants and only realize this when they develop an itch or blisters. Nonetheless, the jewelweed will take excellent care of them and relieve any itch or discomfort within minutes of application.

The preparation and application of jewelweed are both simple. A wise survivalist will always watch jewelweed while in the wilderness, as it may save their life.

Elderberry

People are prone to injuring themselves during times of upheaval, so it would be a brilliant idea for them to stock up on medical supplies. If not, they should know that elderberry works wonders when applied to the skin.

In addition to promoting faster healing, elderberry can be used to manage ailments such as flu, colds, and other common respiratory complications. Elderberry can also be beneficial, especially if you have asthma. It is known to be effective as an anti-inflammatory, treating swelling and mucous membranes.

Elderberry is also known for its anti-cancer properties, implying that everyone, survivalist or not, should consume it regularly. Consuming these useful berries should be done cautiously because they are mildly toxic if not fully ripe. Eating raw while taking laxatives, diuretics, water pills, or diabetic medications may harm your health.

Lavender

Aside from being used as a fragrance today, lavender is still popular among survivalists due to its unique medicinal properties. Lavender, like jewelweed, has been known to provide quick relief from the itches and discomfort that rushes are known to cause. Rushes can grow in difficult areas for various reasons, implying that you should make the necessary efforts to have lavender with you.

Fortunately, you can grow it in your garden to ensure you are on the right track to accessing lavender. If not, you can always watch those growing in the wild and pick them up for yourself.

Lavender, aside from being pleasant to the senses, is also an excellent insect repellent. You'll need the latter, especially if you're out in nature and come into contact with mosquitoes and other disease-carrying insects and bugs. Lavender can also be used to treat minor burns sustained while on your survival quest.

Lavender should be consumed with caution, and pregnant women and small children should avoid it. To be safe, lavender should only be used outside the body.

Lemon Balm

You can drink lemonade while effectively combating the inconvenient side effects of cold sores. Sleep is also essential to a survivalist's life because it allows them to recover and have a better chance of survival the next day. As a result, insomnia can be a terrible disadvantage that lemon tea can alleviate in minutes.

It also aids in relaxation, which is necessary for a survivalist to make life-saving decisions. Lemon balm is also known to treat cold sores and their depressing effects effectively. Researchers discovered that lemon balm is far more effective than the strongest cold medication available over the counter, which also has several side effects.

Lemon balm preparations are relaxing. It would be very convenient for any survivor to have some lemon balm grown in their gardens so they could access it more easily for medicinal purposes. Drink lemon tea as often as possible to avoid cold sores and insomnia-related complications.

Black Walnut

Because of its numerous medicinal uses, the black walnut is another survivalist favorite. First and foremost, its highly medicinal green husks can be used to treat minor bruises, cuts, and wounds. The latter is because these green shells have a clean property that will effectively give you an advantage when clearing infectious microorganisms from your wound, thereby hastening the healing process.

You can also make horrible-tasting tea from the husks in an easy-to-follow process, but you can bet it will be much nastier when the parasites try it, albeit involuntarily. As a result, drinking black walnut extract tea regularly is an excellent idea to protect your body from harmful parasites that can cause malnutrition and further weaken your body.

You can endure drinking at least one cup of tea per day for seven days to increase your chances of successfully expelling these harmful parasites that can easily enter your body while surviving in a difficult environment. A survivalist must also know how to identify black walnut in the wild if they do not have them growing in their home.

CHAPTER 3: HOW TO CREATE A MEDICINE CABINET AT HOME USING NATURAL REMEDIES

Whether you have irritated eyes or a blocked chest, there are some spices in your nursery that people have relied on for a long time. When attempting to use every common fix, these should be the first things you keep in your comprehensive medication cabinet.

Home Remedies for Body Aches and Pain

- **Natural Pain-Relief Balm**

This salve soothes sore muscles with the help of turmeric and cayenne pepper. When you apply it to your skin, it feels warm. Turmeric promotes irritation in your body, while cayenne pepper warms the tissues and combats the irritation. I use it when I get a sore back from gardening.

- **Tub Tea**

An Epsom salt bath is an excellent way to relieve the stresses of the day. Adding spices and different botanicals can also be skin soothing; however, cleaning up after the bath is not too much tomfoolery. Make tub teas for a mending shower splash that won't require any cleanup later.

- **Herbal Foot Soak**

You get sick now and then. When this happens, adding a couple of scoops of this to a bowl of warm water and dousing your feet with it helps you feel significantly better. The steam from these recuperating foot baths also aids in clog removal. Treat yourself to this homemade foot soak made with spices from your nursery.

- **Pampering Peppermint for Feet**

Peppermint is excellent for sore feet. Sugar and dried spices will scour away rough skin, coconut oil will relax breaks, and soothing peppermint medicinal balm will relieve pain.

- **Roll-On Headache Relief**

When I first notice cerebral pain, I use a roller bottle filled with natural oils to relieve it before it becomes energetic. This is usually all I need to get rid of the cerebral pain. Roller bottle remedies are excellent to keep on hand in the medication cabinet.

Home Remedies for Topical Skin Relief

- **Topical Antifungal Treatment**

This homemade tea tree oil antifungal treatment stick assists with calming red spots and rashes in a delicate yet direct manner. It's bundled in a helpful cylinder so you can rapidly treat sore, difficult spots.

- **Drawing Salve Recipe for Bug Bites, Blisters, Splinters**

A drawing salve combines oils and herbal fixings that work to remove poisons from your skin. It can be utilized on mosquito chomps, wasp or honey bee stings, rankles, bubbles, bites, and minor contaminations.

- **Dandelion Salve**

Try not to kill the dandelions in your yard - it could be utilized to make an aggravation-easing salve. These yellow weeds have torment-reducing and mitigating properties. Utilize this salve on throbbing muscles and different afflictions you have.

- **Cold Sores and Little Red Spots**

Lemon balm's antiviral properties make it a well-known spice for treating cold sores, chicken pox, bug nibbles, and other minimal red spots. This recipe for lemon balm lip balm not just has a brilliant and happy lemon scent; however, it likewise is an extraordinary method for forestalling and treating cold sores.

- **Protecting Cuticles**

This alleviating fingernail skin balm is loaded with a natural mix that will patch those breaks and make hands delicate in the future. Treating dry hands while doing a ton of hand washing is vital.

- **Hand & Body Lotion**

Salve might be a wonder item decision instead of a homegrown cure. Yet, this one is produced using skin-calming botanical water and supporting oils that assist in fixing and safeguarding dry skin. Keeping skin delicate assists with keeping it sound, as I'm never without this recipe.

- **Natural Skin Soother**

Use quieting witch hazel to alleviate razor consumption and rashes and cool down aggravation. It's produced using the parts of the witch hazel tree and can likewise be utilized as a face toner.

Home Remedies for the Respiratory System

- **Elderberry Syrup**

This helps with respiratory issues and boosts your immune system all year. Although Lexie's Homemade kit has recently gained popularity, this is still the brand preference among Amazon customers. Children prefer Yum V's Immunity Shield candies. You will appreciate that they are sweetened with glucose rather than sugar, but be cautious if you have a dog, as glucose is highly toxic to dogs.

- **Eucalyptus Essential Oil**

It must be diluted with canola oil and applied to the chest or pajamas so people can smell it all night. When combined with bath salts, you can use them in your volatile oils vaporizer or baths. Remember that children should not be exposed to eucalyptus oil.

- **Humidifier with a Cool Spray**

People use them in their beds to facilitate clean breathing even though they are not strictly medicines.

- **Lymph Rub from Trilight Health**

If you would not want to blend your lavender oil and plants, this is a fantastic massage for inflamed lymph nodes.

- **Diffuser for Essential Oils**

This isn't the same as a humidifier. Diffusing respiratory-supportive oils in the air is beneficial. There is a vast range of diffusers accessible on numerous platforms; however, we have many of this kind that we use in various areas of our house.

- **Respiratory Mixes with Plant Therapy**

These volatile oil mixes are efficient and reasonably priced.

Home Remedies for the Ear

- **Garlic oil drops:** Garlic and liquid silver would be rotated.
- **Colloidal silver:** It will assist if you put a few drops of it in your lobes. It resembles a natural antimicrobial alternative virtually!
- **Trilight Healthy Person's Kit for Ear infection Relief**: This is a great kit to keep on hand.

Home Remedies for the Stomach

- **Peppermint essential oil**: applied to the stomach after being diluted with canola oil
- **Activated charcoal**
- **Probiotics:** These are fantastic for everyday health as well!
- **Ginger tea:** Ginger is great for calming nausea.

Herbal Remedies for Allergic Reactions

Some of the common herbal remedies for all types of allergies or allergic reactions include:

- **Stinging Nettle**: This plant contains healing compounds that might act with effects such as an antihistamine. Concerning some of the studies, stinging nettle has evidence upon its extracts being safe for use by humans. But even more, ongoing research is being executed to validate its efficacy in curing other health ailments.
- **Garlic**: Both onions, as well as garlic, consist of quercetin. It is a specific antioxidant that inhibits histamine production for treating specific types of allergies. When you consume it with an adequate dosage routine, you will eventually help heal the symptoms of allergic reactions.
- **Curcumin**: This is the active compound of turmeric! As far as practical surveys and tests are concerned, oral curcumin supplements ease nasal congestion and all other allergic symptoms. It also reduces the immune response of people suffering from allergic rhinitis problems.
- **Butterbur**: A systematic and purposeful review has proven that butterbur is considered similarly effective to modern antihistamines, especially for treating allergies. The high-quality research is still pending to confirm these properties of the herb. The scientists need to confirm the facts on the safety of this herb for treating allergies without any side effects.

People who are allergic to plants or pollens may also be present. In such cases, they may be allergic to certain herbs, such as butterbur. These herbs have already been discussed in this book in a separate chapter. But the point of repeating them is to focus your attention on the specific health condition that it can cure or treat. So, read it with a fresh perspective to connect these herbs to allergic reaction issues.

Herbal Remedies for Migraine Problems

Migraine is a neurological condition that causes numerous painful headaches. There are a few other migraine symptoms, such as nausea, light sensitivity, and others. Again, some herbal remedies that have the potential to treat or alleviate migraine symptoms are:

- **Feverfew**: It consists of compounds that have the potential to reduce the frequent triggers of migraine symptoms. The experts are carrying out more research into how effective feverfew is for preventing migraine problems.
- **Ginger**: There have been helpful reviews and surveys where people consuming ginger and its remedies have reported reducing their migraine symptoms. They have reported having experienced lowering effects for pain, vomiting, and nausea without any possible side effects.
- **Butterbur**: The extracts of this herb can be used to prepare the necessary remedies to reduce migraine frequency in both adults and children. Butterbur consists of Pyrrolizidine Alkaloids or PAs, which were reported to cause liver damage. Therefore, the use of this herb was restricted to the use of only some specific plant parts. You can consult your herbalist for more details on safely using butterbur.
- **Peppermint Oil**: If you have a different form of headache, apart from migraine problems, then peppermint oil can help, as it consists of menthol and has a cooling effect on the skin. People can use it to apply directly onto the skin and experience relief within a short span. Menthol is not considered safe for kids! Therefore, do not use peppermint oil on them!

Herbal Remedies for Anxiety and Stress

Stress and anxiety have taken control of today's generations' minds. Everything that the average person does not understand is turned into a stress factor. And this can lead to serious health problems! As a result, here are some herbal remedies that can help you deal with stress and anxiety:

- **German Chamomile**: It takes around 1500mg/day of German Chamomile extract for a time span of 8 weeks to reduce the stress & anxiety symptoms. The healing rate for anxiety disorder problems with this herb is the same as that of conventional anti-anxiety drugs.
- **Essential Oils**: Various types of essential oils might reduce stress symptoms. Some of the specific choices include peppermint and lavender oil. People need to make use of diffusers for people to inhale the scent of essential oils. Some essential oils are also ideal for being applied over the skin by diluting with a carrier oil.
- **Lemon Balm**: It is prescribed that consuming around 3 grams of lemon balm every day for around eight weeks might reduce anxiety, stress, and depression.

You can always meditate to calm your mind if you do not want to use herbs or other medications to treat stress, depression, or anxiety. You can always make an effort to avoid depression and anxiety! However, you can always rely on these herbs if it becomes uncontrollable and unpredictable.

Herbal Remedies for Sore Throats and Coughs

Many over-the-counter (OTC) products are available at pharmacies to treat your cough and sore throat. On the other hand, natural herbs can be helpful if you prefer to use natural medications or plants to treat coughs or sore throats. Many medications sold in stores eventually contain plant compounds. These herbal remedies are to blame for this ailment:

- **Eucalyptus Oil**: Around 12 drops of eucalyptus oil with boiling water should be consumed at least three times daily to reduce cough problems. Continue with the dosage until you feel at ease in your symptoms.
- **Licorice Root**: Licorice root has been used since the Native Americans' era to treat sore throats. The remedies are used as lozenges or gargles for ideal treatment outcomes. The licorice root also attends the post-surgery soreness in the throat. But remember not to consume this herb excessively, as it might trigger high blood pressure.
- **Sage**: Sage is accountable for reducing bronchospasm problems, also known as the contraction of airways. Sage has historical evidence of treating asthma and cough symptoms. There is a need for more research on humans to prove its determined effectiveness in healing the condition.

CHAPTER 4: HOW TO STORE HERBS

Herbal remedies should be kept away from children unless directed by a doctor. This is because most herbs have not yet been thoroughly tested on children.

Remember that switching to herbal is more than just a decision; it requires planning! Whether it is a natural disaster that is about to cause health and food problems or a health problem that requires a long-term and permanent cure, you have herbs as a backup. They are not only medicines but also edible in most cases. Most households around the world use them as spices and side dishes.

So, for your initial prepping practices, refer to these ailments and the herbs used to prepare their remedies. However, over time, you will need to broaden your knowledge and investigate other serious ailments that require infusion-based herbal remedies for treatment. A prepper must be aware of the extent of their preparations! As a result, if you decide to enter the world of herbs, ensure you learn everything you can about it over time. You only need to remember that people from all over the world are assisting one another.

You can get better help by discussing your concerns and considerations with a doctor or herbalist! They will be able to provide evidence on which herbs to trust and which to avoid.

How to Keep Herbs Fresh in the Refrigerator

If you need to store herbs for a few days, you can do a few things to help them last longer.

Tougher herbs, such as rosemary, thyme, and sage, with woody stalks, thicker leaves, and short sprigs, can be stored in a plastic bag or wrapped in plastic wrap for up to a week before using. Any moisture trapped inside could cause mold to grow on the herbs you don't want! Real Simple recommends storing them in the coldest part of your refrigerator.

Other, more delicate herbs, like parsley, cilantro, and basil, should not be treated the same way. The volatile oils mentioned earlier will evaporate, leaving you with a handful of flavorless leaves. Instead, treat them as flowers by clipping the ends and placing them upright in an inch of water in a sturdy container to allow them to bloom.

Then, leave them out on the counter instead of storing them in the refrigerator.

Alternatively, wrap fragile herbs in a moist paper towel before storing them to extend their life. Cooking Light recommends storing the ingredients in an airtight plastic bag to extend their shelf life.

How to Keep Fresh Herbs Fresh for Later Use

If you have more herbs than your kitchen can handle, place them in freezer bags and store them in the freezer. Then, to preserve the herbs, place them in an ice cube tray and cover them with water or oil. (If you want to cram even more spices into the compartments, chop the herbs ahead of time.) After freezing, you can use the herbs in various recipes or thaw them before using them in the kitchen.

Another option is to make your herbs into a sauce and freeze it to develop a more robust flavor over time. Then, simply follow the directions for your favorite pesto recipe, substituting your preferred herb for the basil (handy tip: any dark, leafy green with tender leaves works as "pesto," including spinach and arugula).

As before, scoop a spoonful of pesto onto an ice tray and freeze. When ready to use the pesto, simply microwave the cubes or toss them into a skillet or saucepan with the rest of the ingredients.

BOOK 2: MEDICINE TO STOCKPILE

Emergencies may occur without warning. You can be without phone service, electricity, refrigeration, or clean water for days or weeks. You might be advised to stay home in specific circumstances, like during a disease outbreak, for your safety. So, maintaining a supply of medicines is crucial.

Here, you will discover what kind of medications you should always keep on hand and how to store them properly.

CHAPTER 1: MEDICINE YOU SHOULD HAVE ON HAND

Medication Every Medicine Cabinet Should Have

Allergy Medication

Supplied medicine cabinets should include eye drops and allergy medications depending on the season and where you live. Holder also suggests carrying both a "sleepy" allergy medicine (for use before bed) and a non-tired allergy medicine (for use during the day).

Antibacterial Ointment or Cream

Antibacterial creams and salves treat or prevent minor skin infections caused by small pieces, scraped spots, or bug nibbles. "There is a difference between a cream and a salve," Holder explained. "Because creams are water soluble, clients should apply them after washing the injury with a cleaning agent and water." Holder recommends using antibacterial cream when staying indoors, where sweat is more unpredictable. Balms are oil-based and can be applied when the person is in contact with water."

Decongestant

Pseudoephedrine used to make methamphetamine, is commonly found in decongestant drugs behind the drug store counter. As a result, Holder frequently suggests decongestants found on standard drug store shelves; however, decongestants found behind the counter work admirably.

Pain Reliever

When choosing a pain reliever for your medicine cabinet, keep your family's needs in mind. "However," Holder added, "some pain medication should be required regularly." Consider which pain relievers are most effective for your needs and keep at least one on hand; if you have children, keep pain relievers for children on hand as well.

Anti-Diarrheal

"Medicine cabinets, especially for families with small children or even older people, should have an enemy of diarrheal," Holder said. This medication slows the development of the stomach, reducing the number of side effects and making the stool less watery.

Calamine Lotion

Calamine salve is a highly effective treatment for minor skin irritations such as bug bites or minor consumption. The salve can relieve irritation, and if you have a bug bite, Holder says pairing the calamine moisturizer with an allergy medication is also good.

CHAPTER 2: HOW TO KNOW THE MEDICINE YOU BRING WILL SOLVE ANY HEALTH PROBLEM

Medication is important in managing an illness but can be harmful if misused. It's enough not to notice that you take a blue case and a yellow tablet twice daily. You must be familiar with the names of your medications and the critical insights into how they work. For example, some medications may interact negatively with certain foods, medications, or even food supplements, making you extremely ill.

Find a way to learn more about the treatment that has been recommended for you. Feel free to contact your doctor or a drug specialist for assistance in answering these questions.

1. What is the name of the medicine?
2. For what reason do I have to take it?
3. When and how might I take it? With water? With food? While starving?
4. They are sum would it be wise for me to take? How would it be a good idea for me to respond if I missed a portion?
5. What could medication bring about secondary effects? Which ones would it be fitting for me to call the specialist about?
6. Are there any food varieties or medicines I should avoid while taking this medicine?
7. Will this medication change how my different medicines work?

Find these ways to ensure your safety in addition to asking your doctor or a drug specialist for help understanding your medications.

- Fill your prescriptions at the same pharmacy regularly. Your medical history is now on a single document.
- Request a medication reality sheet from your drug specialist.
- Keep a list of the various solutions and over-the-counter medications you use in your wallet or handbag. Make sure to include nutrients, health supplements, and homegrown remedies. When there are changes in your daily schedule, update the rundown. Take down the name of everything, the measurement, why you need it, and when you need to take it.
- Inform your doctor and drug specialist if you have any ailments or allergies to medications or foods or if you are pregnant or breastfeeding.

BOOK 3: PREPPER'S NATURAL MEDICINE

Everyone has access to natural medicine. There is no licensing board, and certification courses are entirely optional. You can learn herbalism on your own or by enrolling in a course.

Natural medicine requires no permission to practice or study.

Natural medicine manufacturing procedures appear deceptively simple compared to pharmaceutical manufacturing standards. I don't know many homesteaders who can make Tamiflu, but I know a few who can make flu-fighting berry nectar. To be honest, there is much to learn about natural medicine before practicing it safely and effectively. There are no quick fixes, and learning is an ongoing process. Students study for many years and devote countless hours to their studies. On the other hand, mastering the fundamental procedures is a simple and enjoyable process that promises long-term benefits for the beginning herbalist.

The ability to reproduce or wildcraft herbs, edibles, lipids, mushrooms, lichens, and waxes year after year is the most apparent advantage of natural medicine for preppers. Having natural remedies on hand to address health issues after the pharmacy's shelves have run dry is a prudent survival strategy.

People will eventually form a social structure and a support network. They will rebuild to increase the worth of their lives.

We can only speculate on what a new currency, whether silver or gold, might look like. Medications and the ability to use them will always be valuable.

Knowledge of which plants can treat bronchitis, how to make a prenatal vitamin supplement from common plants, how to perform lymph drainage on a swollen, injured ankle, and experience with emergency or "ditch" medicine will be in high demand. People will eventually form a social hierarchy and a network of support. They will rebuild to improve people's lives. We can only speculate on the nature of a new currency.

Many plants are medicinal. From the roots to the treetops, every part of a plant can be used to treat a variety of ailments. Plants contain chemicals that can be either beneficial or harmful to the body. For example, most parts of the deadly nightshade (belladonna) are highly toxic and were traditionally used as a poison, as the name implies. On the other hand, the plant's leaves and roots can be used as muscle relaxants to treat peptic ulcers. As a result, this plant possesses both positive and negative traits. Regardless of how appealing it may sound, only take deadly nightshade if it has been prescribed to you. An overdose has the potential to be fatal. Herbal medicine uses plants with positive effects when taken in the proper dosage, serving as the foundation for modern medicine.

Many plants we eat are also effective for herbal medicine and are grown for herbal use. Living outside Western countries, you've probably heard of fruits and vegetables eaten to treat specific illnesses. For example, papaya is beneficial for snacking, deworming digestive issues, and wound healing. Foods that double as medicine in the United States include oats, lemons, onions, and garlic. These are widely available and reasonably priced foods in grocery stores across the United States. They are all useful and convenient to have on hand. Herbal medicine can therefore include both edible and medicinal plants.

CHAPTER 1: BENEFITS OF NATURAL MEDICINE

Learning about natural medicine is essential for becoming a prepper. There is a lot you can do once you know about the medicinal properties of plants and herbs, whether you are looking for common cold and flu remedies or treating allergies; whenever you are learning something new, the motivation to continue learning increases when you become aware of its benefits.

It's not just about learning about the various herbs and medicinal plants used in survival medicine. You should also educate yourself on multiple preparations. In this book, we've compiled the information you'll need for various preparations in the form of recipes. Before you begin, consider the following advantages of natural medicine and remedies:

Natural medicine has numerous advantages, which explains why it has been practiced for thousands of years. As you read the following benefits, you will understand why you should learn more about natural medicine and start stocking up on a home apothecary.

- Natural medicine is far less expensive than modern medicine. Prescription medications are well-known for their high cost. On the other hand, herbal medicines are much cheaper to produce because they are made from readily available natural resources. Because the production cost is low, the retail cost is also common. It will help you save money on upfront costs and by preventing illnesses in the first place. Natural medicine will help you learn more about healing and managing your conditions.
- It will improve your immune system. Natural medicine is vital for improving overall health and assisting you in consuming the right foods and ingredients daily. This helps ensure that your body receives all the necessary nutrients to function correctly. Your immune system is boosted, keeping you healthy.
- It will help your body overcome nutritional deficiencies while supporting healing. Prescription medications function in such a way that they mask your symptoms while not necessarily curing the ailment. You feel better, but your internal condition remains unchanged. Natural medicine teaches you to listen to your body and identify the source of your pain.
- When compared to modern medicine, natural medicine generally has fewer side effects. Because the ingredients are natural, the body responds favorably to natural medicine. You can gradually reduce or eliminate the former's side effects when you replace a prescription drug with a natural remedy.
- Nature provides all the raw materials required to heal your body using natural medicine. You don't have to rely on pharmacies or stores, and you can grow most of the ingredients yourself. It gives you the power to take charge of your health.
- Another advantage of natural medicine is that compared to pharmaceuticals, making medicine at home is less expensive. They are simple to make and use readily available natural ingredients. You can further reduce costs by growing some medicinal plants and herbs at home.
- Herbal remedies encourage self-healing rather than simply treating symptoms. The majority of prescription drugs and pharmaceuticals are designed to treat symptoms first. For example, taking an aspirin relieves the pain when you get a headache. It does not address the source of the pain. When you begin to use natural medicine, you are not only treating the pain or discomfort but also the source.
- Natural medicine education is hugely empowering. When you know you can take care of your medical needs and those around you, you will feel more in control. You have the skills and resources to solve any problem, even in dire situations and emergencies.
- Another advantage of learning about natural medicine is gaining a new skill. Learning how to make lotions and balms, as well as tinctures, are all ways to improve your overall health. This book's list of herbs and medicinal plants will improve your understanding of natural medicine. Knowledge is priceless, and information is powerful. Always keep this in mind. It's never a bad idea to learn something new.

After reading about these advantages, you may want to start incorporating natural medicine and remedies into your daily life rather than just in emergencies. Choosing natural medicine provides a holistic approach to improving your overall health and well-being.

CHAPTER 2: GROWING MEDICAL HERBS

Many plants have healing and regenerative properties. You probably already have some on your spice rack. However, if something unexpected occurs, such as a natural disaster, you may be unable to buy them in a store. Growing them is a great way to ensure access whenever you need them. The recent coronavirus pandemic has highlighted the importance of strong immunity. Many herbs, among others, can help you with this. Spices like pepper, cinnamon, cayenne, cloves, and herbs like oregano, garlic, basil, fennel, and sage should be consumed daily. These herbs can be grown in pots and gardens. Dried onions can be stored if you live in an apartment and don't have enough space to grow your herbs. They can be kept for up to a year if desired. They will keep their healing properties in unopened containers for 12-18 months.

The following are some essential spices with healing properties:

- **Black pepper**: It has a high energy level, which warms the body and improves circulation, but it can also be used to stop blood flow from wounds.
- **Cayenne pepper**: It stimulates the cardiovascular system, increasing blood flow, accelerating digestion, and even stopping minor bleeding. Cayenne may keep the body warm throughout winter and boost immunity to colds and viruses.
- **Cloves**: Because of their analgesic and antibacterial properties, clove oil may be useful in treating tooth and gum infections. Cloves' antibacterial properties make them ideal for including in a topical ointment to treat burns and skin irritations. Cloves may be reduced more efficiently in teas.
- **Cinnamon**: In small daily doses, cinnamon improves digestion, relieves stomach cramps, and stimulates circulation throughout the body.

Here are a few medicinal herbs that you can grow:

- **Bay Leaves**: excellent digestive aid, especially when made into tea. Bay leaves will have a less potent effect when added to your meals. They keep stomach acids at bay when consumed regularly.
- **Basil**: Basil is another well-known sleep aid that reduces anxiety and tension. Its calming perfume can elevate one's spirits and alleviate mental problems.
- **Garlic**: Garlic is a strong antibiotic that can help you fight colds and flu by boosting your immunity and preventing infection.
- **Oregano**: A rich source of antioxidants, which are potent immune boosters that may help you fight infections. Oregano may also help to relieve coughs, settle the stomach, relax the mind, and promote restful sleep when used in tea.
- **Sage**: Sage is recommended for improving digestion and calming cougars, particularly in the winter. It may also be used as a natural antibiotic source and can be taken orally or made into an ointment.

Your garden may also include other medicinal herbs with powerful healing properties. Many medicinal herbs, such as peppermint, thyme, rosemary, and fennel, have potent regenerative properties that should not be overlooked.

Growing and stockpiling medicinal herbs could come in handy in an emergency. Not to mention the money you could save by using natural medicines instead of expensive supplements.

CHAPTER 3: ESSENTIAL OILS

What are Essential Oils?

Essential oil is the essence of a herb, flower, or fruit rind. It is the most effective way to use herbals and other plant materials. They are created by distilling or pressing plant matter. Essential oils are heavily used in aromatherapy blends and preparations.

High-quality essential oils are essential because they contain the components needed to heal your body. The purer it is, the better the effects. A small amount of oil is usually enough; a drop is frequently enough. While they are more expensive than the average essential oil, the benefits outweigh the cost, especially when used correctly.

They are extremely useful pure, highly concentrated compounds. A couple of drops of these oils will suffice for whatever purpose you have in mind. It is far superior to slathering on a thick layer of cream or lotion on your skin. Because they are concentrated, you must dilute them with something before applying them topically. If a strong essential oil is applied directly to the skin, it can cause severe reactions.

You've probably heard of aromatherapy, but it's a good idea to learn more about it before using it. If you are not cautious, you may cause more harm than good. This is why professional aromatherapy practitioners devote so much time and effort to learning how to use essential oils correctly. However, you can learn the fundamentals independently if you proceed with caution. Instead of buying essential oils in stores, we'll show you how to make your own. The most effective and beneficial form is always the purest form. The concentrated oils are the extracted form of each plant's inner essence. These oil concentrations provide plants with hundreds of useful properties. However, most of them must be diluted with carrier oils before use. To save money, you can also try essential oil extraction at home. This will save you money and ensure you get the purest product possible. The oils should then be stored and used as needed.

Essential oils are pure plant extracts used for thousands of years for their medicinal properties. They are extracted directly from plant and tree flowers, fruits, roots, leaves, or resins. They are so concentrated that only a few drops are required to work their magic. They can be applied directly to the skin or ingested, though some should not be consumed. You must exercise caution to ensure that you are not allergic to them. There are thousands of essential oils. There are nearly a hundred letters in the alphabet, so it is impossible to list them all, but here are some of the most beneficial ones and their properties.

List of Essential Oils

Pure Essential Oils

If you haven't already realized it, essential oils are incredibly potent. Not only can certain smells elicit specific emotions and sensations, such as serenity or attentiveness, but many of them are also therapeutic. The following essential oils should be kept in your first-aid kit:

Tea Tree Oil

This is a well-known oil, and tea tree oil is one of the most effective natural remedies for skin rashes. You can dilute a few drops in aloe vera gel or honey and have a perfect mask. Be careful—avoid exposing yourself to the sun after applying it, or you will get spots! It has antifungal, antimicrobial, antiviral, and antibacterial properties, making it a must-have in the battle against all baddies. Additionally, it aids in the relief of pain. Many medicinal uses, ranging from fungal diseases to warts, benefit from this supplement.

Lavender Essential Oil

It has relaxing and analgesic properties, which is why it is widely used in aromatherapy to relieve stress and insomnia. Wonderfully soothing. It may help you fall asleep or relax when you're feeling unwell. It has antibacterial properties as well as is a pain reducer. Skin ailments such as burns or cuts benefit greatly from this therapy. A good tip for a better rest is to put a few drops on your pillow.

Lemon Essential Oil

This is widely used due to its astringent properties. It is also a powerful disinfectant and healer. It can commonly be used as an air freshener at home due to its refreshing aroma.

Rosemary Essential Oil

You can use it in combination with olive oil to relieve discomfort and back pain and also use it for circulation problems. Use it while massaging your legs upwards. Doctors and naturalists use it for scalp problems and to achieve more beautiful hair.

Sandalwood Oil

This oil strengthens hair and smoothes skin. Its strong aroma makes it one of the favorites of yoga lovers. It is also used in cosmetics to moisturize dry skin.

Eucalyptus Essential Oil

This is the base oil for aromatherapy. It is recommended for many people with asthma due to its decongestant capabilities. It is also helpful for coughs, flu, throat infections, and muscle pain. Congestion-clearing properties are excellent. It has antiseptic and antiviral properties. It is exceptionally beneficial for all respiratory problems as well as specific allergies. It is only advised for external usage.

Cinnamon Essential Oil

It has strong antiseptic properties, making it ideal for the skin. Preparing a rejuvenating scrub is a good idea by mixing this oil with sugar, orange juice, and olive oil. Your skin will be perfect!

Thyme Essential Oil

In addition to relieving respiratory problems, it improves memory and stimulates the mind and body.

Clove Oil

This oil is not only effective in combating tooth discomfort but is also remarkably flexible. It is effective against fungi, bacteria, microorganisms, and viruses. Additionally, it has a somewhat sedating effect. Apart from relieving dental discomfort, cloves may be used to heal small wounds and cuts.

Chamomile Oil

However, pure chamomile is ideal for use in a first-aid kit in addition to tea. The oil has a soothing impact on the body and helps to decrease inflammation and discomfort. Exceptional for treating skin problems like eczema and rashes, but also works wonders on other aches and pains, such as cramps and migraines.

Peppermint Oil

Peppermint oil has a jolting effect on the senses with just a sniff. This oil is antibacterial and antiseptic, making it an excellent choice for wound care. During a spell of nausea and vomiting, it is ideal for clearing nasal congestion and soothing the stomach, among other things. Being able to be consumed or applied externally makes it very adaptable.

Now that you are aware of these plants and oils, the following chapters of this book will teach you how to make herbal medicine recipes and a first aid kit.

BOOK 4: HERBAL MEDICINE RECIPES

Rather than relying solely on pharmaceuticals and other manufactured prescription drugs, it is preferable to use natural medicine and remedies. Natural remedies are not only more beneficial, but they are also more readily available in the event of a medicine shortage. It is, as previously stated, empowering. You never know when such abilities will be helpful. After all, the only way to mitigate the effects of adversity is to be prepared.

CHAPTER 1: HERBAL MEDICINE RECIPES YOU CAN EASILY MAKE YOURSELF

1. Colds/Immune Boost Diffuse

Preparation Time: 20 minutes
Servings: 2

Ingredients:

- 4 drops lemon essential oil
- 3 drops eucalyptus essential oil
- 1 drop thyme essential oil

Directions:

1. Add the directed number of drops into your diffuser.
2. If needed by your particular diffuser, add water.
3. Allow diffusing in the room for at least 25–30 minutes.

2. Lavender Marjoram Bath Salt

Preparation Time: 10 minutes
Servings: 1

Ingredients:

- 3 cups Epsom salt
- ½ cup baking soda
- 20 drops lavender essential oil
- 10 drops peppermint essential oil
- 10 drops marjoram essential oil
- 5 drops eucalyptus essential oil
- 5 drops rosemary essential oil
- 10 drops natural food coloring

Directions:

1. Add the specified Epsom salt and the baking soda to a glass bowl and gently mash them with a wooden spoon or spatula.
2. Stir with a wooden spatula to mix the salt and baking soda well, add food coloring and continue to stir to blend the mixture well.
3. Add the essential oils one at a time and stir after adding each one to let it blend well.
4. Use about 3–5 tbsp. of the bath salt in a bathtub filled with hot water.
5. Then step into the bathtub and soak for about 25–30 minutes. Rinse off the body with chilly water.
6. Store your creation in a dark glass bottle or jar and cover it tightly.

3. Goodnight Tincture

Preparation Time: 10 minutes
Servings: 2

Ingredient:

- 3 tbsp. Valerian Root tincture
- 3 tbsp. Chamomile Flowers tincture
- 3 tbsp. Linden Leaves tincture

Directions:

1. Put the tinctures in an amber glass bottle with a dropper lid in the indicated proportions.
2. Label it.

Take 3 drops one hour before bedtime. Then 2 more half an hour before bedtime. Finally, 2 drops before going to bed.

4. Rooibos Tea

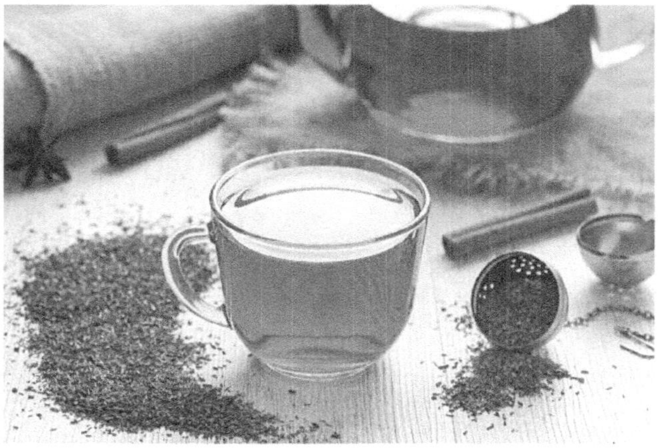

Preparation Time: 20 minutes
Servings: 2

Ingredients:

- Rooibos tea
- cups water
- cubes Brown sugar
- lemon Juice
- Honey

Directions:

1. Heat the water to a medium-high temperature in a medium-sized pot. Once the water has reached a boil, turn off the heat.
2. Pour the rooibos tea into a teapot. Pour the boiling water over the tea. Allow 5 to 6 minutes for the rooibos tea flavor to integrate completely with the boiling water.
3. Half-fill teacups with the prepared tea. To make it sweeter, you can add sugar cubes.
4. Add a few drops of lemon juice and honey to taste.
5. Relax by sipping a cup of hot tea.

5. Calming Vanilla and Eucalyptus Bath Salts

Warm vanilla and invigorating eucalypti are anti-inflammatory and moisturizers in addition to stimulating your sense of smell.

Eucalyptus oil, a natural germicide, has been used to cure wounds for years. In contrast, the aroma of vanilla has been shown to boost the synthesis of serotonin and endorphins, the chemicals responsible for emotions of contentment and fulfillment.

Preparation Time: 20 minutes
Servings: 1

Ingredients:

- 1 cup Epsom salt
- 1/2 cup baking soda
- 3 drops eucalyptus essential oil
- 8 drops vanilla in jojoba oil

Directions:

1. In a big sealable plastic bag, combine the Epsom salt, baking soda, and essential oils.
2. Close the bag and rub the contents with your hands to combine them thoroughly.
3. Transfer the contents of the plastic bag to a lidded glass container.

One tablespoon each bath is recommended.

6. Blistery Rash Poultice

In case of blisters due to contact with an irritating substance, use this astringent poultice to remove the liquid and reduce the itching.

Preparation Time: 20 minutes
Servings: 1

Ingredients:

- 1 cup St. John's Wort flowers and leaves
- 1 cup rose petals
- 1 cup Yarrow leaves

- 1 cup Calendula flowers
- 1 cup Heal –all flowers

Directions:

1. Mix the herbs in a mason jar for easy storage.
2. Create the poultice with some tbsp. of the mixture and a little bit of distilled boiling water.
3. Apply it to the rash.

7. Blistery Rash Quick Fix Poultice

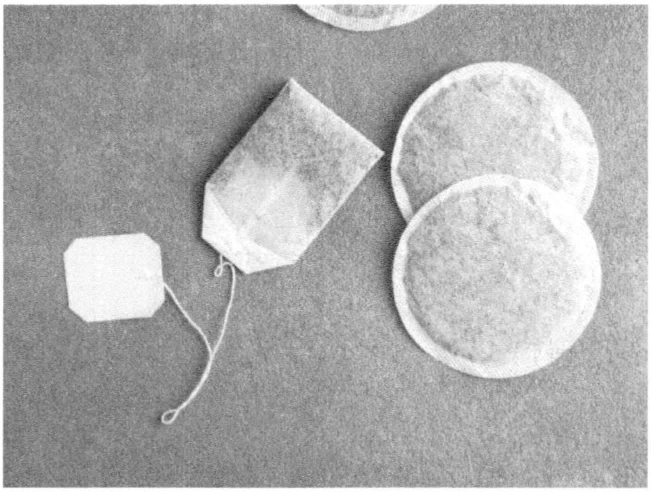

Preparation Time: 15 minutes
Servings: 2

Ingredients:

- 1 Black or Green Tea Bag

Directions:

1. If you are in a hurry or do not have herbs at home, you can prepare a tea and apply the wet, warm tea bag to the rash.

8. Hibiscus Ginger Tea

Preparation Time: 10 minutes
Servings: 2

Ingredients:

- 1 liter of water
- 3 teaspoons of sugar
- 2 heaping tablespoons of dried hibiscus flowers
- 3 thinly sliced ginger slices.
- 1 cinnamon stick

Directions:

1. Bring the water and sugar to a gentle boil in a saucepan.
2. Turn off the heat after stirring until the sugar is dissolved.
3. Combine the hibiscus flowers, ginger, and cinnamon stick in a mixing bowl. Steep for 10 minutes, covered.
4. Pour into the jar.
5. Allow cooling before serving.
6. Serve with ice and a piece of orange or lime.

9. Basil Tea

Preparation Time: 20 minutes
Servings: 2

Ingredients:

- 2 tablespoons of fresh basil finely chopped.
- 1 cup of hot water
- 4 teaspoons lemon juice
- 1 teaspoon grated fresh ginger
- Honey, to taste

Directions:

1. In a small saucepan, heat the basil and ginger until fragrant.
2. Pour boiling water over the top of some ice cubes.
3. Allow for a steeping time of about 5 minutes
4. Sieve the mixture to remove any lumps.
5. Combine with lemon juice and honey.

10. Aloe Vera (Aloe Vera) for Burns

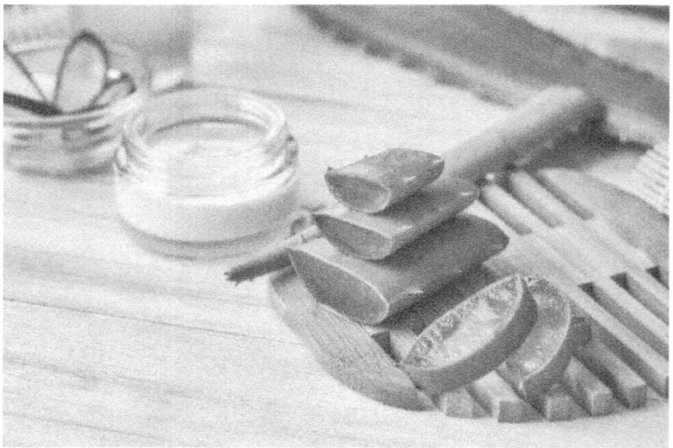

This is probably the most straightforward solution you'll come across. Now is the time to try aloe if you haven't already. To ensure you aren't allergic, test it on a small skin patch first.

Preparation Time: 20 minutes
Servings: 2

Ingredients:

- An aloe Vera plant leaf

Directions::

1. Simply cut the leaf tips off at an angle (but not too steeply straight), leaving at least some leaves.
2. Using a knife, thinly slice the leaf. The gel can be seen by slicing the leaf in half.
3. Directly apply the gel to the burn.

11. Tongue Wash

Preparation time: 5 minutes
Serving: 4 cups

Ingredients:

- 1 tablespoon chamomile
- 1 teaspoon mint
- 1 teaspoon sage
- 4 cups hot water
- a small amount of oak bark

Directions:

1. Hot water should be added to the herbs.
2. Wait for the water to cool down before straining it.
3. A spoonful of salt may be added after that.
4. All that's left for you to do is swirl this water around in your mouth after brushing your teeth twice daily for the rest of the day.

12. Motherwort Tea

Preparation Time: 10 minutes
Servings: 2

Ingredients:

- 1 to 2 tsp. motherwort leaves, dried
- 2 cups hot water
- 1 tsp. honey or other sweetness

Directions:

1. Fill the teapot with 2 cups of boiling water.
2. Allow 5–10 minutes for the combination to steep; the longer it steeps, the stronger the tea will be.
3. Remove the tea leaves with a strainer.
4. Stir in 1 tsp. of honey or another sweetener to taste.

Uses:

- Used to treat inflammatory diseases, but its interior effects are far more obvious.
- Reduces Anxiety.
- Menstruation Relief.
- Reproductive System That Is Healthy.

13. Bay Leaves Tea

Preparation Time: 20 minutes
Servings: 2

Ingredients:

- 3 big bay leaves from the West Indies
- 3 quarts water
- 1.5 to 2 cups of milk
- 1–2 tsp. honey/sugar

Directions:

1. Add three large West Indian Bay leaves to a pot of water to make bay leaf tea (fresh leaves).
2. Bring a pot of water to a boil. Allow the tea to boil for 5 minutes before turning off the heat.
3. Allow the bay leaves to steep for another 3 minutes.
4. Remove the bay leaves from the tea and serve it hot.
5. If you're using a natural sweetener or milk, use it sparingly because the flavor is subtle.

Uses:

- Enhances digestion
- Ideal for sleeplessness
- Promotes heart health
- Stress is reduced.
- Aids in the treatment of diabetes

14. Aloe Vera (Aloe Vera) for Burns

Preparation Time: 10 minutes
Servings: 2

Ingredients:

- The aloe vera plant's leaf

Directions:

1. This is probably the most straightforward solution you'll come across. Now is the time to try aloe if you haven't already.
2. To ensure you aren't allergic, test it on a small skin patch first.
3. Take one of the leaves and cut the tip off at an angle (but not too steeply) straight across, with at least some leaves still on the tree. Using a knife, thinly slice the onion.
4. The gel can be seen by slicing the leaf in half. Directly apply the gel to the burn.

15. Elderberry Syrup

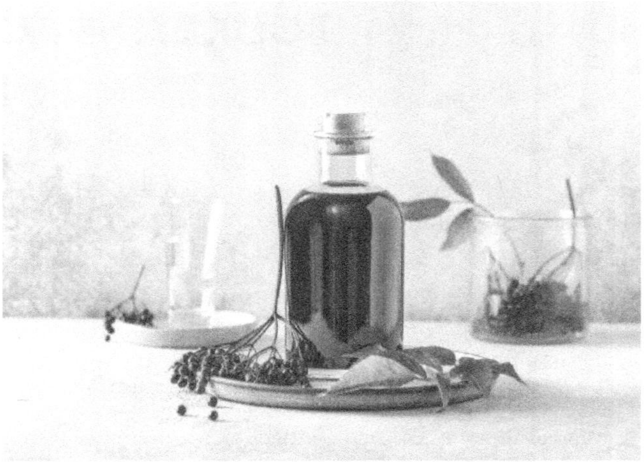

Preparation Time: 10 minutes
Servings: 2

Ingredients:

- 100 g dried elderberries
- 1-2 quarts of cold distilled water
- a half cup of honey (raw)

Directions:

1. Combine the water and berries in a large stockpot. Soak for 30-60 minutes.
2. Bring to a boil, occasionally stirring, over medium heat.
3. When you're dealing with a rolling boil, cook for 30-45 minutes, stirring occasionally and removing the pan from the stove. Toxins that could be harmful are removed during the cooking process.
4. Strain the mixture and measure it. For these purposes, it should be remarkably close to 2 cups.
5. In a mixing bowl, combine the honey and the lemon juice.
6. Place the pot back on the stove.
7. Refrigerate for up to 2 weeks before serving.

To get one dose, divide your total amount by one. If you're healthy, you can take 1 tablespoon every 3-4 hours (up to six times a day), and children over one should take one teaspoon per dose.

16. Honey with Sage Infusion

Preparation Time: 20 minutes
Servings: 2

Ingredients:

- A cup of honey (raw)
- 1 cup sage leaves, fresh

Directions:

1. Wash and dry the sage leaves.
2. Remove the leaves from the stems if you haven't already.
3. In your glass jar, place the sage and fill it up to 34% of the way with water.
4. Pour honey into the jar.
5. Heat destroys many of the medicinal properties of raw honey. Stir the honey in your jar once it has reached the desired consistency. The jar must be labeled and sealed.
6. Store the container in a cool, dry, and dark location. It will be at its peak for a year. Always use a clean spoon to avoid contamination when taking honey out of the jar.

17. Elderberry Extract/Tincture

Preparation Time: 20 minutes
Servings: 2

Ingredients:

- Dried or fresh elderberries
- Cover with menstrual clots (vodka or liquor of choice).
- 1 oz. to 16 oz (470 ml)

Directions:

1. Fill a 1-16 ounce (470 ml) container with dried material to 33% capacity before adding fluid (menstruum is the specific term for the dissolvable or liquid).
2. Fill the jar with herbs to the top.

BOOK 5: THE PREPPER'S SURVIVAL KIT

First aid is the prompt care given to a person who has been injured or is sick until complete medical therapy is available. For minor injuries, first aid treatment may suffice. First aid should be used for serious issues until more advanced care is available.

Many situations may necessitate first aid, and many countries have regulations, guidelines, or instructions determining a basic level of first aid arrangement in specific situations. This can include explicit training or hardware available in the workplace (such as a mechanized external defibrillator), expert first aid cover collection at public social events, or mandatory first aid training inside schools. In any case, first aid requires no specific hardware or prior knowledge and can include the act of spontaneity with materials available at the time, frequently by undeveloped individuals.

Suturing an injury is a thrilling aspect of the prepper lifestyle. In a primitive environment, however, this would be futile because it would increase the risk of infection. Bandaging the wound will keep it clean in this situation. Herbal poultices are another great way to reduce inflammation and stimulate tissue regeneration. The Basics of First Aid and Medical Herbs for Survival Prepping will be a useful addition to your bug-out bag if you're camping.

Reading the directions on the packaging is one way to ensure that you have the right medical supplies for any situation. Even if you believe you do not require a specific item, it is still a good idea to have detailed instructions on hand. This will boost your confidence and give you peace of mind in an emergency. You can save money on shipping by purchasing first aid supplies in bulk, and you'll be ready for any unforeseen event.

CHAPTER 1: FIRST AID KIT

First aid is the first and most immediate assistance given to anyone suffering from a minor or major illness or injury to save a life, prevent the condition from worsening or promote recovery.

When putting together your first aid kit, list the items you're most likely to use. Next, rate each item on a scale of one to five, with one being the least likely to occur and five being the most common. Depending on the risk, you can make your first aid kit or buy one ready-made. This way, you'll always know what you'll need.

Storage of First Aid Kit

When preparing for a disaster, it is critical to have a basic first aid kit on hand. You don't want to be caught without this vital medical equipment. Planning ahead of time will save you time in an emergency. If a disaster strikes, you will not have time to go through all medical supplies. Instead, you will be given a time limit to obtain a specific medication. Everything you need should be easily accessible.

There are numerous types of first aid kits. Pillboxes, for example, are compact and practical. These are available online as well as in retail stores. They can be reused or recycled and are designed to store medical supplies. Others are more expensive, so go with the least costly option. Whether you buy a plastic or metal container, you should buy a zippered bag. Zipper bags are available in various sizes, shapes, colors, and designs.

Remember that the contents can be replaced when storing a survival first aid kit. Keep first aid supplies in a waterproof container to keep moisture at bay. You can even bring your baseball equipment if you go camping. If you have enough room, a first-aid kit can be useful. It will, however, be invaluable in a survival situation.

A great first aid kit can be customized to meet your specific requirements. You can customize the kit for a specific purpose by purchasing the necessary items. Whether you need a bandage or not, a first aid kit can be useful. A survival medical kit can save hundreds of dollars, but an EDC model will set you back less than $100. You will, fortunately, have enough money to upgrade your supplies if necessary.

The primary goal of first aid is to prevent death or severe injury. The abbreviation 'the three Ps' sums up the critical points of first aid:

- Preserve life
- Prevent deterioration
- Promote recovery

Instruments for First Aid

Starting your survival first aid kit with the things you already have at home is a smart idea. These things are suggested for treating small cuts and scrapes that are common in everyday life.

This harm includes:

- Abrasions
- Burns
- Cuts
- Splinters
- Sprains
- Stings

These injuries can occur even after a disaster, so having items to treat them in your survival kit is a good idea. You must supplement it with a few additional injury-specific items and personal medications.

In your supply, don't forget to include some medication to relieve the symptoms of respiratory and gastrointestinal infections, such as coughing, fever, stomach pains, and diarrhea. If you have children, keep medications in dosages appropriate for their age and current prescriptions on hand.

The following are the items and utensils that should be included in your first-aid kit:

- Bandages and self-adhesive tape
- Anti-diarrhea and antacid medications

- An antiseptic used to clean wounds and hands
- Oral and topical antihistamines
- Antibacterial cream or spray for minor cuts and scrapes
- Antiseptic lotion or spray for insect bites and rashes
- Aspirin or any pain reliever that can also be used to prevent heart attacks
- Bandages for sprains and splints, as well as securing gauze to wounds
- Relief gel or relief cream
- Cough suppressant drugs
- First-aid guidelines
- Ibuprofen or a pain reliever, fever reducer, and antibiotic
- Knife
- A mask for CPR
- Moleskin is applied to minor burns and blisters
- Instrument sterilization
- Asthma and cold nasal decongestant
- Non-adhesive sterile gauze pads for cleaning and covering wounds and burns
- Medications on prescription
- A phone card with at least 60 minutes of talk time, spare change for pay phones, and an emergency contact list
- Other significant phone numbers, such as 911 and poison control.
- plastic resealable bags
- Safety pins for splint removal and bandaging
- single-use gloves and ice packs for infection treatment
- Solar screen
- Scissors (optional)
- A small flashlight
- Topically applied corticosteroids to treat rashes
- Tourniquet bandages and triangular slings
- Tweezers for extracting stingers, splinters, or ticks

All these items are readily available at any well-stocked drugstore, but it is up to you to put them together in an orderly manner. Remember to place the items in a resealable nylon bag with good visibility. You don't need to buy a special case; a nice water-resistant makeup bag will suffice. Drying adhesives and sterilized items are critical. Because this collection is much larger than a standard first-aid kit, labeling and categorizing everything is a good idea. Each category of items can be divided into smaller bags and stuffed into a large backpack. This allows you to keep everything in one place and check to see if anything needs to be restocked regularly.

Make sure you understand how to use all the items in your kit and teach your loved ones how to do the same in case you need first aid. Keep the first-aid kit handy for anyone who is staying with you.

First Aid Herbal Kit

This list is a great place to start if you want to make a natural first-aid kit. It should be noted that these items should only be used to treat minor injuries and should not be used in place of medical treatment provided by a licensed physician or other qualified health care provider. Natural treatments may be less dangerous than conventional medications, but this should not be used as an excuse to avoid rigorous research in pursuing holistic health care. Essential oils can cause severe reactions in some people, particularly children, and pregnant women. As a result, extreme caution is required.

You should keep these items on hand to have a medicine kit ready in an emergency.

These natural products should be stored in glass jars, preferably wrapped in thick flannel, to prevent them from mixing. Other items stored in a first aid kit compartment include aloe vera gel, elderberry capsules, lavender oil, and tea bags.

These are the herbs that cannot be missing from your home kit:

- ***Green Fennel*** strengthens the stomach, promotes digestion, and calms or eliminates gastrointestinal spasms. It is a plant for combating gas, bloating, flatulence, and bad breath.
- ***Calendula*** is probably one of the best herbs to treat skin conditions such as insect bites, dermatitis, minor sunburns, scalds, abrasions, or scratches. In addition, it helps relieve ear infections and, as an eye drop, can be used on the eyes and a stye.

- The main use of ***Milk Thistle*** is liver protection, an excellent digestive resource, and an intravenous supplement. It is an excellent digestive resource that helps stimulate the appetite and fights heavy digestion, indigestion, and the feeling of an upset stomach. It is an intravenous tonic for varicose veins and hemorrhoids.
- ***Dandelion*** is used for hepatobiliary diseases, indigestion, and food poisoning, such as preventing gallstone formation and promoting urination.
- ***Echinacea*** is one of the well-known plants for strengthening the body's defenses and preventing respiratory and other diseases. It activates the formation of white blood cells, blocks the action of bacteria and viruses, and prevents infections from spreading.
- ***Eucalyptus*** has hypoglycemic properties and can be used to support conventional or natural remedies for mild diabetes or in its early stages. Vaporizing with its leaves is the best solution to combat congestion caused by mucus in bronchitis and other respiratory diseases.
- ***Bearberry*** is the best herbal remedy for urinary tract infections. Therefore, it is suitable for problems such as cystitis or prostatitis. As an astringent, it is used to stop diarrhea.
- With ***Ginkgo***, the leaves of this legendary tree are the main herbal resource to treat the effects of aging at the vascular level. Herbalists recommend it to stop dementia, increase brain irrigation, and help stop memory loss and concentration.
- ***Devil's Claw*** has become one of the pain's most famous herbal remedies. It is mainly used to combat rheumatic pain and inflammation, arthritis, knee, and hip osteoarthritis, low back pain, and neuralgia. Its use can reduce or replace the consumption of cortisone and NSAIDs, which can damage the gastric mucosa in the long run.
- ***Hypericum*** has antidepressant properties that rival chemical antidepressants that contain MAOIs. It is widely used to treat mild to moderate depression, early depression, non-acute anxiety disorders, night terrors, states of sadness, nervous palpitations, insomnia, and autonomic disorders related to menopause.
- ***Malva*** relieves inflammation of the mucous membranes, calms irritating cough, and eliminates mucus. It is suitable for common colds, flu, rhinitis, or sinusitis respiratory allergies. It is also used for stomach irritation, stomach ulcers, diarrhea, and mild constipation.
- ***Chamomile*** is one of the most consumed plants and one of the most used in the pantry. It is effective in promoting digestion after a heavy meal. It is also helpful in calming menstrual cramps or PMS.
- ***Passiflora*** combats insomnia and is a great muscle relaxant. It provides restful sleep, although it does not affect everyone equally. It is also designed to combat neurological arrhythmias, palpitations, mild anxiety, hyperactivity, and migraines.
- ***Licorice*** is an excellent resource for treating digestive disorders. It has a strong sweetening power and can be used to remove the bitterness of many herbs. It can make bronchial secretions more fluid and helps reduce inflammation of the mucous membranes of the respiratory system. It is also used to treat inflammation of the mouth to reduce swelling of the eyelids and around the eyes.
- ***Rosemary*** has a great stimulating effect on the central nervous system. It helps fight weakness and fatigue and provides post-rehabilitation support. It is thought to protect liver function.
- The ***Butcher's Broom*** tones the veins and promotes blood flow. It treats poor peripheral circulation problems caused by poor circulation, such as varicose veins, phlebitis, hemorrhoids, and numbness in the hands, feet, or legs.
- ***Sage*** helps relieve symptoms of premenstrual syndrome, the crampy pain that accompanies menstruation, and fights weakness. The external parts are used as a mouthwash or as a gargle for mouth ulcers and wounds, gingivitis, stomatitis, and pharyngitis.
- ***Linden*** calms nervous palpitations and arrhythmias and is suitable for the whole family. It is an excellent resource for natural stress control and is also used to treat insomnia.
- ***Thyme*** is a Mediterranean plant that treats colds, sore throats, and other respiratory problems. Its use is also aimed at eliminating intestinal parasites.
- ***Valerian*** is the best herbal remedy for the treatment of insomnia. It is an excellent ally for young people, children, and athletes who maintain a high level of physical activity because it helps to relax muscles and combat discomfort caused by overwork.

CHAPTER 2: IMPORTANT FIRST AID PROCEDURES

In catastrophic scenarios, injuries are virtually unavoidable. Depending on the nature of the disaster, you may be injured in various ways. If you are not injured by falling debris, fire, or water, you may be injured due to panic in an emergency. Learning basic first aid techniques can help you prepare for these scenarios, whether they affect you or someone close to you.

While these goals may appear straightforward, worry may cause you to lose sight of what you need to do to help someone you care about. The "Three P's" are the primary goals of first aid. Here's how to implement them.

- **Preserve Life:** The overarching goal of all medical care, including first aid, is to save lives and reduce the risk of death. First aid performed correctly should help reduce the patient's pain level and calm them down during the assessment and treatment process.
- **Prevent Deterioration:** Preventing deterioration includes tending to external factors such as creating some distance from any source of harm and using first aid methods to prevent deteriorating conditions, such as using strain to keep a drain from becoming dangerous.
- **Promote Recovery:** First aid also includes attempting to start the recovery cycle from the disease or injury and, at times, may have finished treatment, for example, by applying a mortar to a bit of hurt.

Fractures and Sprains

Sprains can occur if you spend a lot of time outside. This danger primarily affects hikers and rock climbers, but it could affect anyone.

Ankles, knees, and elbows are the most sprained joints. The RICE method is the most effective for treating minor sprains. This stands for rest, ice, compression, and elevation. Apply cold packs to the injured area for the first 24 hours after the incident. After that, heat packs may be helpful for pain relief.

Keep an elastic bandage and over-the-counter pain relievers in your first aid kit to relieve the discomfort. Knowing how to treat sprains before they occur is critical to controlling the pain as soon as possible.

Sprains and fractures can be difficult to distinguish. If a body part looks strange, cannot be moved, or screams for several hours, it is most likely a broken bone rather than a sprain. Sprains usually heal independently, but there are ways to accelerate the healing process. This is accomplished by applying ice to the skin, constricting blood vessels, and reducing blood flow. To avoid contact with sensitive skin, wrap the icing bag in a towel. After icing the injury for a few minutes, rest for a few minutes before repeating the icing. Keep the area elevated and avoid putting any weight on it. If you suspect someone has broken bones, a splint may be used to stabilize and prevent the bones from moving. Straightening the bones should be avoided because it may cause more harm than good. To reduce swelling, apply an ice pack to the injured area and give the person pain relievers.

Hypothermia

Hypothermia, the second leading cause of death, can cause death in the outdoors. Hypothermia can occur when the body's temperature falls below 90 degrees Fahrenheit, resulting in death. It is a medical condition caused by prolonged cold exposure. Symptoms include shivering, a weak pulse and coordination, confusion and slurred speech, and loss of consciousness.

Hypothermia is a condition that requires immediate treatment as soon as it is discovered. Before venturing outdoors for the first time, it is critical to understand hypothermia and how to avoid it. When exposed to cold temperatures or damp conditions, it is possible to become hypothermic.

Being submerged in cold water may intensify this disease. Experts believe that if you fall into cold water and cannot get out within 10 to 15 minutes, you may be unable to get out without assistance. Depending on the temperature of the water, hypothermia can cause cardiac arrest within 90 to 180 minutes. If a person is submerged in cold water, remove them from the cold and wrap them in blankets and heat packs until it is safe to move. Be gentle with them, as any sudden movement in their body could cause cardiac arrest. To avoid scorching, do not apply heat directly to their skin. If they are aware, offer them warm drinks. If the person's clothes are wet, remove them from the cold ground.

You are also susceptible to hypothermia when you are outdoors. You must drink no alcoholic beverages. Alcohol dilates blood vessels, which is hazardous and impairs judgment. Because your blood isn't getting to the rest of your body as quickly as it should, you're losing valuable body heat faster.

Hypothermia has some obvious symptoms. Here are some examples: For most people, shivering is the first sign that their body is becoming too cold. That is the way the body attempts to warm itself. If you are having difficulty speaking or walking, seek immediate assistance. The Wilderness Skills Institute can teach you more about hypothermia and how to avoid becoming ill from it.

Allergic Reactions

Allergic reactions happen when the immune system's response to a foreign substance is exaggerated. Anaphylaxis, a potentially fatal condition, may occur if the reaction is severe enough. If you see someone having an allergic reaction, inquire about their allergies. If they do, they might have a pi-pen, which you could use to help them feel better. Allow the individual to lie on their back with their feet elevated. They should remove their clothing to allow them to breathe more freely. No water, food, or medication should be given to them orally. Check to see if the person's clothing is loose and if they can breathe. If you used the pi-Pen, wait about 15 minutes. If the reaction persists, you should administer a second dose.

Infection Control

Before touching any wounds, use antibacterial hand wipes to disinfect your hands. Avoid using public restrooms to avoid spreading bacteria and causing an infection. You can also use hand sanitizer gel or spray before touching anything.

For assisting with wound care, a total body cleansing station stocked with lancets, alcohol swabs, alcohol wipes, a thermometer for checking body temperature, and a thermometer tape measure would be ideal.

A portable foot bath can disinfect and clean foot wounds. It is suitable for cleaning but lacks antibacterial properties, resulting in infectious damage.

Any FDA-approved medical tape or bandage may be used. Please ensure they are free of latex and safe to use on human skin or wounds. You should also choose a specific brand of medical tape because some contain silicone. This substance can cause skin irritation or burning if you don't notice it immediately.

Heart Attack

If someone has a heart attack, it is essential to call emergency services immediately. When emergency personnel arrives, they will give the person oxygen and CPR if necessary. They may also give medications to dissolve blood clots or unclog blocked arteries.

Burns

One of the most dreadful accidents that can happen to anyone is burns. Burns are, unfortunately, a common occurrence when camping outside. If this happens to you, you must know how to treat burns effectively and safely.

You should understand the distinction between healing chemical burns and treating burns caused by heat sources like a fire. To avoid spreading fire, ensure everyone in your group understands how to stop, drop, and roll. The brief motion reduces the increased body surface area caused by the exercise. Moderate burns are easier to deal with in the woods than severe burns, which can be fatal. On the other hand, anyone who suffers a severe and painful burn should seek medical attention immediately.

Treatment of burns can be complex depending on the nature of the injury and what caused it. The first thing you should do if you come across someone with a burn of any kind is to remove the source of the burn. Next, assess the extent of the burn. A first-degree burn affects only the skin's surface layer. A second-degree burn damages the skin's deeper structures and causes visible damage. Third-degree burns are the most serious and can have long-term consequences. They require immediate medical assistance.

For first-degree burns, apply a cold compress to the burn and secure it in place. To treat the burn, you can use a variety of substances, such as burn cream. Soak the wound in warm water and, if necessary, take a pain reliever.

Second-degree burns necessitate more immediate action. The skin's surface will blister and become damaged. The area must be kept clean. Applying a light dressing is an option. The longer it takes to treat a burn, the more severe it becomes.

The most serious of burns, the third-degree burn, may necessitate intensive medical treatment due to the extent of the burn and its location on the body. These burns are thought to be the most painful due to their severity. However, this is not guaranteed because many nerve endings in and beneath the skin will have been severely damaged. As a result, the affected area may have no sensation. If you have such a burn, seek expert medical attention, make sure your clothing does not stick to the burn and do not attempt self-care. Elevate the injured area above the heart if possible. There is no timetable for recovering from a third-degree burn, but severe scarring can occur if the burn is not treated.

Minor burns can be treated by applying cold (but not ice) water to the affected area, followed by a moisturizing ointment. Keep the blisters and the injury away from the sun. Medical attention should be sought as soon as possible if a person has suffered a severe burn. Avoid applying anything to the wound to prevent infection; instead, cover it with a loose cloth. Give the injured person pain relievers if they are in a lot of pain.

If a person is burned, call 911 immediately and try to stop the burning process. Remove all contaminated clothing and gently flush the burn with running water until it stops steaming if the person cannot stop the burning or chemical exposure. Then, cover it with a clean bandage and follow all other emergency responders' instructions.

Seizures

If someone has an epileptic seizure, ensure they are safe and wait for them to stop shaking or convulsing. Then, after the seizure has passed, check their breathing and pulse rate, which should be normal. If they are injured or are still having difficulty breathing, dial 911, and an emergency medical technician will provide first aid until a doctor arrives.

Fall

Remove any clothing that could restrict a person's movement if they have fallen and may have broken bones or other injuries. Then, as gently as possible, transfer them to a flat surface while applying pressure to any open wounds. Inquire about any neck or back pain if the person is awake and responsive. If this is the case, gently press both sides of these areas and have them wiggle their toes to check for numbness. Finally, gently move the joint to check for swelling or discoloration around the joints.

Treating Shock

Shock is a condition that occurs when blood pressure drops due to severe blood loss. If you cannot stop the bleeding from a severe injury, you may need to administer shock treatment. Place the victim on a comfortable but flat surface and gently raise the affected or injured limb above the heart, allowing blood to flow back towards the heart and relieve pressure on it. Ascertain that the victim is breathing. If not, start CPR right away. Adjust any tight belts or clothing. Ascertain that the victim is warm. If the victim is choking, try to clear the airway by removing the obstruction. If the victim's airway is not clear, turn them on their side.

It can cause serious complications, so it must be treated right away. Take a blood pressure reading if someone is in shock. If their blood pressure is low, start giving them warm liquids intravenously. Then, try to keep the patient as calm as possible to avoid a seizure or cardiac arrest.

If someone has diabetic shock, go to the hospital immediately. Then, examine their airway, breathing patterns, and mental state. Check their blood sugar levels every few minutes to see if they improve, and to keep them hydrated as much as possible when you arrive at the hospital, dial 911. Once there, emergency personnel will administer oxygen to the individual to increase their oxygen intake. They may also administer medications such as insulin and intravenous fluids until they stabilize.

Broken Bones

In survival situations, broken bones are common. They can occur due to trips, falls, and other accidents. The main concern with a broken bone is that it may shift into a dangerous position. As a result, the critical issue must be securing the bone in place. If a fractured bone shifts by accident, it may press against a blood vessel or nerve, causing damage. This could obstruct blood flow and potentially damage a limb in the long run. If the fracture is open, it may become infected. The first step is thus to address this open wound. The bone must be secured after the wound has been closed.

Stopping Bleeding

If someone is bleeding, you should first keep them from losing too much blood. Locate a bandage or clean cloth immediately and apply it liberally to the wound. Apply the bandage to the wound and check if the bleeding has stopped after 20 to 30 minutes. If this occurs, clean the wound with a damp towel and an antiseptic. Do not apply soap to open wounds. Apply an antibiotic spray to the wound and cover it with a bandage. Never use a spray or ointment to a cut that appears to be too deep or isn't stopping the bleeding. Cover it loosely with a towel to prevent infection. Maintain pressure and seek medical attention. For a simple nosebleed, lean slightly forward and press a tissue or cloth against the person's nostrils until the bleeding stops.

To stop the bleeding, elevate the affected area above the heart. You must stop the bleeding and excessive blood loss from that wound. Applying pressure to the affected area is another way to avoid or stop blood loss. Another option is to use a tourniquet on the affected limb. By doing so, you are limiting blood flow and allowing the wound to clot.

Concussion

A concussion occurs when the head or skull is traumatized, resulting in brain injury. A concussion is a serious condition in which everything appears normal to the onlooker, but severe bleeding or damage has occurred inside the brain. Despite popular belief, rest is one of the most effective treatments for concussion. Confusion, dizziness, or a lack of ability to complete simple tasks should be looked for. If there are signs of more severe brain damage, expert medical attention may be required. The patient must be kept calm and well-rested for the most part. If there are external head injuries, treat them as best you can in the given situation.

Making a Splint

Making a splint allows broken bones to rest and heal without being jolted out of place. It also strengthens the affected limb and keeps it straight, preventing bones from healing in a crooked position. Splints can also be used to support sprained or dislocated limbs. A splint is a piece of wood, metal, plastic, or another stiff material tied to the affected limb to prevent further damage. You can make your splint using whatever materials you have on hand.

First, if any bleeding occurs, it must be stopped. Next, wrap some padding around the wound and secure it. Finally, secure the splint beneath the injured area. Make sure not to put too much pressure or press on the injured area.

Dehydration

Dizziness, lack of concentration, and profuse sweating are the first signs of dehydration. When you notice these symptoms, you must immediately determine whether you drank enough water during the day. You will lose more water if you engage in physical activity, so drink more. Dehydration is not always evident at first. But this is the risk of dehydration. You are not always aware of when you are approaching this stage. As a result, you must take the necessary precautions to avoid becoming involved in a dangerous situation. If you're far from home and find yourself in a desert or a precarious situation, you'll have to devise a method of obtaining water when more obvious solutions aren't available. One of the options available to you is a hydration bladder. This plastic bag has an inner sleeve that allows you to store water and place it in the victim's mouth if they cannot swallow. The fluid is accessed through a hose connected to the bag. Drinking is the only way to treat all types of dehydration, but if you can't find any, have passed out, or are unconscious, you may require more immediate medical attention.

You can easily get dehydrated when you're out in the sun and heat, especially moving around. This illness is deceptive, with symptoms appearing at any time. Dehydration occurs when you lose more body fluids than you take in. It's easy to forget to drink enough water or sports drinks when you're busy outside, which can lead to dehydration. This means your body is dehydrated, especially after peeing and sweating. Dehydration can affect anyone, but children and the elderly are especially vulnerable. There are several early warning signs and indications that someone is dehydrated.

These symptoms include an inability to produce tears, a dry mouth, skin that sags when squeezed, and dried eyes. It is critical to keep newborns and small children hydrated even when you are outside. The most effective way to treat dehydration is to avoid it in the first place.

Dehydration is a potentially fatal condition. If you notice any early warning symptoms or signs of dehydration, seek medical attention as soon as possible to avoid serious consequences.

Wounds

Cleaning and dressing wounds is a situational task because it depends on the situation and the wound. If the wound is superficial and not bleeding heavily, you do not need to treat it as quickly. If, on the other hand, a wound is excessively bleeding, it may indicate a severed underlying artery or vein, and immediate assistance is required. If the wound is superficial, treat it as follows:

1. To begin, put on gloves to reduce the risk of infection.
2. Next, ensure that the wound is clean. Gently scrub it with a gauze or cotton pad, soap, and water. If something is stuck in the wound, use tweezers to remove it without causing pain to the victim. You can also use a syringe to clean a wound without touching it.
3. Next, make sure that the water you use has been disinfected. Iodine tablets can be used for this.
4. Finally, use a clean cotton or gauze pad to pressure the injured area and stop bleeding. If the injury turns out to be more serious than you first thought, more drastic measures may be required.

After cleaning the larger wound, you must bandage it. Minor wounds may also require this, but they usually only need a lighter dressing. Apply antiseptic ointment to the wound. After that, wrap the wound gently but firmly. If the bandage is not adhesive, you may need to secure it with duct tape or a safety pin. If the dressing becomes wet or dirty, it must be replaced. Make it a habit to check it every day. Splinting may be required if a joint is injured. After bandaging the wound, assess the patient's ability to move the injured part without pain. If they can move, blood flows to the area. If the bandages are numb, they may be too tight. They can be slightly loosened or removed and reset.

If you find yourself on a disaster scene, there are numerous things you can do to help. One method is to provide victims with immediate medical attention. Natural disasters can result in widespread and severe injuries. If you know what to look for and how to respond, you can make a difference in the lives of others. It should be noted that treatment facilities will quickly become overcrowded with injured people who do not have access to medical care. You may have to act as a doctor until additional medical personnel arrives.

Snake Bites and Insect Stings

The days are getting longer, the weather is warming up, and we can finally enjoy being outside. However, as we all know, increased outdoor activity increases the risk of injury. And it's not just accidents with sharp objects or treacherous terrain that pose a threat these days; plenty of poisonous creatures lurking nearby can inflict serious harm if they decide to strike.

A snake bite usually results in a puncture wound through which venom is injected into the skin and surrounding tissue. Here's what you should do in case you or someone you know gets bitten by a snake:

- **Do not pull:** You should not attempt to pull and shake off the snake clutching your body. Instead, remain motionless and seek medical attention. That is correct, and you should maintain as much stillness as possible until you can see a doctor.
- **Calm the bite area:** Maintain as much stillness and calm as possible in the affected area of your body. Going somewhere you can rest and relax for a few hours is best to allow the venom to work out of your body.
- **Do not rush to breathe:** One common fear of snake bites is that the airway will become blocked (due to the swollen bite area), and the victim will die from a lack of oxygen. But don't worry; your body will react naturally to this situation. To aid in healing, the body will send more blood to the area and produce more mucus. So, if your airway feels swollen, it could be (though you should still see a doctor).
- **Stay calm:** You might be surprised to learn that panicking or freaking out can worsen your symptoms.
- **Do not rush to an emergency room:** Some people are afraid of hospitals and doctors (or any medical care, for that matter), but for snake bites and other minor wounds, this is unnecessary.
- **Leave the area immediately:** It is best not to stay in the vicinity of the snake or the incident. For example, if you are bitten, and there is a sign warning people not to touch poisonous snakes, you should leave the area immediately.

Assume you were bitten by a snake or something else that could be venomous and pose a threat to your health (such as bees, wasps, bull ants). This reduces the possibility of death from the injury or other medical conditions later on.

CHAPTER 3: SURVIVAL EQUIPMENT

It makes sense to be ready for an emergency. Having essential survival gear on hand can help you survive, if not thrive, in any situation.

Essential Survival Gear You Should Always Have Prepared

Paracord

Paracord is a lightweight cord that can bind objects together, make clothes, or rescue people from dangerous situations. To be adequately prepared to deal with any potential problem, you must have a paracord. You can also choose from a variety of colors and lengths of paracord!

Knife

While it is not true that bad guys only appear at night, a knife can provide some protection during the day and when no bad guy is present. Having a Swiss Army knife (or other multi-tool) on hand would be useful while traveling and camping.

While an air horn isn't exactly survival equipment, it can still save your life.

Water Filter

Water is essential for survival, and you must purify the water yourself if you cannot drink from natural sources. A water filter is one of the best ways to ensure your water source is safe to drink. It's helpful if you end up in an area with polluted water, and it's also great for purifying natural water sources.

Portable Cell Phone Charger

Cell phones are great when they're charged but not so great when running out of power.

Seasonal Clothing

This is especially important if you'll be outside during a season change. When the temperature drops, you must dress appropriately or risk freezing to death. If the temperature rises, you must remove your layers as you may risk overheating and suffering from heat stroke.

Two base layers are required for cold weather survival clothing. The first should cover the entire body, while the second should cover the lower half. The wrists and ankles should be covered, and the shirt should fit over the back and overlap at the waist. Merino wool, which wicks moisture away from the body and is odor resistant, should be used. It also has natural antibacterial properties. You can wear synthetic or cotton clothing if you don't want to spend much on winter clothing.

One of the first things you should consider when planning your cold-weather survival clothing is the temperature of the environment you will be in. It is critical to stay warm to avoid frostbite, hypothermia, and even death. Layering clothing aids in heat retention and the prevention of cold-related illnesses. Layers are the most fundamental approach to clothing: the base layer should wick away moisture, the insulating layer should keep you warm, and the outer layer should protect you from the elements.

Hatchet

While not quite as versatile as a knife, the hatchet is still a great survival tool for chopping wood, making shelter, and starting fires. If you don't have a hatchet, then the next best thing is a good multi-tool.

Paracord Bracelets

Paracord bracelets are great for holding things together that are prone to coming loose or getting caught on other objects. Because it is lightweight and versatile, paracord is ideal for these applications.

Folding Shovel

While not precisely survival gear, this is another handy tool you should consider for redirecting water, digging holes, etc. You may also not carry a standard shovel, but if you can, go for it.

A Good Map and Compass

Knowing where you are is critical, especially if help is on the way or if you are attempting to find your way back home. If you're hiking, ensure you have a good map and compass because one without the other can significantly slow you down.

A map is one of the most essential pieces of survival equipment. It is also beneficial to big game hunters. If you're in the middle of nowhere, you need to know where the nearest road is. A map is also helpful for determining alternative routes if you are in an area with no roads. A good topographic map is worth its weight in gold. Check with local authorities to find the best map for your situation.

A printed map is the least expensive option, but it will eventually wear out after repeated use. Using a waterproof zip-top bag can help keep your maps dry. A plastic Ziploc bag is another less expensive option. It is not waterproof, but it will keep your survival gear safe. Many of these bags are available online. You can even buy them from local hiking/mountaineering clubs. You can prepare your survival gear once you've found the right map.

Compasses are essential survival equipment, but they have limitations. For example, the military compass lacks a declination adjustment. The compass also lacks a thumb loop, making it difficult to adjust the needle properly. The compass is intended to be accurate and reliable, but some users have complained that it is not accurate enough for outdoor activities.

While GPS is simple to use, it may not be the best option in an emergency. If there is no electricity and the signal is weak or absent, it will fail to provide you with accurate directions. A compass can save your life in such a situation. Having a compass with you can also assist you in navigating the wilderness. However, never intentionally put yourself in a survival situation. Seek an expert to teach you how to use a compass for survival.

Energy Bars

These are a great way to gain the energy needed to hike back home if you become lost. Not only that, but they're also pretty tasty to eat.

Flashlight and Extra Batteries

If it gets dark, a flashlight can help illuminate dark areas.

Choosing a flashlight as survival equipment is critical. Regardless of the various types and features, finding one that provides enough light is vital. A tactical survival flashlight is an excellent choice for this purpose. A flashlight's beam can temporarily blind or scare an attacker into hiding. Furthermore, light deters would-be attackers. It isn't the only reason to carry a flashlight, but it is an excellent piece of equipment.

A flashlight is one of the most useful pieces of survival equipment. It can be used to communicate and provide comfort in difficult situations. Unsurprisingly, flashlights are an essential component of any survival kit. Until the invention of fire and incandescent bulbs, humans struggled with darkness. Fortunately, modern LED lighting has eliminated this risk. A flashlight can mean the difference between life and death in an emergency.

Pen and Paper

Take down important details such as where a person is going or why they went somewhere. A pen and paper are also ideal for taking notes for yourself or a loved one.

Whistle

This is a great way to get help if you're trying to call for assistance when lost. Ensure you pack a whistle with a solid sound to attract as many people as possible.

A Water Bottle

It's easy to overlook items in your pack, but a water bottle is essential if you're stuck or lost. Staying hydrated is also particularly important; you'll want to stay as hydrated as possible to avoid dehydration. If you've forgotten your water bottle, make sure you have another way to stay hydrated without having to stop and drink too much.

Food and Snacks

Food and snacks are critical, and if you are stranded, lost, injured, or otherwise in a bad situation, these will help you survive. Always bring enough food to last for the duration of your trip, plus some extra in case of an emergency, such as being caught in the rain. Keep in mind that your survival food must be light and easy to transport, so keep the amount of food to a minimum.

Even if you don't feel hungry or have a lot of energy, when you're lost, food will help. Pack enough food, so you don't have to go out looking for food or risk getting hurt if hunger strikes late at night.

Firestarter

Many people are unaware of how inexpensive and simple it is to include a fire starter in their survival kit. Dip a cotton ball into petroleum jelly to make this simple survival tool. Although less effective, this item can be purchased at a pharmacy or made at home. Patience is essential for a successful fire starter. If the fuel does not ignite in a timely manner, the product can be prepared ahead of time and bagged for protection.

A magnesium bar is another option for starting a fire. To start a fire, these tools combine combustion with tinder. They measure three inches long and half an inch thick, and one side has an embedded ferrocerium rod. The magnesium shavings are ignited by the rod. Because of their small size, they make an excellent backup fire starter. Firesteels are simple but not a good substitute for traditional tinder.

Sleeping bags

Sleeping bags are now an essential piece of outdoor gear. They can be unzipped and unpacked to allow for cooling. Down insulation is made from the feathers closest to the dermal layer of ducks and geese. This material traps air, which aids in body temperature regulation. Female birds pluck these feathers from their bodies to use as nest lining. Down insulation is the most effective type of insulation; it keeps you warm in cold weather.

This may seem obvious, but when it comes to camping, you may forget about having a sleeping bag until the night arrives. A survival blanket is an excellent way to stay dry on a rainy night and can protect you from insects or animals if there is anything outside at all. You also don't have to pack a sleeping bag unless you get caught while traveling and are forced to do so.

Another useful piece of survival equipment is mylar emergency blankets. They are cheap and will keep you warm even in the coldest weather. They can also assist you in quickly heating up if you get wet. These bags fit easily in the glove box and protect you from the elements. These blankets can be used for a variety of activities and scenarios. Sleeping bags are essential survival gear whether you're going camping or backpacking.

HERBAL GLOSSARY

- **Achillea:** It is a popular herb, which is also known as the yarrow plant. It is also preferable for the common cold, hay fever, menstruation problems, appetite loss, etc. Some people also prefer to chew the leaves of this plant to heal toothache problems. It has the properties to deal with gastrointestinal discomfort.
- **Agrimony (Agrimonia Eupatoria):** Agrimony is a powerful prepping herb that has the properties of alleviating menstrual discomfort, managing diabetes, improving bladder control, supporting body detoxification, and promoting skin health. When consumed in an ideal remedy form, this herb also helps revive respiratory health.
- **Alder (Alnus Rubra):** The leaves and bark of this herbal plant are used for medicines. People consume alder as remedies to prevent bleedings, heal a sore throat, swelling, arthritis, constipation, and even suppress cancer symptoms. People use it in gargles to ease sore throat conditions.

- **Aloe Vera**: Aloe Vera comprises special health compounds that accelerate wound healing, reduce dental plaque, lower blood sugar levels, prevent wrinkles, reduce constipation, and treat many other problems. The good news is that aloe vera is easily accessible around several spaces, and it is also convenient for you to grow this plant in your backyard.
- **Amaranth (Amaranthus retroflexus):** The nutrient contents in the Amaranth herb allows you to add it to a healthy diet. It is a rich source of Vitamin C, vital to your body's healing process. It is because that helps form the blood vessels, process iron, repair the muscle tissue, and help maintain collagen levels.
- **Chamomile**: It's a good idea to have a supply of high-quality dried chamomile on hand for brewing tea. Do your research on dried chamomile and get the finest you can afford. Dried chamomile flowers may also create soothing poultices for various wounds and ailments. Chamomile is one of the medicinal plants known for its floral properties. Its role is significant in the treatment of gastrointestinal complaints.
- **Cayenne***:* A cayenne powder sachet is highly recommended since it has excellent wound-sealing properties when applied topically to exterior wounds. Make your cayenne capsules by filling up empty gel capsules with cayenne pepper. Due to its ability to increase blood flow, cayenne may assist in speeding the healing process following sickness.
- **Comfrey***:* Comfrey is a beautiful plant that may be used as a poultice to relieve pain. This herb seems to aid in healing numerous ailments, but it is particularly beneficial for fracture repair.
- **Ginger**: Ginger is useful in the first-aid box and a tasty spice to use in cooking. Perhaps you've heard the suggestion to eat ginger snaps or drink ginger ale if you have an upset stomach. Ginger has a calming effect on digestive disturbances of many kinds and is particularly useful for nausea.
- **Aromatic Clove**: The aromatic clove comes with antimicrobial properties for killing bacteria. It acts as a pain reliever for specific conditions like muscle pain and toothache. The aromatic clove properties are accountable for healing stomach aches and digestive problems. The essential oil derived from aromatic cloves is also used for relieving respiratory conditions such as asthma and cough.
- **Bach Flowers**: The Bach flowers are accountable as powerful remedies for dealing with depression, anxiety, emotional trauma, physical trauma, and stress. Not just that, but the ideal remedies made out of these flowers have also replicated the ideologies of healing HIV and Cancer. There might be fewer research pieces of evidence to prove these facts, but the practical reviews of consumers have stated positive results.
- **Beeswax**: Beeswax is more of a hair-healing herb! It moisturizes the hair and smoothens it out. It works upon sealing the strands and promotes the healthy growth of hairs. The scalp conditions are also improved to serve the overall healing purpose.
- **Beech (Fagus Grandilolia):** This herb's most crucial benefit is stimulating hair growth and protecting the immune system. Moreover, it also improves skin health and boosts the health of a newborn. If you or your family members have any kind of respiratory distress, kidney toxicity, chronic disease, or pain symptoms, then beech can help ease its symptoms.
- **Black Cohosh (Actaea Racemosa):** This is commonly preferable for healing menopausal symptoms, night sweats, hot flashes, and other conditions. Women mainly use it for treating vaginal dryness symptoms and irritability around intimate areas. With proper blend and infusions, black cohosh reduces body pains and muscle aches associated with perimenopause, post-menopause, and menopause conditions.
- **Valerian**: This plant is widely used in phytotherapy. It has countless benefits, but perhaps the most famous is helping you to relax. This plant is proven to reduce anxiety and help you sleep. But it is also good for diarrhea, reduces mild tremors, and relieves headaches and menstrual tension.
- **Poppy**: It is a medicinal plant with therapeutic properties, mainly found in seeds. With these, it is possible to prevent cardiovascular diseases, anemia, or skin diseases.
- **Eucalyptus**: One of the most famous properties of eucalyptus is the relief of cold symptoms, especially respiratory diseases (cough, bronchitis, pneumonia, asthma, etc.) It is an all-around beneficial plant for health.
- **Ginkgo**: Research has established the Ginkgo tree to be the oldest surviving tree on Earth, and it is one of the most important healing plants. Its fan-shaped leaves are characteristic, and as for its benefits, Ginkgo has antioxidant properties that improve concentration and memory.
- **Sage**: Clary sage or sage is one of the most famous plants in cosmetics, but it also has other functions. The main one is to relieve the symptoms of menopause. It has thermoregulatory properties that can help women control hot flashes, excessive sweating, and hormones at this stage.
- **Dandelion**: Dandelion has been extensively used as a natural remedy to prevent digestive disorders. In addition, the plant contains a good amount of B vitamins, which help rebuild the intestinal flora and reduce joint pain and gas.

Herbs are the same as medicinal plants. The only difference is that their stems are more tender. Amongst the most important ones are:

- **Lavender**: In addition to its calming properties, lavender regenerates cells, fights inflammation, and heals. It treats burns, wounds, allergies, and conditions such as rheumatism or arthritis.
- **Rosemary**: This is among the most widely used medicinal plants. For example, it has anti-inflammatory properties and can be used to fight dandruff and repel mosquitoes, among other things.
- **Mint**: Mint is a digestive, analgesic, and antiseptic medicinal plant. As well as being an excellent nasal decongestant, it has antispasmodic, antiemetic, diaphoretic, and choleretic properties.

- **Calendula**: Calendula is one of the most popular and versatile medicinal herbs. It is traditionally said that it lifts the spirits. It has proven excellent in treating eczema, dermatitis, ulcers, burns, wounds, pimples, acne, delicate skin, and itching.
- **Dandelion**: Dandelion is a medicinal plant with leaves and roots used in natural remedies as a diuretic, mild laxative, and liver detoxifier. It is a hepatic and digestive tonic that stimulates the pancreas and the bile ducts.
- **Nettle**: One of the most common and abundant plants, nettle is an herb rich in minerals and circulatory stimulants. Likewise, it has astringent, diuretic, tonic, nutritional, hemostatic, hypotensive, anti-scurvy, and antiallergic effects.
- **Garlic (**Allium sativum**):** This powerful immunostimulant antiviral protects against infections. It works as an antibiotic to treat colds, flu, and respiratory infections.
- **Arnica**: Arnica is the drug of choice for muscle or joint damage, bruises, strains, or sprains. It can be used in creams and dip oils or ointments.

CONCLUSION

Thank you for taking the time to read this book. For thousands of years, people have used natural or herbal medicine. Pharmaceuticals have only recently entered the modern world. While allopathic medicine is critical, learning about natural medicine is also advantageous. It is a helpful skill that can help you in various situations and, in some cases, may be a better alternative to traditional drugs.

Nature's pharmacy contains thousands of herbs with powerful medicinal properties. Learning how to use these natural ingredients to promote healing and relieve discomfort is essential for someone who likes to be prepared. It will allow you to treat minor ailments and regain health control. While some conditions may necessitate medical intervention, natural medicine can assist you in treating them so that they do not worsen before you can get more help. Many medical professionals advocate for the use of both complementary and alternative medicine as well as conventional medicine.

Preppers should understand the significance of medication storage. Make a list of the medications that your family takes daily. Include some over-the-counter medications as well in your kit. Keep the kit in a cool, dry, and dark place. You should be familiar with medicinal plants and herbs and how to use them, and stock up on standard medications. If you become lost in the wilderness and lack medical supplies, you can always use plants and herbs as medicine. Finally, assemble a basic disaster supplies kit. Everything you might need in the event of a disaster should be included. Keep multiple copies of the kit on hand. It should be kept at home, work, and even in your car.

Natural medicine is based on the knowledge of our forefathers. Our forefathers were aware of nature's healing properties. The dependability of traditional medicine's ingredients and methods is one of its advantages. This is backed up by centuries, if not millennia, of practical experience. For centuries, knowledge has been passed down from generation to generation, and it has been improved and expanded so that we can confidently apply it in the modern world.

It's important to remember that many cultures worldwide have long understood natural medicine. The same illness can be treated in several ways. As a result, learning as much as possible before putting what you've learned into practice is critical.

Good luck.

PREPPER'S

WATER SURVIVAL GUIDE

INTRODUCTION

In a disaster, having access to sufficient water supplies can be the crucial difference between life and death. Water is so important, that often separates flourishing societies from those who fail. It is an enormous health necessity in the twenty-first century is providing everyone with safe, inexpensive drinking water.

Water is an absolute necessity in our lives. Science proves a person can last up to 3 weeks without food but wouldn't last 3 days without water. Also, the consumption of contaminated water can cause serious illness. It's no news that people living in places with little or no access to clean water suffer from various illnesses which would be nonexistent to them if they had clean water.

Worldwide, wastewater treatment plants typically use conventional methods to filter pollutants. These methods must be more effective and reliable to guarantee that food is free of disease-causing microorganisms and is safe for human ingestion. Therefore, creating materials capable of decontaminating water throughout a broad spectrum is crucial, especially for preppers.

CHAPTER 1: THE DANGERS OF DEHYDRATION

Dehydration most often results from inadequate fluid replacement. Reducing your body's regular water content disrupts your body's delicate mineral balance (salts and sugars). A healthy human body is more than half water. It helps digestion, flushes out waste and toxins, lubricates the joints and eyes, and maintains a healthy skin barrier. The body will become dehydrated if fluid loss is not replaced.

Dehydration is a severe problem for everyone, but infants and the elderly are particularly vulnerable. As a result, dehydration can occur in older adults from even relatively mild conditions, such as respiratory or urinary tract infections. Anyone, regardless of age, can become dehydrated if they don't drink enough water while exercising in hot weather.

Lowered strength and stamina are additional side effects of dehydration. It's a significant contributor to heat stroke. Increasing your fluid intake at this point should help you recover from dehydration.

Long-term (chronic) dehydration has been linked to impairments in kidney function and an increased risk of developing kidney stones. Constipation and muscular injury are also possible outcomes. Although light to moderate dehydration is usually reversible by consuming additional water, severe dehydration requires urgent medical attention.

Condition Related To Dehydration

It is possible to get dehydrated if you expend more fluids than you replace, leaving your body lacking sufficient water to function normally. When fluid loss exceeds a certain percentage of body weight, mild, moderate, or severe dehydration sets in.

Dehydration can be caused by the environment, the quantity and intensity of your physical activity (especially in hot weather), and food. Illnesses such as prolonged vomiting, diarrhea, or excessive perspiration due to fever can also lead to dehydration. Other conditions associated with dehydration include excessive sweating, alcoholism, diabetes, and some illnesses.

Several factors may contribute to dehydration. For example, diarrhea and vomiting that lasts for days or weeks are the leading causes of dehydration in little children. The body's water content decreases with age, and several medical conditions and medications might further raise an older adult's susceptibility to dehydration.

Thirst and dark color to the urine indicate impending dehydration. The body balances its fluid levels by increasing consumption and decreasing loss. The signs of dehydration include thirst, dizziness, dry mouth, dark, pungent urine, and less frequent urination.

CHAPTER 2: WATER CONTAMINANTS

Any material or substance other than water molecules found in water is considered a contaminant, whether physical, chemical, biological, or radioactive. There could be trace quantities of pollutants in your drinking water. Specific contaminants in drinking water may be dangerous at high enough concentrations, whereas other contaminants may be innocuous at those levels. Even though contaminants are present in water, that doesn't mean drinking is unsafe. The following are broad classes of contaminants in water and some common types of each:

Biological Contaminants

The purity and safety of drinking water may be compromised by contamination. Most people know that drinking water directly from a body of water like a lake, river, or pond can cause severe gastrointestinal disease or even death. Microorganisms can be washed into the wells system or seep underground if rainwater or snowmelt runoff is not managed correctly. They are present in human and animal excrement and can be found all over Earth's surface.

The presence of microorganisms in water wells can be traced back to the introduction of sewage and other waste products from leaking underground tanks and septic leach fields. Bacteria, viruses, and protozoan cysts are the three most common biological pollutants.

Public health officials call the presence of harmful organisms in water waterborne pathogen contamination. Animal waste, farm runoff, sewage breaks, floods, and earthquakes are ways this contamination can make its way into our drinking water. These biological pollutants are too tiny to be seen with the eye but pose a significant risk to human health if consumed. Waterborne microbes can cause diarrhea and other gastrointestinal problems for those who drink them.

Heavy Metals And Water Turbidity

Regarding relative density or atomic weight, metals with higher values tend to be classified as "heavy metals," which are also known for their toxicity. Humans are particularly vulnerable to heavy metal exposure due to water drinking, leading to the bioaccumulation of harmful metals. Inducing cancer and other harms to human health. Incorrect household and commercial garbage disposal is a significant contributor to water pollution.

Many human activities and industrial processes, including mining, petroleum refining, electronics production, municipal sewage disposal, cement production, and natural mineral deposits, can all contribute to the leaching of heavy metals into drinking water. Arsenic, cadmium, antimony, chromium, copper, lead, selenium, and many more are all examples of heavy metals.

Due to the mobility of groundwater and the seepage and runoff of surface water, heavy metals can pollute private wells. Heavy metal consumption is associated with chronic and acute toxicity, kidney, anemia, liver and intestine damage, and cancer.

Groundwater Contamination

When artificial substances like gasoline, oil, road salts, or chemicals find their way into groundwater, the water becomes contaminated and unusable. Subsurface water can become contaminated with substances from the land's surface. Groundwater can get infected with harmful substances like pesticides and fertilizers over time.

Additionally, groundwater contamination can be caused by the seepage of road salt, harmful compounds from mining sites, and spent motor oil. Further, dangerous compounds from underground tanks and seeping landfills might contaminate groundwater if proper precautions aren't taken. Storage tanks, septic systems, unregulated hazardous waste landfills, airborne chemicals, and road salts are all possible causes of groundwater contamination.

There can be severe consequences for your health if you drink contaminated groundwater. Disposal of human waste in septic tanks has been linked to spreading diseases like hepatitis and dysentery. Toxins that have seeped into well water could potentially cause poisoning.

Groundwater contamination also poses a threat to wildlife. Exposure to dirty water may also cause other, more serious long-term problems, such as cancer.

CHAPTER 3: DIFFERENT WATER SOURCES FOR SURVIVAL

Many things could suddenly impair our access to clean municipal water sources. For human beings, water is a must-have commodity. When preparing for an emergency, have you thought about where you could get clean water to drink?

Knowing how to locate and safely collect water is crucial in a natural or artificial disaster. The water you have stored is always the best bet in a crisis. Nonetheless, many people may find keeping vast quantities of water difficult.

Therefore, when the water you've stowed away runs out, where can you go to replenish your supply? In this chapter, we will discuss some of the options for obtaining water in an emergency. You may find some of these unexpected such as the liquid in canned fruits and vegetables and water from the water heater, which are all excellent sources of water to collect. All of these options may end up being life-saving for you.

Finding Water Sources

Most of us take accessibility to clean water for granted since it's so easy to come by. It's tough to conceive of a world where people cannot access clean water at the touch of a button. Sadly, water can be consumed or destroyed in seconds, depriving you of a life-sustaining resource.

In case of an emergency, the safest source of water to consume is water that has been previously stored. Your water supply may run out if the crisis drags on longer than expected, so you'll have to get creative with the solutions we discussed below.

Bottled Water

Bottled water from a store is a great option. It may be easily transported and stowed away without any hassle. There is a storage area in the basement where we keep our bottled water, and it keeps for a long time. Heat accelerates the plastic seeping into the water, making it smell and taste terrible; therefore, bottled water stored in a garage or hot car will require frequent rotation.

Be careful to stock up on high-quality bottled water in heavier plastic if you intend to keep the bottles for an extended period. If you plan to use all your water bottles within a year, you can get away with the thinner plastic ones. Keep water bottles on hand in case of a power outage or other unexpected circumstances.

Canned fruits and vegetables

Additional sources include canned vegetables and fruit broths, and ready-to-eat soups. Do not throw away the drained liquid; it can be used as a beverage or as a substitute for water in cooking. Oatmeal and pancake batter are excellent vehicles for the fruit liquid from a can. The juice from the vegetables can be used to boil noodles or added to canned soups. Try not to waste any of it by not using your imagination.

Ice

The freezer section of many homes has ice. Once melted, it might provide a valuable water source. You can save some water if the power goes out by melting the ice in a clean container. The water can be saved, and the container can be returned to the freezer so that the other food within can maintain its frigid temperature for longer.

Beverages That Can Be Stored at Room Temperature

Part of your daily water intake can come from beverages other than water, such as fruit juices, vegetable juices, pouch drinks, milk cartons, sports drinks, and canned milk. Carbonated drinks do not qualify as safe drinking water. Beer, like other alcoholic beverages, causes dehydration and calls for more water consumption.

Toilet Tank

Without chemical treatment, the water inside the toilet's flush tank might be considered "safe to drink." You could have anywhere from 3-5 gallons depending on your tank size. However, you'd have to filter it before drinking it or use water from the toilet tank. It's important to know that water in the toilet bowl should not be consumed.

Water Heater

Storage tanks that keep water at a warm temperature are a reliable supply. Depending on size, twenty to fifty liters of potable water may be stored there. In an emergency, you should turn off the water supply valve to avoid contaminating your home's water supply. In addition, make sure the tank's power or gas supply is disconnected.

Water in Household Pipes

Even after turning off the main water supply to a multi-story residence, water in the pipes can be collected via gravity flow. Turning on a faucet's highest setting lets air into the plumbing system, which helps water accumulate. The water will slowly leak out. The purified water for drinking is then retrieved from the sink or tub that is the lowest in the house.

Building A Rain Catchment System

It's safe to assume that rainwater is free of contaminants because it comes straight from the sky. One can quickly and easily set up a catchment system to collect rainwater for later use. As an easy solution for preppers, a rain barrel could be a good buy.

Save the rainwater in sanitary containers. Water is assumed to be contaminated if it touches the Earth or other unclean surfaces, such as roofing sheets and trees. While you might be able to collect in clean containers directly as it falls from the sky, you may need help to accumulate a large volume of water. Most rain catchment systems channel the rainwater as it falls on the roof into a barrel, making it unsuitable for consumption without proper detoxification. However, you can still collect direct rain into clean containers for drinking. Here are some things you must consider when creating a rain catchment system:

1. Roofing Sheets

Any roofing material will work if you use the collected water for household chores or outdoor gardening. You should know that asphalt shingles can leach pollutants, so runoff shouldn't be used to irrigate your garden or make drinking water. To collect drinkable water, roofs composed of slate, copper, terra-cotta tile, concrete, untreated wood shingles, and epoxy-painted metal are appropriate.

2. Select a container made to hold water

It might not be successful to gather rainwater in an old rubbish can. The wall thickness of rain barrels is made to endure freezing, the expansion of freezing water, deformation from the volume of the water, and the impact of continuous intense sunshine. Barrels used for collecting and storing water should have the following characteristics:

- Be transparent to avoid the formation of algae.
- Do not leach dangerous substances.
- Be securely covered to prevent small children, pets, animals, and insects from drowning.
- Be screened to keep out debris.
- Be easily washable.

3. Find a barrel while keeping safety in mind

Never put a rain barrel close to any stairs or other features, allowing a kid to climb up on top of it. Additionally, it's important to stop children from playing close to the rain barrels.

4. Raise the barrel from the ground

Rain barrels should be put at or near floor level on a flat surface to avoid tipping over when the barrel is full. While the rain barrel can be placed straight on the ground, lifting it a little bit will provide you more space to place a small bucket underneath the outflow fixture near the bottom of the barrel.

To prevent cross-threading damage:

1. Screw in the spigots straight when assembling the rain barrel.
2. Only tighten screws until the fitting is finger-tight.
3. Avoid using a wrench or pliers since the extra strain may break the thread, leading to leaks.

5. Routine maintenance includes clearing up the gutters

Cleaning and inspecting gutters twice a year is recommended, especially before a wet period. Water supply is optimized when gutters are sloped so that water flows continuously and does not pool in low locations. And if there are any depressions, debris will eventually decompose, contaminating the water and the filter screen. Older gutters which have soldered seams are questionable since they may leach lead. Additionally, channels that have riveting seams are better.

Indications Of Water Sources From Wildlife

One way to find water, especially if you are away from home, is by watching wildlife or animal tracks, which may lead you to a water source. Lush, lush foliage is another indicator that water is close by. Insect swarms might be annoying, but they usually mean fresh water is nearby. Following birds' morning or evening flight routes, you can find your way. Here are some tips for indications of water sources from wildlife.

1. Making Use of Animals to Scan for Water

The presence of a wide variety of life forms is usually taken as a sign of water in the area. A source of water is essential for the bees. Big, yellow, and black, hornet-like mason flies need mud and water to construct the tunnel where they'll keep the paralyzed spider. All birds that eat grains, like pigeons, need water, while birds that eat meat, like crows, hawks, and eagles, can survive for extended periods without drinking.

2. Using Various Plants

To gather the free-flowing fluid from the roots and branches of many trees that can be used to quench thirst, just cut the roots or stems into 3-foot lengths and hold them upright in a trough (made of bark), from which the collected water will drain to the pannikin. When some plants are cut, the water they've stored inside of them physically gushes out.

Survival in the Wilderness: Tips for Locating and Collecting Water from Plants

- You can't keep this "drinking water" for vegetables for a day. If the fluid is held for too long, it may begin to ferment or go wrong, making it unsafe to consume.
- There is no correlation between the characteristics of the plant's leaves and the safety of the fluids that make up the plant's sap.

CHAPTER 4: PURIFYING WATER

Preppers find it very crucial to purify their water before use. This is because water can be obtained from multiple sources, most of which may be subjected to contamination. In this chapter, you will discover the most critical steps to water prepping, including different methods of water purification, storage facility, and creating your emergency water supply.

Different Methods To Purify Water

Water purification can be accomplished in several ways, including physical procedures like filtration, sediment, or distillation; biological processes like sand filters and active carbon; and chemical processes like flocculation, chlorination, and the use of ultraviolet radiation. The method employed by preppers would be determined by the source of the water, available resources for purification, and the state of the water. This section will look at some key factors when storing water.

How To Build Your Own Water Supply

There are different options for building your water supply, especially if you live in a city without one. Having more than one water supply system around your home is essential in emergencies. Furthermore, building a water supply system depends on your location and how much money you can invest.

Some water supply options you should consider developing include:

1. City Water Supply
2. Dig a Well
3. Purchase a solar-powered pumping machine
4. Go wind-powered
5. Have extensive storage facilities to ensure water
6. A hand pump system
7. Store rainwater

Developing your water supply system involves utilizing more than one option to generate water for your household constantly.

Why Store Water For A Long Period?

Keeping water on hand is a good idea for a variety of reasons: Disasters of a natural nature (flood, hurricane, earthquake, etc.), If the water supply in your area becomes poisoned or polluted, When it is necessary to turn off the water supply (frozen pipes, local emergency, a broken water main, etc.).

Remember that you can't go very long without eating or drinking anything if you're a person. Ten days is the most time a human can go without water, and four to six weeks without food. These figures may change under different conditions, such as high temperatures or levels of activity.

How Much Should Water One Store, And For How Long?

Each person in your household should have at least one gallon of water daily. Consider stocking up now to ensure that your family has enough water to drink for at least two weeks. Even though public water supply water, if properly maintained, should last forever, it's preferable to replenish it every 6-12 months for optimal flavor. Water from a spring, private well, or another untreated source should be purified before storing to eliminate contamination.

Water storage tanks should be emptied and refilled every six months. It's best to keep water in storage at a cold (50-70 degrees Fahrenheit) temperature. Keep water out of the sun if you can. Keep water containers away from places with fuel or insecticides.

Creating An Emergency Water Supply Strategy.

Step 1: Consider how much water you will need to keep.

Half of that gallon (4 liters) is used for drinking, and the other half is used for cooking and personal hygiene. Children, nursing mothers, the chronically ill, and those living in extremely hot or high-altitude regions should drink an additional half a gallon (1.5 liters) per day. Using these estimates, aim to have enough supplies to last your family for two weeks. Prepare for a possible evacuation by stocking three days' worth of supplies in lightweight, portable containers.

Step 2: Select storage containers that are safe for use with food

Food and drink containers made of HDPE plastic, or those with the recycling symbol #2, are excellent choices. Stainless steel and plastics #4 (Low-density polyethylene) are other secure options. Never use a container that has held anything other than food or drink again; instead, get new containers designated "food quality," "food safe," or have a knife and fork emblem on them.

Step 3: Keep things like that away from plastic containers because they might be harmful

Check the number printed beside the recycling symbol on plastic containers; this is the resin identification code. Containers with the numbers 3 (for polyvinyl chloride), 6 (for polystyrene), and 7 (for Styrofoam) should be avoided (for polycarbonate). These substances may be harmful to human health.

Step 4: Decontaminate drinking water before using it.

Disinfect healthy water or water that has not been treated for safety before being stored. One minute at a rolling boil is ideal for this or three minutes at altitudes above 5,000 feet (1,000 m)

Containers That Store Water For Long-Term

When it comes to storing water for a long time, you want to consider different storage containers to store water for other purposes. For example, the best options for storing drinking water are in glass containers as glass contaminates water. Plastic containers are also viable alternatives for glass. If you are confused as to how many storage options you have, below is a list of containers that can store water long-term:

- Collapsible Water Storage Container
- Stackable Containers
- Water Tank
- Stainless Steel Containers
- Plastic Water Barrel or Drum
- Glass Jars
- Water Bladder
- Reusable Food Containers
- Water Jugs
- Backyard Pool
- Plastic Water Bottles
- Water Filtration system

Cleaning And Disinfecting Of Water Storage Containers

- First, clean the outside of the tank. Scrub inside surfaces with soap and hot water. Pole-mounted brushes or power washers can remove sediment, algae, rust, or biofilm. Clean and rinse loading and emptying hoses, pumps, and pipelines. Only skilled personnel with the proper PPE can securely enter a tight place.

- Next, power washes the tank until no detergent remains. If high-pressure hot water isn't accessible, the tank can be filled with hot water and left for several hours. Drain the tank and pipes. Use a handheld pump to clean the storage tank.
- Calculate the tank's volume. Quarter-fill it with potable water. Mix in bleach. 1 Online instruction differ based on the storage tank. Use the table below to prepare 50 mg/L free chlorine (parts per million or ppm). While filling the tank, mix well. Open all taps until you smell chlorine to disinfect plumbing lines and fixtures. Allow chlorinated water to remain for 12 hours to disinfect. This 50 ppm solution is toxic.
- Drain the tank and piping away from plants, not into a septic system (which might kill "good bacteria"), stream, or pond. Fish and plants may die. Check local and state laws first. Chlorinated waste should be disposed of in a sewage system. Fill the disinfected tank with clean water. Open the distribution valve and run tap water till the chlorine smell is gone. Clean and disinfected water tanks provide safe drinking water.

How Is Water Kept Safe Once The Container Is Opened?

Once a container of water has been opened, there are a few majors you can employ to preserve It. Refrigerating an opened container will kill any remaining bacteria if power is available. When refrigeration is not an option, store the container in a safe, out-of-reach location. If feasible, drink the water within a day or two of opening the bottle.

CHAPTER 5: HOW TO TEST WATER QUALITY

After successfully storing water, it's best to test its quality to know if it would suit consumption or other domestic activities. Preppers test water quality by examining its chemical and physical attributes. This chapter will delve into these testing methods and why they are essential.

Types Of Water Testing

As mentioned above, there are two essential testing parameters: the water's physical and chemical qualities. As the terms suggest, the physical attributes refer to the water's visible appearance, including its color, temperature, taste, etc. On the other hand, the chemical properties of water are related to its alkalinity and ph. level, and so forth.

Physical Water Quality Parameter

1. Turbidity

Turbidity is cloudiness. Turbidity sensors measure light transmission through water. Silt, clay, and organic compounds can cause high turbidity. Turbid water looks terrible. Cloudy water could be more appealing. High turbidity also causes:

2. Temperature

Temperature affects fragrances, solubility, palatability, chemical reactions, and viscosity. Temperature affects oxygen consumption, sedimentation, and chlorination. 50-60 degrees Fahrenheit is the optimal water temperature.

3. Color

Decomposing organic debris, primarily flora, can change the hue of the water. Rocks, dirt, and stones can also impact watercolor. These color changes may affect the water's appearance but not its taste. You can measure watercolor using color glass disks or standard color solutions.

4. Taste and Odor

Water for consumption should be tasteless and odorless

5. Solids

Water can suspend or dissolve solids. When water is filtered via a glass fiber filter, suspended particulates remain on top. Dissolved solids stay in the water. Total dissolved solids are commonly used to measure water solids. Total dissolved solids measure organic substances in water.

6. Electrical Conductivity

Electrical conductivity evaluates how well water or a comparable solution conducts electrical currents. As water ions grow, so does conductivity.

Chemical Water Quality Parameter

1. PH

pH is one of the primary measures of water quality. A pH sensor or test kit measures the acidity or basicity of water. More hydrogen ions are in acidic water. Essential water has more hydroxyl ions.

2. Acidity

This is a solution's acidity. Water's acidity is its ability to neutralize a base at a certain ph. Mineral acids, hydrolyzed salts, and CO2 cause acidity. Acids in moisture can affect biological activities, chemical reactions, and corrosion. pH sensors measure water's acidity.

3. Alkalinity

Alkalinity shows acid-neutralizing ability. Alkalinity is measured to determine how much soda and lime must be added to water for softening. Water softening reduces boiler corrosion.

4. Chlorine

Chlorine is added to wastewater to disinfect it. The aqueous solution of elemental chlorine is safe for humans. A modest level of chlorine signifies clean, contaminant-free water. Spectrophotometers or color comparator kits measure chlorine residual.

5. Hardness

Hard water is mineral-rich. Unchecked, dissolved minerals in water can scale hot water pipes. High-mineral shower water might make it hard to lather soap. Calcium and magnesium ions from rock and soil generate water hardness. Groundwater is typically more complex than surface water. Colorimeters or test strips measure water hardness.

6. Dissolved Oxygen

This parameter determines how filthy lakes, rivers, and streams are. High dissolved oxygen levels indicate high-quality water. Oxygen's solubility causes dissolved oxygen. Dissolved oxygen in the water relies on salinity, temperature, and pressure. Colorimeters and electrometers may measure dissolved oxygen.

What Is The Most Important Water Quality Test?

For drinking and cooking water, it's vital to test for both physical and chemical parameters. However, checking for and checkmating physical qualities is enough for most domestic activities.

CHAPTER 6: WASTE DISPOSAL IN THE OUTDOORS

Proper waste disposal is crucial to keeping water quality accessible in our environment. Generally, wastewater can be disposed of into gutters. However, it's more challenging to dispose of solid material. Recycling is an effective method but not all solid waste can be recycled. Burning can also be effective, but this activity must be carried out far away from water bodies. Some matter may also be left to decompose as a method of disposal safely.

Improper waste disposal can have harmful effects on the water in our environment. This threatens our health if we consume or come in contact with polluted water.

Cholera, dysentery, and leptospirosis are just a few of the waterborne illnesses that have been shown to spread rapidly across a population. Soil contamination, which happens when harmful substances come into touch with the soil, is another example of the detrimental impacts of incorrect waste disposal. These pollutants may seep deep down and pollute the water supply. Therefore, it's imperative to dispose of waste properly.

Water Waste Reduction For Every Individual

1. Spend less time in the shower

Reduce shower time and avoid baths. Most baths consume 35-50 gallons of water, whereas showers use about 25, especially with a low-flow head. Consider buying one if you don't. Significantly if you rent, a new leader might alter your shower routine. It's kid-friendly.

2. Check for leaks and amend leaking pipes

Check outdoor faucets and pipelines. Hopefully, you'll notice an interior leak, but an exterior one can be missed. Check them every six months. Watch your water bill. If it rises, you may be leaking.

3. Avoid wasting water in sinks

Consider how long you wash your teeth with running water. Check for leaky sinks. You can waste a lot of water if you have a leaking faucet in your house.

4. Check for Toilet leaks

Before you turn in for the night, add some food coloring to the aquarium. Check to see if any dyed water has made its way into the bowl before you use it in the morning. If that's the case, you've got a leak in your system that needs to be sealed.

5. Only run full laundry or dish loads

I know you only have so many delicates. You can still fill it up with dirty but washable items. Having a full load means chores go faster, detergent lasts longer, and you never run out of clean underwear.

Common Waterborne Illnesses

Waterborne infections are those contracted via drinking polluted water or touching human waste and are caused by microscopic organisms like viruses and bacteria. Preppers can avoid these diseases by giving proper treatment to water before use. Some of the most common waterborne diseases include:

- Typhoid Fever
- Cholera
- Giardia
- Dysentery
- Escherichia Coli
- Hepatitis A
- Salmonella

CONCLUSION

It is better to prepare before a water shortage occurs in your area. However, when unexpected events happen, preppers can better survive the water shortage by effectively utilizing the water sources in their environment.

Clean water is essential for the physical health of communities and the prevention of diseases related to inadequate water, cleanliness, and hygiene. Diseases including cholera, typhoid, Hepatitis A, giardia, and dysentery are spread either by ingesting contaminated water or being in contact with someone who has these illnesses

Being able to source water isn't enough preppers must learn to make the water usable. We hope this guide provides you the essential information to equip preppers to source for, accumulate, purify and store water in times of emergencies or otherwise.

PREPPER'S

WILDERNESS SURVIVAL GUIDE

INTRODUCTION

You don't have to be a participant in the television show "Survivor" to learn how to survive in the wilderness. Our forefathers knew this information instinctively many generations ago. However, we have lost touch with nature and forgotten how to provide for such basic needs as food, water, and shelter in today's high-tech civilization.

But given that we have modern conveniences at our disposal, why should we learn how to make a fire without matches or obtain clean water to drink? There is a simple fix. One needs to consider Hurricane Katrina in the past to understand how swiftly a natural disaster may hit and rob residents of the electricity they need to get by each day. Even less predictable than hurricanes are other types of natural disasters like sudden earthquakes and tornadoes that can form in a matter of minutes.

According to many scientists, there is a substantial chance that a global disease pandemic similar to the Spanish flu, which wiped off people all over the world in the first quarter of the 20th century, may occur. For instance, a bird flu epidemic may put a strain on local infrastructures, rendering residents unable to rely on services like ambulances, hospitals, police, or fire departments, leaving them to fend for themselves. Furthermore, given today's increasing unpredictability, it is not impossible that a terrorist attack may destroy power plants, water reservoirs, or other public infrastructure.

Because of this, the sensible person will spend time learning how to make a fire, get water, build a shelter, gather food, and prepare food with only essential equipment. Instead of seeing acquiring this knowledge as a tedious duty, it should be seen as an exciting opportunity to become more independent. Additionally, should a calamity happen, these talents can be more valuable than any insurance.

Therefore, this book is designed to be a quick and practical resource for learning wilderness survival techniques. It provides numerous examples of creating a fire without matches, constructing a shelter in the wilderness out of solely natural resources, recognizing edible plants, and hunting wild animals for meals.

With a small knife, compass, matches, fishing hooks, and possibly a thin, metallic "space blanket," you can create a pocket-sized wilderness survival kit for a few dollars and a few minutes. If you ever find yourself in a survival situation, stop by any sporting goods store or camping equipment store. The acquisition of wilderness survival skills, however, is more crucial than survival gear. This is due to the fact that your mentality, not your technology, is the most valuable resource in an emergency. Someone with the proper knowledge and abilities can survive far more easily without any tools than someone with a lot of survival gear but is not skilled in using it.

HOW TO BUILD A SHELTER IN THE FOREST

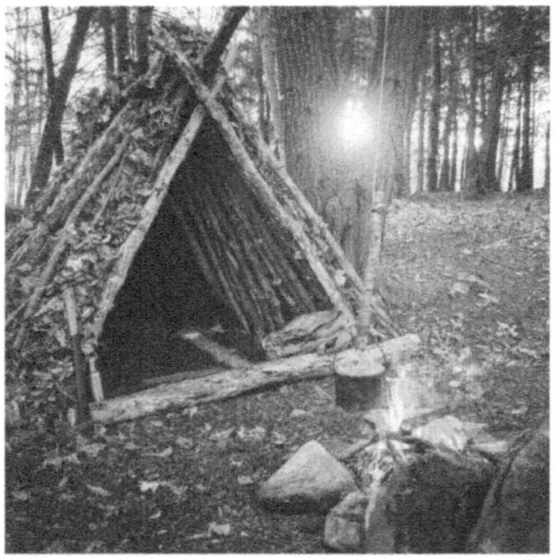

Many people in a wilderness survival situation focus too much on food, water, and fire when they should be considering shelter. Most individuals generally have enough food to last for a month or longer; however, you could feel a bit hungry throughout that time. Water is undoubtedly essential, but you can survive without it for a few days unless you're in a scorching desert. Although fire is also quite wonderful and enjoyable, you may live without it if you have a good shelter. Therefore, only a person's mentality is more crucial when it comes to factors that can help you live in the wilderness.

In a wilderness survival situation, your worst opponents in terms of attitude are fear and panic. You'll be fine if you can retain composure and a curious attitude toward your surroundings rather than viewing them as adversaries. Instead of acting as though nature were your enemy, the secret is to live in peace with it.

Let's look at the shelter right now. With the supplies at hand, building a shelter is a simple process. Shelters should be well-insulated to keep you warm and, ideally, dry if it should rain. They do not need to be complicated. Almost everything you find in the woods can be used to make a shelter. Pine boughs, sticks, and dry leaves are all commonly found materials that work well to construct a temporary debris hut.

The simplest type of shelter to construct is a hut made of debris. Making it just the proper size is the key. You want to build a debris hut that is spacious enough for you to fit inside without being too enclosed in a large volume of frigid air. A framework made of larger branches should be the first step in creating a debris hut. A layer of smaller branches should then be added on top of the framework. The ideal scenario would be locating an 8-foot-long tree branch and a two- to three-foot-tall tree stump. A tree branch could be leaned against the stump such that the short end was on the ground and the large end was on top. Your debris hut's foot would be where the tree limb met the ground, and the stump would serve as the entrance to your shelter.

The next step is to create a framework in the shape of an A on both sides of the tree limb using smaller branches. It's time to start accumulating the leaves now. Use any nearby materials, such as ferns or pine boughs. The better the insulation, the better. Not too thick; it is two or three feet. You will require a lot of insulation if it gets chilly at night in order to maintain your body's natural warmth and keep the cold away.

This essential information on constructing a debris cabin in the bush can help you maintain your composure. It can avoid panicking if you ever find yourself in a true wilderness survival emergency.

Part 1 of Constructing a Survival Shelter in The Forest

You often bring a sleeping bag, pad, and tent with you whenever you intend to spend the night outdoors. But what should you bring if you don't want to stay the night? Several portable substitutes can save your life in an emergency. For example, a decent emergency shelter can be made from an 8' by 10' to 12' tarp. Another option is to erect a tube tent in between two trees rapidly.

The first step is choosing a suitable location between two trees. If there are no nearby trees or branches, you might have a pole or walking stick that can be used to support one end of the tent. To secure your lines, make sure you have a couple of tent stakes. Here are a few suggestions for good website selection.

- Never pitch a tent over an animal burrow or an ant nest.
- Avoid pitching your tent near a river or gully because a flash flood could obliterate you.
- On a shoreline, never erect anything below the high-water mark.
- Avoid setting up camp on top of a hill or along a ridge line since lightning can strike more frequently in these places.
- The tallest trees in the forest or a single tree should not be used as a base for your tent because these are equally vulnerable to lightning strikes. Affixing your tent to shorter trees surrounded by taller trees will be safer.
- Dead branches and trees may break off at night and fall over your tent, so avoid securing your tent underneath or to them.
- Avoid putting your shelter close to a dead tree that could collapse on it.
- Always erect your shelter during the day so you can view your surroundings and steer clear of these potential issues.

Keep in mind that lightning is not a friend. Determine the windward side or the overall direction the wind will come from. You may determine the overall direction the wind is blowing from by observing the surrounding grass and the order in which it is lying down. The shelter's fold should face the direction of the wind. You might come upon a little hollow that can shield you from the wind, but it needs to slope downward because you don't want water to accumulate there overnight. Verify that the area where you intend to sleep is free of pebbles. Nothing is worse than spending the entire night curled up on a rock. You should also dig a little hole to make your hips more comfortable. If it's cold outside, gather some grass or leaves to create a layer of insulation between you and the ground. You'll be warmer the deeper the pile. There are two types of shelters for survival that you can build. The other is open on one side to receive fire heat, while the other is shaped like a triangle tube. Given that most tarps are combustible, keep your distance from the fire.

Part 2 of Constructing a Survival Shelter in The Forest

Let's start by making a tube tent. Overlay the location where you want to sleep with 1/3 of the tarp. Place a line at roughly 2/3 of the tarp's width from the tarp to a tree on either side of the area where you plan to sleep. The ridgeline, also known as the shelter's ridge, will be formed by this. The final third of the tarp is lowered over the bottom third of the tarp. In case of rain, ensure it reaches past the outer edge of the bottom tarp. You don't want the entire rainwater to end up on the ground beneath your shelter. To avoid your shelter from collapsing in the middle of the night if it is windy, be sure you tie the corners down and teach. To make the tent a little cozier, you can close one end.

How do you attach the lines to your tent if your tarp's eyelets have torn off? First, pick up a tiny rock with a diameter of about 1" and set it inside the tarp. Next, wrap the tarp tightly around it. The rock inside the tarp will now be captured by the rope that has been tied around the rock on the tarp's exterior. This should save the need to make holes in the tarp that will likely rip out over time and attach the line to the tarp.

You can accumulate garbage on the tarp's exterior when it's chilly out to aid the tent's insulation. In freezing temperatures, you should keep your tent's volume as tiny as possible to reduce the volume your body will need to heat. In what position should I sleep? Wear as many layers as you can to stay as warm as possible. You could wrap yourself in an emergency space blanket if you brought one. A space blanket-material all-weather emergency pack is another portable solution that you should always have with you. The metalized mylar will reflect heat from your body, which will keep you warm.

A tube tent is a quick-to-assemble, easy-to-use, portable shelter. It is made up of a plastic tube threaded through a line. Similar to constructing a tarp tube tent, you tie the line to two tees to create the tent's ridge line. Crawl inside after sealing the opening. Remember to place debris under the tube to protect your body from direct contact with the ground, which will drain it of heat.

One other design for an emergency shelter places half the tarp on the ground and the other half at a 60-degree angle to form the roof. This design includes a single fold on the windward side. To serve as an insulating layer, the ground sheet must be staked to the ground, preferably over a pile of garbage. It will be necessary to tie the roof taut between two trees. A metalized space blanket that will reflect heat from a fire behind you may be added to the roof's interior if you're lying down. A twisted loop of 550 paracords strung over the top border of the emergency shelter and fastened between the two trees can be used to secure the space blanket. The two twisted paracord strands serve as a support for the space blanket. Near the tarp's fold, the other side of the metalized mylar is similarly fastened. Put the fire in the emergency shelter's opening center, but far enough away, so it doesn't pose a fire hazard. Make sure there is no combustible debris close by and that the fire is entirely confined in a ring of rocks. Debris can be used to build the shelter's side walls and to add a layer to the tarp's exterior on the windward side.

If you don't have a tarp, you can make a ridge line between two nearby trees or with a stick supported by two forked branches. To make the roof, you could lean more branches against the ridge line stick at a 60-degree angle. You may cover the top supports with evergreen boughs to serve as a roof and shield you from the wind and rain. Finally, you can create a pile of debris on the shelter's floor to protect you from the earth. If you don't have a tarp, this is one of the simplest shelters you can build.

HOW TO HUNT

Hunting is one activity that calls for a particular level of proficiency to be performed competently. However, if you have the correct abilities, hunting game for food can keep you and your family alive for a long time. Learning how to hunt is essential for survival when you are trapped in the woods or when your city's infrastructure has been damaged due to a calamity. You can locate the game in many urban areas or a few miles outside any city. In an urban setting, you can anticipate seeing pigeons, ducks, geese, and squirrels.

It does not guarantee you can provide for yourself just because you have a hunting rifle. You must learn how to hunt to be able to utilize that weapon. In addition, you must learn how to use your weapon, the game you are tracking, where to find the prey, recognize their traces, and prepare the game after it has been killed. Although you can use many different weapons, a pistol is the most versatile and precise weapon for a beginner.

Before you need to hunt to feed yourself and your family in an emergency, you must practice to do it well and not go hungry. Stress and a lack of skills are a surefire prescription for failure in a survival crisis. Therefore, hunting is one of those things you would never attempt without the necessary knowledge.

Before to going on a successful hunt, it is essential to train with a weapon and improve your hunting techniques. If you decide to use a bow and arrow, you must practice shooting targets for a long time to become confident and skilled. To prepare for hunting, you must be extra careful with weapons and attend safety classes.

You can probably join groups in your region to receive instruction in archery, shooting, and trap setting.

After you have become proficient with your hunting tool or strategy, you should go into the woods and hunt. Still, you should do so in a manner that is under close supervision. You want to get the necessary training before a crisis occurs so that any mistakes you make won't negatively affect people's lives. It will take time, patience, and learning through trial and error before you can master the game you are hunting. However, suppose you are ever in a position in the future where you are expected to produce food via hunting. In that case, the time and effort you put into improving your hunting skills will be well worth it.

Survival Traps: The Most Popular Types

Traps can be used to catch animals in a survival situation, giving humans valuable calories from their meat and fat. Imagine them as tiny hunters that you send out to complete your work while you are away completing other duties. There appear to be as many different types of traps as there are animals to capture. So, learning to trap is one of the most essential survival skills.

For prepper survivalists, trapping is a crucial component of most survival plans. You may save a lot of energy by setting up numerous strategically positioned traps that you check frequently. It is better to set up your trap line a little bit away from where you plan to bug out, as with most hunting and gathering techniques. You will only have finished the game in the nearby area if a perimeter that extends from your bug-out spot becomes too dangerous. Additionally, even if hunting can be successful, it also consumes the necessary calories you cannot afford to lose in a survival crisis. You need therefore learn how to make a variety of hunting traps to increase your chances of locating food.

You can catch wild games using any one of hundreds of different types of survival traps and snares. For anyone who spends any amount of time outdoors, having a rudimentary understanding of how to use them is crucial. At their most basic level, they are intended to entangle, hang, or crush wild animals.

The most important thing for preparedness enthusiasts to understand about trapping is that the best survival traps are fairly easy to create and can typically be made using natural materials if you know what you're doing. This means that to be effective, you must practice these talents before a scenario arises where they are essential to your survival.

Where to Place Traps

In a survival situation, your odds of capturing food increase with the number of traps you place. Unfortunately, that implies that you must constantly create new ones, maintain and repair current ones, and search for suitable locations to set them.

Be sure to keep an eye out for these things while you're hunting for locations to plant your traps:

- Game paths and runs that are well-known.
- Watering holes and feeding grounds that are well known.
- Traces of animals, such as prints and droppings.
- Nesting places and den holes.
- Chewed vegetation.

The most challenging aspect of the equation is deciding where to lay your traps, especially if you don't have a strong understanding of tracking and animal behavior.

A good trap placed incorrectly is a bad trap!

Types of Survival Traps

Snares and deadfalls are the two primary types of traps that are typically utilized in survival situations. Even if there are a few more categories, most of the traps you employ will likely be a variation of either of these two primary groups.

1. **Setting up a Survival Snare:** A trap is a little noose that gets tighter around the neck of an animal as it moves through the opening in the device. In most cases, they are planted on animal pathways that are already well-traveled or just outside of existing dens.
   Check that the hole in the noose is big enough for the animal's head to fit through it before you use it. The snare must get tighter around the animal's neck as it goes through the trap. The animal's efforts to get free will cause the snare to become even more constricting for it.

2. **Setting up a Deadfall Trap:** Unlike snares, designed to cause the animal to suffocate, deadfalls are intended to cause the animal's body to be crushed after the trigger is pulled.

   Getting all of the parts to function as a whole:

   - Carve a tip resembling a flat screwdriver on one of the sticks; this will be the post that goes vertically.
   - Carve a second screwdriver point into one end of a stick, and then carve a notch close to the opposite end; this will be the diagonal stick.
   - On one end of the third stick, carve a notch, and on the other end, cut a point for the bait.
   - Arrange the sticks to resemble the number 4, then place the vertical post correctly. Next, cut a notch in the horizontal bait stick so that it catches the carved square edge on the vertical shaft.
   - Join the three sticks together so that the notches on each one grab onto the others to support the deadfall weight.

Using a Crossbow for Hunting

The next time you go hunting, consider utilizing a crossbow for a more challenging experience. This is a terrific approach to increase your heart rate and offer additional hands-on experience before you hunt your preferred game.

Most people have used a gun for hunting at some point in their lives, so you may be familiar with the procedure. Kill the animal with a shotgun, then take the meat. The only significant difficulty in the procedure is shooting the game. However, you have a high chance of bagging an animal as long as you can point and aim.

However, using a crossbow makes this process more difficult. Consider how important the wind and other natural forces are to your success. You must adjust for the wind's direction if it blows away from the animal. This requires you to carefully contemplate the shot you will take and all the elements that contribute to the effectiveness of the kill.

Because it provides the animal with a chance at survival, many people believe this is a superior method of hunting. Additionally, you will experience a high that a gunshot will never be able to match when you get your shot in and strike your target. You will be elated and pumped since you were able to successfully harvest the animal you were hunting while also utilizing natural resources. It enhances the experience's satisfaction.

Crossbow hunters also have the advantage of seeing more games than rifle hunters, which is a wonderful feature. During bow season, animals prefer to stay outside for longer, giving you more opportunities to encounter wildlife. In addition, you won't have to worry about coming into other hunters during this season because there are fewer bow hunters, which also increases your chances of catching wildlife.

Naturally, you'll also need to be stealthy during this process. You must ensure you can get close to the animal you aim to kill unless you can pull back on your bow and strike hard at a long distance. This could become troublesome if they detect you in any way, such as by smelling you. Due to this, you will also need to hone your stealth abilities, which could add to the thrill of the hunt.

Remember that these are only a few of the fascinating issues that crossbow hunting can expose you to. You should find that you have a heart-pounding experience you will never forget if you take your time to learn about your game and start training with targets to master the art of hunting.

Crossbow Hunting: Safe and Successful Hunting Advice

Consider these suggestions to ensure a safe trip before leaving for your next bowhunting excursion. After all, a risk-free journey can result in a fruitful hunt.

- Check your crossbow for hunting to make sure everything is in functioning order.
- Use crossbow arrows designed for your particular crossbow type and support its draw weight and length.
- Hold the safety position until you are prepared to fire.
- Wait to pull the trigger until you are prepared to shoot.
- Never load your crossbow before you are prepared to shoot and have your target in sight.
- Never aim a crossbow at something you don't want to shoot, such as a person. Always take a safe course of action.
- Keep your fingertips below the cables' and bowstring's travel paths to protect yourself from harm.
- Check to see that there are no obstacles in the way of your bow limbs before you shoot. For example, if you are in a tree stand, ensure no tree branches are blocking your shot.
- The crossbow's hunting range is 40 yards and less. To ensure that you preserve this piece of bow hunting gear's efficiency, stay inside this range.
- Practice! You will be ready for your next hunting trip if you spend a lot of time practicing with your crossbow and know how to use it. Regular practice makes a crossbow hunter a safer hunter almost by default

HOW TO SURVIVE IN THE WILDERNESS

You must learn several fundamental skills before setting out on any outdoor adventure. To survive, one needs to fulfill four basic needs. For survival in the woods, you must have access to warmth, drink, sleep, and food.

It cannot be easy to keep warm at night in some places. It would help if you were well-prepared for every journey or circumstance that could put you in a chilly climate. The temperature range of the human body is minimal. For survival, you must keep your temperature within that range.

The majority of the human body is made up of water. So even while you can do without water for one or two days, you should immediately start looking.

Lack of sleep can have a significant impact on your cognitive function. You can have hallucinations and be unable to decide how to survive in the outdoors.

Humans are capable of going without food for a few weeks. Although eating may not be your first concern, you will need enough food to keep yourself stable because your walk will burn many calories.

It takes a lot of preparation to survive in the wilderness. To be safe, you must plan for the worst-case situation. Make sure you are carrying the proper equipment. Find out what gear would be best for your trip. Your needs for a week-long backpacking trip will differ significantly from those for a short hike. It would be best if you were ready.

Ensure you have a map of the area on you. Before visiting, learn about the area. Refresh your navigational knowledge and be able to use a good compass and a map. Your primary priority is to survive in the wilderness. Your adventure will be much more pleasurable if you familiarize yourself with the area before you go.

Never leave on a trip without informing someone of your plans. They must be aware of your travel route, intended destination, and anticipated return time. If you don't arrive as expected or within a fair amount of time, some services will phone your family and/or friends.

In favorable conditions, survival is significantly simpler. Check the local weather forecast online before you leave for your trip, or at the very least, watch the forecast on the evening news the night before. Make sure you are prepared and review your winter survival abilities if you venture out into the woods during the colder months.

Your preparation can save your life, and your odds of survival will increase as you learn more. For example, it's not a good idea for a beginner to go backpacking or hiking in a chilly area during the winter. Additionally, it is advised to go on a couple of day hikes before attempting the longer survival treks that last a week.

Continue to learn about survival techniques. Before you go on the expedition into the wild, put your talents to the test as often as possible. It's crucial to remember that the traveler is primarily responsible for wilderness survival.

The Top Six Tips for Surviving in the Wild

Recent times have seen a rise in interest in wilderness survival. Whether this is due to a sense of impending doom or a morbid obsession with a zombie apocalypse, the fact remains that people are interested. In anything but the harshest wilderness conditions, even your pet dog would survive, thus wilderness survival doesn't have to be entirely secret. Seven suggestions to aid in a survival crisis are provided below.

1. **Understanding the "Rules of Three":** Even the most inexperienced survivalist may identify the survival priority spectrum using the "rules of three." A person will most likely pass away without oxygen after three minutes. Around three hours pass before life processes cease in an extreme climate without shelter. Without water, the human body can survive for three days. Without nourishment, you'll typically need three weeks to pass away. When a survivalist is familiar with the "rules of three," planning tasks to ensure survival is considerably simpler.
2. **Recognize the Value of Cordage:** Any size and shape of rope or string are considered cordage. You can construct a weapon or a shelter by lashing together branches with cordage. At the U.S. Army Special Operations Survival school, they spend days learning how to make cordage out of objects found in the environment. Most survival bands and reminder bands are constructed from 550 lbs. of test cordage since making cordage takes time, and there never seems to be enough of it. Building a fire-starting bow with cordage can be more effective than simply rubbing sticks together. If you have enough, you could use a fishing net or make a fishing line out of cordage. If you have cordage, your only creative constraints are your own.
3. **Stay Healthy:** This advice may seem very clear, but people frequently take unnecessary risks when trying to survive. Avoid it to stay healthy if you can't tell if something is safe to eat. Look before you leap, and if it's dark or difficult to see outside, don't move quickly or at all. The best judge of what is dangerous and what is not is each individual; if something makes the hairs on your neck stands up, don't do it. Recognize your limitations and respect them.
4. **Go Ugly Early:** Food may not seem essential for a short period of survival, but you won't have much energy if you don't eat. When people lack energy, they often become lethargic and make blunders. If you find yourself in a survival situation, you should begin identifying edible food as soon as possible because you will need food for sustained survival operations. When someone has a food aversion, they won't eat simple foods like grubs and termites. When you're ready to eat them, however, you might not have the energy to get them if you wait too long. Going ugly early means overcoming your aversions to food and starting to gather food as soon as you realize you are in a survival situation.
5. **Have the Resources to Start a Fire:** If you've ever tried to start a fire by rubbing two sticks together, you'll be familiar with how challenging and time-consuming it can be. However, in a survival situation, fire can help cook spoiled food, lifting your spirits, and keeping you warm on a chilly day. In addition, with fire, there is a possibility of calling for help or heating water for drinking. So, whenever you go into the wilderness, you should have fire-making gear because it is extremely useful and takes up almost no space.
6. **Survival Is Not a Sprint. It's a Marathon:** You must maintain your composure and frequently wait it out in the attrition struggle that is survival. Waste results from unnecessary haste, whether you're waiting for assistance or moving slowly over the countryside. Working at a very high energy level only leads to energy waste and higher calorie and fluid intake needs. Survival typically involves making the most of scarce resources. You will quickly run out of resources if you race at top speed or fight through river rapids.

The advice mentioned above is straightforward, so the impending zombie apocalypse shouldn't be an issue if you follow it.

The Top Nine Survival Skills for Living in the Wilderness

One of the greatest blessings our planet can give the human race is nature. In addition to being full of beauty and exciting possibilities, the natural world has been shown to be good for our physical and mental health. But there is a big difference between enjoying the outdoors and staying alive when it comes to doing so. Going camping for a weekend is one thing, but if something goes wrong, it's another to stay alive in the wilderness. For example, could you survive if you got lost during your upcoming unscheduled outdoor event? What would you consume? How might you collect water? Would you possess the abilities required to guarantee your security and subsistence?

I have compiled a list of the top 10 survival abilities that every person needs to succeed in the wild. So, read on if you have what it takes to live in the vast outdoors.

1. **Water:** Without water, humans are unable to thrive. You need to learn how to gather and purify water to survive in the wilderness. There are several ways to accomplish this. One method is to catch rainwater in pots or tarps. Another approach to get water is to dig a foot-deep hole in some mud and wait for the water to bubble up. Finally, you must cleanse your water after you've collected it. You can accomplish this by heating your water to a boil in a glass jar, a plastic bottle, or a tin can over an open flame.
2. **Food:** For your body to survive, you need to provide it with nutrients. Your body gets the water, energy, and attention it needs from food to function effectively. How is this possible to accomplish? Knowing which plants and insects are edible is a fantastic place to start. When cultivating plants in the wild, a basic rule is to steer clear of anything that looks milky, hairy, bulbous, has three leaves, or has pink spurs; these are telltale signals that the plant is dangerous. Common and edible wild plants include clovers, dandelions, and sorrel. Your body won't be able to exist on just greens, though. To thrive, you need both protein and fat. In the wild, insects are your go-to source of protein because almost all of them are edible, including ants, grasshoppers, worms, and even bees. You may also give survival hunting a shot. All that is needed for a primary snare is a noose, which can be made from wire or rope. Wait for your next meal while the noose is fastened to a tree close to an animal's den.
3. **Learning first aid** is a quick and easy approach to increasing your chances of surviving in the wild. Knowing how to make splints, slings, and correctly bandage wounds could mean the difference between life and death in the woods.
4. **Learn How to Mending Your Garments:** Although keeping your clothes will provide much-needed warmth and safety when surviving in the wild, clothing repair may seem like a dated skill to master.
5. **Starting and Maintaining a Fire:** Fire is necessary for heating and purifying water. Therefore, one of the most crucial survival skills to survive in the wild is the ability to start and maintain a fire in dry and wet conditions.
6. **Self-Defense:** If you're forced to survive in the wilderness, you'll probably come across a circumstance where you must defend yourself or risk losing your life. You can protect yourself in the bush by studying self-defense techniques and remembering to bring a pocket knife on your expedition.
7. **Grooming:** Although it may be the last thing that comes to mind when considering wilderness survival, learning some basic grooming techniques might help you stay alive and in good health.
8. **Worldly Awareness:** Be conscious of your surroundings, including their advantages and risks. You can become a more competent and fruitful survivor by increasing your awareness.
9. **Expect the Unexpected**: Develop the attitude of accepting and expecting the unexpected. Your morale and ability to live are both significantly influenced by your cognitive approach.

In the end, surviving in the wild is unavoidable, regardless of how many safeguards, preparations, or intellect you develop. Continue to create a survivalist mindset by learning to scavenge, seeing the opportunities that natural objects present, and increasing your resourcefulness. No matter how grave the situation, keep going, and you'll be well on your way to becoming a true survivor.

Making Fire in the Wilderness

If you intend to spend any time outdoors, you must learn how to make a fire. Shelter is the most crucial survival necessity, followed by fire. Once found, fire may be utilized for various purposes, such as boiling water to make it drinkable, hardening wood for spears, and arrows, digging tools, pottery, keeping you warm, and so on.

This section will go over the various ways to make a fire that you should be aware of before going into the wilderness. The topics of flint and steel, Ferro rods, lighters, matches, and various drill techniques will be covered. Although not all fire-making techniques will be covered in length, you should be able to get enough information about the advantages and disadvantages of each to help you make an informed decision about how to start a fire when setting up camp.

Hand Drill Technique

The drill methods for starting a fire use friction between two pieces of wood to produce coal that may be blown into a flame. A spindle is moved back and forth upon a hearth board laid on the ground. The dust created by the contact between the two pieces of wood heats up enough to turn into an ember or coal. Then, you can place this ember inside a tinder bundle and blow it into a flame. When employing the hand drill technique, a dry piece of wood or plant material (such as a mullein or cattail stem) with a soft, pointed center is typically utilized as the spindle. As the name suggests, the spindles are turned by the force of the hands. A bow (similar to the kind used to shoot arrows) is used in the bow drill technique to spin the spindle. This makes it possible to crank the spindle with greater force and speed while decreasing the likelihood of hand blistering. Once you have the talent, these drill techniques are incredibly reliable, but they can be laborious to prepare.

There have long been flint and steel. The basic idea is that you have a piece of steel, similar to what metal files are made of, and a piece of flint. Sparks are made by striking the two things together. Your tinder then catches these sparks, which can be blown into an ember and eventually into flames. It is a relatively simple method to utilize, as well as portable and lightweight. Charcloth is the only item you require in addition to flint and steel. When a natural fiber, like cotton, is heated to the point where its chemical composition changes, the air is kept away from the threads so that it does not catch fire but chars. Charcloth is necessary because it ignites sparks very quickly. Afterward, you can insert your charcloth into your tinder bundle and ignite it with a match. Typically, you may produce charcloth in the same altoid tin in which you carry your fire gear. Put the natural fiber inside the container, secure it, and place it over an open flame. When you eventually remove it, it will be black but not burned.

The ferrocerium rod or Ferro rod is the next development in the flint and steel evolution. When a piece of steel (such as the rear of your knife blade) is run down the rod, it will produce a lot of sparks. These sparks can then be ignited by blowing them into flames over charcloth or another type of tinder. The Ferro rod is easy to use and comes in a smaller container than flint and steel.

You can start a fire without the "spark" step and go straight to the flame with matches. Even though matches typically function well, they won't light if damp. They are also easily breakable. Carrying some is not bad, but don't rely on them.

A step up from matches are lighters. However, they have the advantage of having a considerably larger fuel supply, allowing them to produce more flames for extended periods. In addition, if they are wet, some can be dried out and used. A lighter is always a good idea to carry about you, just like matches, but don't rely on it.

It doesn't hurt to bring a lighter, matches, Ferro rod, flint, and steel with you if you're going into the wilderness. You'll have four alternative ways to start a fire, and everything fits neatly into a little bag. To start a fire by friction, even if you are alone in the woods without anything, it is also very beneficial to know how to produce an ember using one of the bow drill techniques.

Wilderness Survival: Sourcing Drinkable Water

Water is essential for survival and may be more crucial than food and fire combined. Perhaps it is evident, yet much of it is found in our bodies.

There are numerous ways to obtain water. Free-flowing water might not always be accessible unless you have many ponds and lakes, like Minnesota (the Land of 10,000 Lakes) or Michigan (the Great Lakes State). If you need a test kit or a technique to filter the water, you should look for standing water elsewhere because it can be a little dubious.

Some of the most accessible and dependable sources of pure water are plants. Numerous have raindrops stuck to their leaves, and others have plenty of moisture stored in their stems.

Avoid consuming water from sewers, storm drains, and puddles with a rainbow sheen. Instead, use your other senses to help you identify whether or not it is water because not everything wet is made of water.

The groundwater might be contaminated if a plant grows on soil close to populated areas. In this scenario, your chances of locating healthy sources are better the more rustic the setting. Naturally, this is to your benefit because you are already relatively remote from civilization if you are in a survival situation.

Be cautious when getting water from wild plants. Only utilize a plant if you are sure whether it is toxic. Do you recall the unfortunate camper who ran across the poison ivy while wearing shorts? Consider attempting to scratch your throat while it is itching.

You can rely on grapevines, birch tree sap, maple tree sap, and thistles most of the time—some plants, which you don't want to employ for water collecting, resemble other plants. Be careful since the Canada Moonseed vine, which resembles grapevines, is poisonous.

Instead of trying your luck by squeezing what might or might not be grapevines, clench your fist with the fibers of birch trees and point your thumb in the direction of your mouth.

Remember that there are many natural places where you can find water. Still, it would be best always to use caution and never make assumptions.

Survival Backpack

Here are some of the things you should store in your survival bag if you are worried yourself and looking to start putting one together:

1. **Emergency rations of food and water:** You may go three days without water and four to five weeks without food before dying from famine. However, you could also pass away from digestive problems if you consume something infected. You don't want to contract cholera or typhoid illness following a disaster. Gather non-perishable foods, such as canned goods and energy bars. At least two liters of water should be stored aside for later use.
2. **Camp Tools:** Additionally, you would want lodging and equipment to enable you to resume something resembling your previous way of life. A sleeping bag, tent, tools for digging, chopping, and cutting wood, cooking utensils, a fire starter, communication tools, and some ropes are included in this particular set. They will keep you safe from harsh, tangible, and intangible elements and are essential to survival in a chaotic atmosphere.
3. **Medical equipment:** A survival kit would be incomplete without the necessary medications and first aid supplies. Medication is the most essential item you'll need to survive in a post-apocalyptic world where accidents will happen frequently.

4. **Garment:** It wouldn't be too bad to have a change of clothing in your survival kit since that would help you cope with adversity comfortably. It may not be an urgent need. But you should consider these products since they contribute to your sense of security and safety and meet the second of Maslow's five basic human needs for persistence.
5. **Armaments:** You'd naturally want something to fend off bodily dangers, whether they came from untamed animals, lawless people, or the unfathomable otherworldly. So, you can arm yourself with a 45-caliber handgun with five boxes of bullets, a BB gun, or a tranquilizer gun to take out anything that threatens your life.

You may get things prefabricated online if you need more clarification. You can gather all the necessary supplies and have a reliable backpack to carry your survival kit. However, you may access several resources over the Internet if you prefer to choose all the articles yourself.

How to have electricity in the wilderness

While camping outdoors, many survivalists and adventurers take advantage of their home comforts. They enjoy having the ability to use their cameras to record those special moments and their iPod systems to continue listening to music. Likewise, preppers want solar power for various reasons, not only portable power while camping. I'll talk about a few solar goods in this section that are necessary for having electricity in the wild.

A flashlight is the first and one of the most crucial items that survivalists and anyone out in the wilderness should own. In the past, flashlights weren't just expensive; they also needed pricey batteries, which frequently needed to be changed 3–8 times every few months. If you never used it, you could never get a flashlight whose batteries you wouldn't need to swap out every few years.

While some of the more powerful, larger flashlights are pricey, they are now being provided with solar power technology as producers become smarter and realize what consumers want. As a result, they have a variety of models available, ranging in price from affordable to expensive. The difference in brightness is due to the internal light source. Still, unless you are a military member or want unbelievably brilliant lighting, you can get most solar flashlights at affordable costs.

Hybrid Solar Flashlight is one of the solar flashlights you may purchase. It is available in 4 different colors, costs 19.99, comes with a lifetime warranty, and floats for campers who want to boat.

The goal of zero goods is the next piece of solar-powered equipment that survivalists can purchase. But, again, there is a solar option for everyone, whether campers, hikers, mountain climbers, or survivalists. For example, the Scout 150 Explorer Kit has a solar backpack and can produce up to 150 watts. The Sherpa 120 Explorer Kit is another option; it comes with all the necessary parts and can produce up to 120 watts of electricity while fitting easily into a backpack or duffel.

Another kit, the Guide 10 Adventure Kit, is available for people who require portable power for their iPhones, iPods, and GPS devices. Although many more solar products are available, these are the most popular ones that sell out rapidly each week.

Serious long-term adventurers will soon be investing in solar power equipment that is more powerful, has long run periods, and is portable. The Power source 1800 Solar Generator is the first solar device. Everything needed to have power and plug it in is included with this solar generator. It may conveniently be hauled in the back of your truck or car and provides up to 1800 watts of power. Additionally, a 50-foot wire and a rolling solar panel are included.

The Base Camp Solar Equipment is a different solar generation kit that outdoor experts and survivalists enjoy. It includes an inverter, two 350-watt battery packs, four lanterns, and four 30-watt solar panels. This is the ideal equipment for users who want to customize the setup and take what they need. It's also great for users who require significant power for extended travel.

These are the best solar devices that outdoor experts and survivalists use when out in the wild. They power everything from pumps to computers to cell phones.

CONCLUSION

In conclusion, it's always preferable to be prepared for survival in the wilderness, whether you dare to challenge the brave outdoors where Mother Nature herself sets the laws, or you end up in a scenario of dire outdoor hazards. Making the best of a terrible or uncomfortable situation in the wild usually starts with a survival handbook, even for the most experienced survivalist.

Implement and ingest all the guidance in this book, and I'm confident it will make you a better wilderness prepper and survivor.

PREPPER'S

WORST SCENARIOS SURVIVAL GUIDE

INTRODUCTION

In recent years, the phenomenon of prepping has grown significantly in popularity. This has progressed to the point where TV programs with a preparation theme have been created. The public's attention has been drawn to well-prepared individuals for any disaster that may strike the earth.

Equally, it's given that to endure a crisis, we must be physically capable of handling the difficulties. And in the end, the struggle for existence may be won by the strongest. This is because they have psychologically prepared themselves to battle and survive. Although such a survivor has strong mind, they cannot stay alone for long on their mental fortitude.

As a result, this book is a survival guide for preppers' worst-case scenarios. It discusses how to survive, how long an emergency might last, and how to handle each disaster's main issues. Additionally, it discusses the typical approach to being ready for each type of disaster listed in this book.

What does "prepper" actually mean? A prepper is a general phrase for someone who always keeps himself ready for any emergency. Such survivalists are commonplace. They not only survive disasters but also aid in the survival of others. And as a result, a large number of individuals can survive the catastrophe and escape the death trap. Every day, a variety of emergencies take place all across the world. Some of them are artificial, while others are created naturally. Such circumstances are inescapable, yet nobody wants to find themselves in them. Therefore, it is wise to be ready for such disasters and have supplies for yourself and your fellow humans. An emergency can frequently linger for a long time and put you through the wringer.

CHEMICAL DISASTER

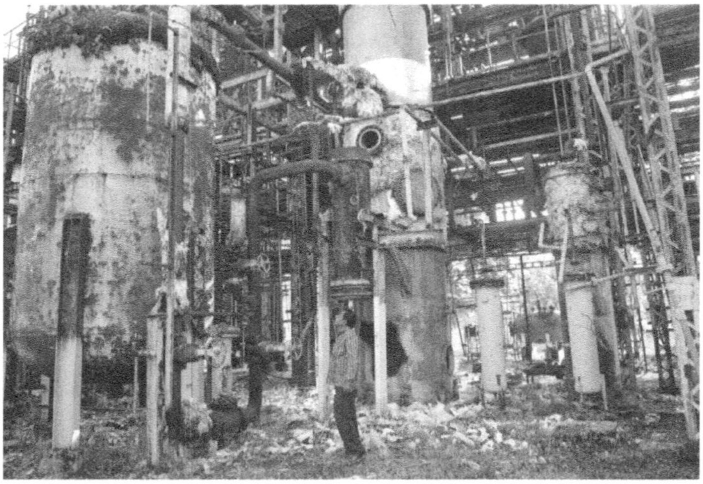

A major chemical disaster that causes widespread environmental damage and the severe injury or death of many animals, plants, or humans is what we mean when we talk about a chemical disaster. A condensed version might read something like this: dangerous to all forms of living cells and the fundamental components of life.

Chemical disasters could occur in:

- Manufacturing and formulation of equipment, including during process operations and commissioning, maintenance, and disposal.
- Warehouses, goo-downs, tank farms in ports and docks, fuel depots; material handling and storage in manufacturing plants; isolated storage.
- Transport (road, rail, air, water, and pipelines).

Among other factors, it's important to emphasize the improper analysis of hazard reviews, the installation of pollution control equipment, the use of defective or poorly built equipment, the use of incorrect process condition indicators, and the failure to heed warnings. Other factors include operator error and inadequate training.

Rarely is it thought that a single operator's conduct or inactivity was the only or even the leading cause of the vast majority of severe chemical disasters.

Effects of a Chemical Disaster

A chemical catastrophe/disaster results mostly rely on the accident's type (a leak, spill, or "runaway" response, such as a powerful explosion or fire). They may differ from target to target.

Depending on the level of a person's exposure to a chemical and how it might affect his anatomical structures and physiological processes, chemicals have been known to cause a wide range of biological reactions in humans. As a result, chemical disasters may cause clusters of diseases or immediate death as adverse effects.

How to Stay Safe in The Event of a Chemical Disaster

Wear a protective suit first, even though gas masks are less effective. You can also construct a protective room to can store food and water. For a shelter for disaster relief, experts advise Hughes Shelter Systems.

However, you should seek medical attention immediately if you are exposed to a chemical accident. Before you show up, think about calling first to prevent the disease from spreading to others. Be psychologically prepared to act on whatever cues are presented to you. Acting quickly is crucial to preventing the sickness from affecting all of your organs.

The Top 5 Chemical Disasters

Chemical substance production, storage, and transportation are inherently dangerous operations. Chemicals have the potential to be toxic, corrosive, and react violently. As a result, chemical accidents can have catastrophic effects on people and the environment. Various factors, including reckless handling of hazardous chemical substances, outmoded equipment, and human errors, can cause such catastrophes.

In 1984, a pesticide facility in the Indian state of Madhya Pradesh experienced one of the deadliest chemical disasters. Over 500,000 people were exposed to toxic gases and byproducts at midnight on December 2nd and 3rd due to a combination of factors ranging from the risky handling of hazardous chemical substances to the use of old and broken industrial equipment. This incident resulted in nearly 3,800 officially confirmed human deaths.

At a chemical facility near Toulouse that belonged to one of the top fertilizer manufacturers in France, an explosion occurred in a shed housing roughly 300 tons of downgraded ammonium nitrate in September 2001. The explosion in the vicinity resulted in 31 fatalities, over 4,500 injuries, and 27,000 destroyed buildings.

The worst industrial disaster to affect the US was a catastrophe at a significant petroleum refinery in Texas City, United States, in 2005. Explosions happened when a hydrocarbon isomerization unit was restarted and a distillation tower was filled with hydrocarbons. As a result, 15 people died, and 180 people were hurt.

An incident in June 1974 close to the British community of Flixborough resulted in a considerable tightening of the UK government's regulations governing risky industrial activities. While fixing one of its chemical reactors, a locally owned chemical factory leaked of 40 tons of cyclohexane in less than a minute, creating a vapor cloud with a diameter of around 200 meters. The factory was completely destroyed by the cloud explosion, which also caused damage to approximately 1,800 houses within a radius of more than 1,5 km.

A toxic chemical spill in the Romanian city of Baia Mare in February 2000 decimated animals and fisheries while endangering the water supply of 2.5 million people throughout Central and Eastern Europe. A reservoir wall at the nearby mine collapsed, releasing some 100,000 m3 of cyanide, used to extract gold, into the river Somes. The incident was considered the worst calamity to hit Europe since Chernobyl.

The development of modern industry demonstrates that companies working with chemicals cannot be too vigilant, swift, or well-equipped when attempting to control the impacts.

Chemical Disaster: How to Prevent It

Natural or man-made, a disaster is typically a cruel occurrence. Death and destruction are typically the results. The singularity and scope of the catastrophe that leads to tragedies profoundly impact the human soul.

Chemical, biological, and nuclear calamities are inventions of the 20th century. These items continue to pose a risk to people despite already being accountable for many crimes. The catastrophe was the fifth and last act of the tragedy, just like in the Greek theatre.

Disasters, unlike accidents, entail new considerations regarding how they can be avoided or averted. Human error, such as the unintentional use of one product instead of another or the incorrect understanding of work practice, is to blame for most accidents. Therefore, all hazardous products must be clearly labeled to indicate potential risks, such as toxicity, inflammability, or reactivity. In addition, all of the equipment, particularly the heating and cooling systems, and the security and control devices, must undergo routine inspections.

A few common-sense guidelines must be followed to avert a chemical disaster in an establishment or business where chemical compounds are present. First, less hazardous alternatives must be used in place of high-risk goods. The use and storage of hazardous materials must also be kept to a minimum.

With sufficient technical and organizational measures, the effects of a potential disaster can also be controlled and minimized. Technical methods include making a list of every accident that could happen and making an inventory of all the security equipment already in place. Application of intervention plans, evacuation, coordination of intervention services, and notifying local authorities are organizational procedures intended to produce adequate reactions during a crisis. Establishing a team in charge of emergency circumstances is also crucial. The team members must be directed to ensure that all planned safety measures are adequate, efficient, and understood by all staff.

Suppose a company that is vulnerable to chemical disasters requires better security. In that case, it can enlist the support of experts from businesses that create emergency plans, offer disaster relief, and provide training for such situations.

NUCLEAR DISASTER

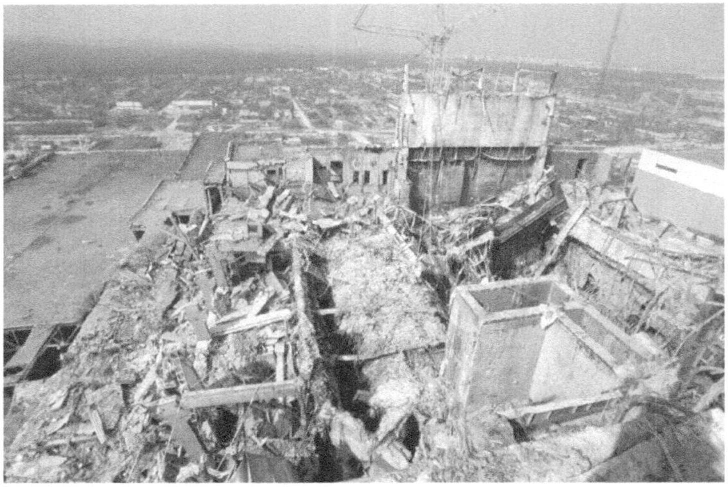

Nuclear explosions can cause significant damage and casualties due to blasts, heat, and radiation. Still, you can protect your family from harm if you know what to do in such an emergency and are well-prepared for it.

A device that causes an explosion through a nuclear chain reaction is referred to as a nuclear weapon. There is a broad spectrum of nuclear weapons, from something small and portable that a human may carry to a bomb that is carried by a missile. An explosion caused by nuclear fission could occur with or without warning for a few minutes.

Getting Ready for a Nuclear Disaster

Although it's difficult to imagine, a nuclear catastrophe may occur at anytime, anywhere in the world. The good news is that you can be entirely ready for a nuclear disaster if you are well-informed. Thus, what you should do in the event of a nuclear catastrophe is reviewed here, along with steps you can take to protect your family and yourself.

What to Do Right Away

It is recommended that you do this activity with your family on multiple occasions throughout the year to ensure that you are well-prepared to collaborate well to achieve the desired outcomes.

1. Take potassium iodate KIO3 pills, which are a thyroid blocker and will help prevent radioactive damage to the thyroid if authorities inform you that there is an impending nuclear threat or radioactive exposure via plume or fallout. Make sure that every member of the family and any pets consumes the recommended dosage following the instructions on the bottle's label.
2. Lock all the vents, windows, doors, and other open spaces that lead outside. Anything with an exterior opening need to be covered and closed. Work swiftly. You must completely seal off the outside air space to the best of your ability. Pet owners should bring their animals inside with them. Nuclear material will irradiate any living thing outside.
3. Turn off any equipment that brings outside air into your home, including your air conditioner. If you don't, the radioactive fallout from outside can enter your home more easily.
4. Put your family in the room closest to the heart of your house that doesn't have any windows. The ideal location is a bathroom with no windows. For added safety, babies can be put to sleep in the bathtub. If you have a basement or bunker, remain against the walls and away from any windows. By doing this, "ground shine" exposure will be reduced. You need to be in a secure room with no outside air access.
5. Use a battery-operated portable radio or television to access the local media. You can follow the instructions of emergency officials to determine whether it is safe to return outside. Be ready to stay two weeks at your place of safety if an EMP has damaged your communications.

What You Can Do in Advance

1. Bring along at least one accessible emergency kit. Potassium Iodate KIO3 tablets, which will aid in preventing radioactive thyroid damage, must be included in your emergency kit. Also, bring supplies of any prescription medications you need to stay alive so you will remember to take them. Additionally, the kit should have all the necessary supplies you could require to survive for an extended period without access to food, water, or electricity. Include any additional emergency supplies

you might need, such as bottled water and tightly sealed, non-perishable food for emergencies, flashlights, batteries, a battery-operated radio, headlamps, and a first aid kit with plenty of bandages and skin disinfectant. Due to the likelihood that you won't have electricity, everything you need to prepare food must be battery-operated.

2. Fill clothing storage containers with additional sets of clothing and foundations so that you and your family may stay as fresh and clean as possible without access to showers.
3. You and your family will not be able to use the water in your home, so bring hand sanitizer and wet wipes you may use to wash down your bodies and clean yourself.
4. So that your family may sleep and be as comfortable as possible, pack pillows and mattresses or cots in a clean, secure area of your basement or windowless room. You will have all the resources you need in one place. You could feel less anxious because everything is available to you and your family if you pack these goods in a convenient location in the room chosen as the meeting room.

A nuclear disaster could occur in the United States and other parts of the world at any time since the country has nuclear power facilities close to residential areas, or that could affect residential regions within a specific distance of the facility. However, you may take steps to protect yourself and your loved ones in the event of a nuclear disaster, even if you cannot live in the constant terror of one. Review this helpful advice to examine the precautions you may take, and bear in mind these suggestions in case a nuclear accident occurs around you.

EPIDEMIC DISASTER

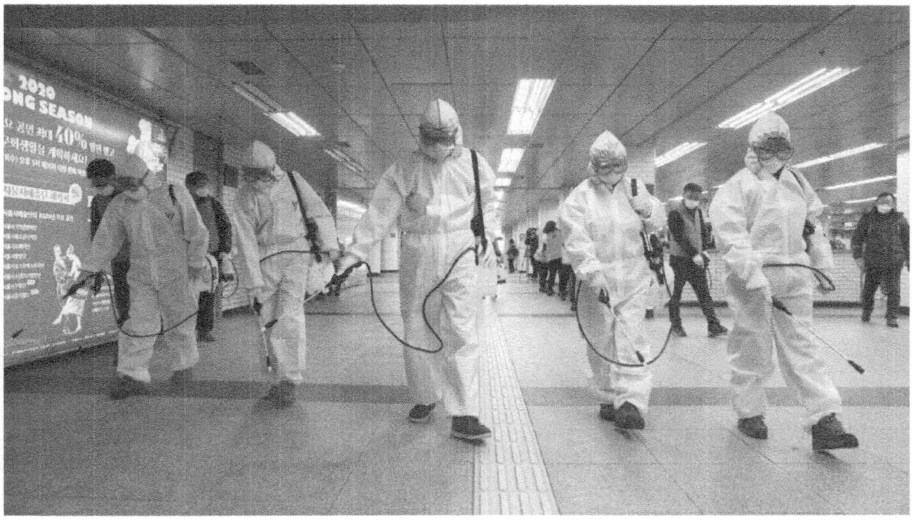

The word "epidemic" comes from the Greek words "epi," which means "upon or above," and "demos," which means "people." It is a term used to describe a situation in which a disease spreads rapidly to a large number of people within a given population within a short time.

The phrase "epidemic" refers to more than merely infectious diseases. It is also applied to any situation that raises harmful health hazards in society.

There have been a lot of horrific epidemics in human history. In the 1300s, the plague killed some 25 million people in Europe. It was given the moniker "Black Death." There were sporadic plague outbreaks in European cities for 300 years or so. Then, the dreadful influenza (flu) pandemic struck between 1918 and 1919. More than 20 million people died all across the world.

Epidemics have been less frequent throughout time. The spread of illnesses has been curbed by improved healthcare and cleaner living conditions. Malaria and cholera epidemics, however, continue to spread around the world. In the 1980s, AIDS initially appeared, and it spread swiftly, especially in Africa. SARS, a widespread influenza-like illness, first surfaced in 2003. SARS swept from Asia to every continent in a few months. A brand-new virus type brought on the COVID-19 disease in 2019. It also quickly spread across the entire world.

Control of Epidemics

Taking proper control measures, such as treating the sick to lower the reservoir of infection, and disseminating health information to prevent the spread of the disease to others, are all part of epidemic management operations. Higher-level health professionals will need your assistance in stopping the spread of the disease, like giving medications to community members and distributing health information.

Once the appropriate authorities recognize an epidemic in health, you might participate in its management. The kind of infectious agent, the mode of transmission, and any additional causes of the disease will all affect the control measures you need to put in place. The infectious agent, the source of any infection, and the care of people who become unwell should generally be the focus of your control actions. Keep in mind that the source of an illness could be an animal, a human, or something in the environment that is not alive.

The disease could spread farther in your area if you don't put the proper control measures in place. For instance, if contaminated food is the cause of an outbreak in your neighborhood, you'll need to contain it by educating residents about food safety to prevent them from coming into contact with infected food. You should warn them not to drink the water until it has been chlorinated if the problem is due to polluted water. You will need to educate the locals on how to eliminate mosquito breeding areas if they cause an epidemic of malaria.

Differences Between Pandemics and Epidemics

Both the terms "epidemic" and "pandemic" describe the spread of infectious diseases among a specific population. However, epidemics and pandemics differ primarily in two ways. First, a pandemic impacts a significantly larger population and a larger area, and it occasionally has the potential to harm everyone on the planet.

The distinction between an epidemic and a pandemic is that an epidemic often happens when a disease spreads to a larger-than-expected or unusually high number of people. In contrast, a pandemic affects a far more considerable portion of the population than an epidemic does.

For instance, a city or county may have a spike in the flu in a specific region. This spreads like wildfire. A sickness or illness becomes more widespread when it affects multiple nations, even different continents, and fans across numerous populations. In this case, the swine flu virus is doing this.

The incidence of concentration of disease transmission can also be used to distinguish between an epidemic and a pandemic. A disease or ailment may have taken hold across the country, but the concentration level could be clearer. So, there is an epidemic here.

However, suppose the prevalence or concentration rises to such a level. In that case, even if the outbreak is contained in a single nation, it can already be classified as a pandemic. When a disease's transmission becomes uncontrollable, it becomes a pandemic.

Disease Outbreak Causes

Numerous circumstances cause infectious illness outbreaks. Transmission through humans, animals, or even the environment can result in contraction. For example:

1. The environment. For instance, measles typically shows in the winter, whereas whooping cough arrives in the spring.
2. Chemical or radioactive substance exposure. For instance, mercury exposure can cause the illness of Minamata.
3. Various environmental elements, including access to clean water, food, healthy air, and sanitary facilities, can promote the spread of infectious diseases.
4. The social fallout from natural disasters like hurricanes, earthquakes, and droughts can result in a high disease transmission rate.
5. The cause of a disease may also be unknown. There are numerous potential causes of these disorders, including:
   - A newly discovered or altered pathogen
   - Organic poisons
   - Chemical emissions that go unnoticed
   - Overexposure to unknown ionizing radiation

To safeguard the health and safety of the general public, the science of epidemiology works to identify the origin of these unknown outbreaks.

NATURAL DISASTER

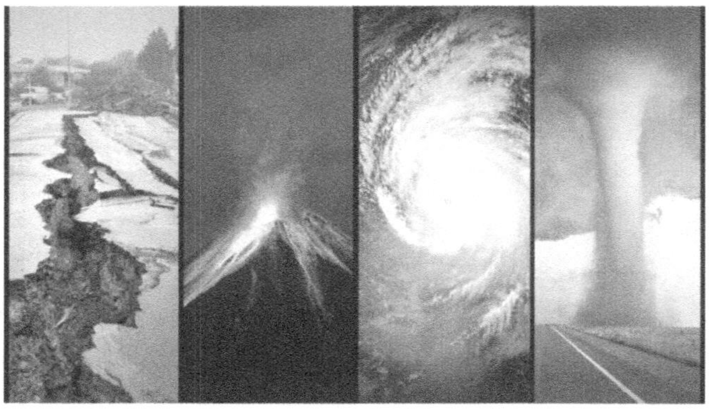

The next time a natural disaster occurs, will you be ready? Unfortunately, many people still need to take easy and affordable precautions to support them during a natural disaster. What happens if a tornado, earthquake, or hurricane hits? Your home could be completely destroyed by the direct devastation these natural disasters bring. Most people are unaware that these catastrophes can result in significant power disruptions. Due to these outages, supermarkets, ATMs, and other important companies may close, depriving us of the essential goods and services that we typically take for granted.

Investing a little time and money may protect you from these catastrophes. Having the right emergency food and water supplies, communication devices, and survival kits will assist you and your family get through any challenging situations. These kinds of kits are affordable compared to the cost of purchasing the necessities you would need to survive. In addition, your family and pets will be protected with these supplies for disaster preparedness, and everything is within your reach.

One of a natural disaster's most pervasive effects is the loss of electricity. Anything electrical that a different source of electricity cannot power will not be operable. The length of the power outage could vary depending on the severity of the natural disaster. When the power goes out, you should make sure that you have easy access to the necessities. This will ensure that you and your family have everything you need up until the electricity is restored and neighborhood shops can open again.

When the electricity goes out, a flashlight is an obvious option. Most folks ought to have one on hand. Contacting for assistance will require other tools like a cell phone and an emergency radio. The radio is crucial because it will keep you informed of what is happening around you. Although a battery-operated radio is convenient, the batteries will eventually run out. A hand crank radio that you wind every 30 minutes or so would be a better option. You can use this radio for as long as you need to.

Freshwater, non-perishable food, and prescription medications that will last you for a particular time are other necessities. The number of essentials required will depend on where you reside and the natural calamities that affect your neighborhood. Not being ready for a disaster is the worst scenario.

Natural Disaster Survival: Preparing for the Event

People frequently feel gloomy after a natural calamity despite their most significant efforts to shield themselves from external problems. Although weather forecasters frequently predict hurricanes days in advance, it is challenging to foresee what will happen when the natural disaster strikes and how it will affect particular homes. Despite the ambiguity, there are steps you may take to get ready for a natural disaster.

1. **Plan beforehand:** Making a plan is the first step in tackling any emergency. For something that might be sudden and unavoidably unexpected to be handled smoothly, a strategy that has been planned, prepared, and put in place beforehand is essential. Your plan may include meeting locations, emergency phone numbers, and what to do if you become separated. It might outline who is in charge of what, where to get key resources, and how to prepare for a disaster step-by-step.
2. **Purchase plenty of emergency supplies**: People frequently lack access to food, medical supplies, and other essential requirements after a significant natural disaster. Stock up on non-perishable food items, clean water, medications, and supplies like toilet paper to prevent panic. Generally, it would be best if you had enough to get by on your own for a week. Consider building up your food storage with water, powdered milk, canned meats, beans, fruits, and easy-to-prepare meals such as pasta, soups, etc.
3. **Get a generator:** The importance of power is frequently only understood once lost. People rely on electricity to prepare food, log into their computers to work, and stay warm during the winter. A backup generator can help you stay safe when a natural disaster strikes and get your lives back to normal.
4. **Networking:** Connect with a network set up to aid one another in times of need, whether through a church or another local organization. Depending on the network you join, your only responsibility is ensuring everyone is safe and has access to all they require. In an evacuation or protracted power loss, you may also put together a combined supply of emergency goods.
5. **Maintain a full tank of gas:** In the aftermath of a natural disaster, the gasoline supply quickly runs out, much like food and water. Experts usually advise filling up your tank whenever it is halfway complete. If necessary, you can leave a damaged area thanks to this.
6. **Have emergency funds:** Have enough money to get by for a week or travel to a secure location. This doesn't mean storing your entire bank account under your mattress. Additionally, open a savings account to aid in financing any unexpected costs brought on by an unforeseen event.
7. **Have Home insurance:** If you do not have the proper insurance to cover your losses, losing your house could be the most devastating result of a natural disaster. Make sure your plan addresses typical natural occurrences in your area.
8. **Safe location to resort to:** Having a safe place to go might imply several things, depending on where you live. Some people may think of it as an attic above flood waters. Others might find refuge in their basement, which is tornado-proof. Make sure everyone knows the location of the safest spot to go in case of a natural disaster by discussing it with your family. It's crucial to agree on a meeting location in case of separation.
9. **First Aid:** Having the appropriate first aid supplies in your home can be the difference between life and death of a natural disaster. Unfortunately, when a tragedy happens, you might be unable to get the essential first aid items to the hospital or the store. So, ensure your medicine cabinet is fully equipped with all the painkillers, bandages, and antiseptics you require in an emergency.

Questions to Ask About Your Natural Disaster Survival Kits

The first four major natural disasters are as follows: Although they give advance notice, hurricanes can continue for hours or days. Tornadoes strike suddenly, swiftly, and without warning. Tsunamis and floods can occur suddenly or gradually. Earthquakes are brief occurrences. There is neither a warning nor a way out. Let's now list the essential kit components.

1. First of all, are you organized?

Consider the scenario when you desire a single, enormous bug-out bag. You could manage anything with it. Yet it would be huge. As a result, you modularize your kit to solve the issue. Each container stands for a specific specialty. Using Gear Pods is one remedy. These are containers made of translucent plastic. Simple screwing of the lids is all that is required to join them.

The use of CD sleeves made of plastic is an option. In addition, you can create a kit specifically for your situation using modularization. For instance, you can grab the communications kit if the phones aren't working.

2. Do you have checklists?

A collection of checklists is another thing you should always have available. Remember the operating procedures and decision lists. Make judgments and plans for your response in advance. You will free up mental space and be able to concentrate on other things.

So how do you implement this concept?

Use laminated cards to begin. Make a few with contact information. Next, create cards with destinations for bug-outs. The third option might be the communication channels that your group decides to use. Let's go to our third main question while still talking about communications.

3. Do you have access to communications?

We will rely on something other than cell phones for communication as our first line of defense. So, it won't be functioning. Why? Because they will have spoiled.

Furthermore, we are still determining how long the consequences will last. As a result, I've included four communications tools that can work well to get you going in the correct direction.

- When service is lost, everyone's initial instinct is to use their cell phone or SMS. Battery-free radios use a wind-up or dynamo mechanism.
- CB can manage a radius of 1-2 miles. Here, cigarette lighters can charge your batteries.
- FRS/GMRS is widely used but loses its usefulness with too many users. Ham radio is adaptable and has portable models but needs a license.
- Shortwave is a receive-only technology, yet you can hear signals from all over the world. So, say goodbye to batteries if you can locate a wind-up.

Finally, you can assume that the necessary survival equipment is the same for all-natural calamities. That is not accurate. These three questions will assist you in creating a plan, setting priorities, and being prepared at a moment's notice.

What's coming up? Consider which of these catastrophes occurs more frequently in your location. Then, plan your disaster supply now.

List of Natural Disasters That Could Occur

Earthquakes, droughts, floods, mudslides, tsunamis, tornadoes, high heat, volcanoes, and wildfires are just a few examples of natural catastrophes that can occur. Unfortunately, anywhere in the world, these catastrophes are possible. But, even if we are powerless to stop these catastrophes, we may plan and be ready to lessen their impact.

1. **Earthquakes:** Earthquakes are sudden shaking of the ground brought on by a sudden displacement of one of the earth's plates. They can destroy even the most robustly built house. Tsunamis and volcanic eruptions are mostly caused by earthquakes, which can happen anywhere in the world. One of the most recent nations to experience an earthquake was Haiti, where the death toll and material damage were practically incalculable.
2. **Floods:** Excessive amounts of rain cause flooding. Both humans and animals can perish when suddenly surging seas overtake their habitats. Because of the damage they cause to crops, food shortages directly result from these floods. Furthermore, floodwaters carry dirt from the sewage drainage system; as a result, this area is contaminated with diseases that are spread through water.
3. **Drought:** Water availability for home and agricultural use becomes limited during a drought. This results in flora's death, making it impossible for animals and people to obtain food. Most African countries continue to use rain-fed agriculture rather than adopting technological crop production methods, which contributes to the continent's high incidence of drought.

4. **Tornadoes:** Thunderstorms can produce powerful storms called tornadoes. In their wake, tornadoes can leave a path of devastation and mortality. They frequently travel at a speed of about 480 km/hr. Damage may extend over a vast area, as much as 80 km long and 2 km wide. They are renowned for having powerful winds that may instantly topple skyscrapers and lift trucks. The suddenness of tornadoes catches many people by surprise. In North America, it is relatively prevalent.
5. **Mudslides and landslides:** These calamities typically happen on high ground. Houses, trees, soil, rocks, and other items gradually cover the base of the hill. Landslides are generally brought on by earthquakes, whereas mudslides are brought on by prolonged, intense rain. Mudslides and landslides can bury people, animals, and property, making them highly dangerous.
6. **Tsunami:** Tsunamis are caused by the ocean, lake, or lake's water being displaced. They frequently take place on a considerable scale and swiftly. Undersea earthquakes cause tsunamis. Areas close to coastlines and seas are vulnerable to this kind of catastrophe. The tsunami, with the most recent memory, struck the Indian Ocean, affecting nations like Singapore and Indonesia.
7. **Wildfires:** One-of-a-kind natural disasters are wildfires. These flames typically occur in a hot, dry atmosphere. They usually appear in wooded or otherwise bushy areas. Extreme heat and lightning are two natural ways that they might begin.
8. Human lives, vegetation, and wildlife can all be seriously endangered by wildfires. In addition, the wind can accelerate the spread of a fire. This type of fire is extremely challenging to put out and requires the use of advanced tools. Firefighters frequently employ helicopters to put out this kind of fire.
9. **Intense heat:** Extreme heat is brought on by the environment's rising carbon levels interacting with the sun. Carbon makes the climate warmer than usual by preventing the sun's heat from escaping into the atmosphere. As a result, the mercury can rise as high as forty degrees Celsius. Both humans and animals may get sick from the heat due to this.
10. **Volcanoes:** Mountains with an opening at the top are called volcanoes. These openings extend to the molten rock of the planet. While some volcanoes are dormant, others are active. Active volcanoes provide the most significant risk. When the pressure below is high, volcanoes may erupt suddenly. Lava spills from the eruption into the soil through the vent.

This may produce toxic fumes that could be harmful to all types of earthly life. Flying pebbles are also frequent, and the eruption's ash plume can travel hundreds of kilometers. The ash can hamper air transport. The situation in Europe after ash smoke from mountains in Iceland forced air journeys around the continent to stall, notably in Western Europe, serves as an example of this.

Preparedness for Natural Disasters with Pets

Natural disasters can sometimes strike without warning, but there are steps you can take to get ready before that happens! Continue reading to discover more about disaster pet care.

Pets should be evacuated along with the family.

This may sound apparent, but you can forget about everyone and everything besides you and your family in a natural disaster. Saying, "we'll go back and get him/her," won't help because you'll probably forget, or it'll be too late, and if you leave your pet behind, they risk getting hurt, lost, or even worse.

Whom to call?

Prior to the occurrence of a natural disaster, there are a large number of individuals as well as organizations that should be notified. To begin, the local animal shelters in your area are the finest source of information and advice regarding local safety precautions. If you cannot care for your pets and need assistance, they may not be able to take them in themselves, but they can direct you to someone who can. Therefore, the first thing you should do to ensure that you are ready for a disaster is to educate yourself about the measures your community takes to care for animals in emergencies.

Look for pet-friendly shelters.

Research pet-friendly shelters in advance to know where you may and cannot take your pet. The most crucial thing to be aware of is that dogs are not permitted in Red Cross disaster shelters. So, plan and find a different shelter for your pets if you must go to one of these. Also, it would be helpful to find out in advance whether hotels, boarding houses, and veterinarians accept pets in case of emergency. Additionally, you can find friends, family members, or other people outside the neighborhood to care for your pet while your family gets back on its feet.

Create a pet emergency supply kit

A pet first aid kit, durable leashes, harnesses, and/or carriers should also be included in this list of essentials for transporting pets safely and preventing escape from your pet. If your pet goes missing, send recent pictures of them. The kit should also include food, potable water, bowls, cat litter or a pan, and a can opener. Ensure that everyone in your home knows where this kit is placed and is easily accessible.

How to handle a missing pet

Losing a pet in a natural disaster is a terrifying experience. The first thing you can do is get in touch with the local police department, vets, and animal shelters to see whether they have ever taken in a pet similar to yours. If unsuccessful, try contacting boarding houses or any other place where your pet might end up. Photos of your pet can help people know what to look out for, which is why having them in the disaster pack is helpful. In addition, it is advantageous to get your pet microchipped in advance and to ensure that they are wearing an identity collar and tags.

Natural catastrophes are terrifying but can be even more alarming for our pets. Because of this, it is crucial to be ready for a disaster, even if it is unlikely to occur. Keep in mind that your pet only has you. The finest action you can take is to be organized!

CONCLUSION

In conclusion, the popularity of preparing has grown significantly. However, over the past few years, some things have happened that were genuinely rather frightening. Events like earthquakes, storms, rising oil prices, and more have caused a threat to the food supply. Furthermore, market failures brought on by such events resulted in numerous people losing their houses and retirement savings. As a result, most individuals are distraught and decide to learn more about preparation because of the current occurrences.

Before, being prepared was a way of life. We have grown so reliant on the contemporary comforts and technologies we have created. All those fundamental abilities, like farming and hunting that were freely acquired before the advent of technology have been lost. One had to be independent in the past. People are starting to reevaluate their exact plans in the event of a natural disaster or an economic collapse due to recent disasters. This is what has caused today's preparation culture to boom.

I hope that this book helps you become a better prepper!

Made in United States
Cleveland, OH
05 November 2026

47663999R00160